OBEDIENCE PILLS

ADHD AND THE MEDICALIZATION OF CHILDHOOD

Expert Endorsements

"Patrick Hahn has provided another lifesaving book on the dangers of psychiatry. This is an outstanding and painstakingly researched treatise on ADHD that clearly exposes the hazards waiting to destroy your child. It should be in every pediatrician's office and in every graduate student's library."

> ***Michelle Barrett***, *M.Ed.*,
> *Founder and CEO of Del Dios Counseling Service.*

"Dr. Patrick Hahn is one of top researchers in the field of psychiatry and his book on ADHD is among the best. As a psychiatrist, I confirm his warnings—a diagnosis of ADHD and medication leads many children into disability and lifelong dependence on psychiatric or street drugs. Read this book and save your loved ones."

> ***Peter R. Breggin M.D.***, *author of Medication Madness and*
> *COVID-19 and the Global Predators*

"*Obedience Pills* recounts the shocking story of psychiatry's abandonment of scientific evidence in favor of professional power and profit. As expertly discussed here by Patrick Hahn, the bizarre transition from some musings on youth morality in the nineteenth century to the current drugging of millions of kids with highly dangerous substances for a non-existent condition would be almost laughable if it wasn't so utterly tragic and devastating for so many young people and their families. A must-read for anyone currently living with or considering a diagnosis of 'ADHD'."

Bruce Cohen, Ph.D., *Associate Professor of Sociology at the University of Auckland and author of* **Psychiatric Hegemony**

Also by Patrick D. Hahn

Madness and Genetic Determinism:
Is Mental Illness in Our Genes?

Prescription for Sorrow:
Antidepressants, Suicide and Violence

OBEDIENCE PILLS

ADHD AND THE MEDICALIZATION OF CHILDHOOD

PATRICK D. HAHN

Samizdat Health

Samizdat Health Writer's Co-operative Inc.

Cover Design: Billiam James / Illustration: iStock, alashi
First Printing, 2022
Title: Obedience Pills: ADHD and the Medicalization of Childhood

ISBN: 978-1-989963-24-1

Publisher: Samizdat Health Writer's Co-operative Inc.
www.samizdathealth.org
www.meliponula.wordpress.com

Acknowledgments

Grateful acknowledgement is made to each of the following:

To the experts who so generously gave of their time to make this book possible: Peter Breggin, David Healy, Jay Joseph, Linda Logdberg, and Deborah J. Rhea;

To Anne, Michelle, Rick, Debbie, David, and Dara, who courageously shared their stories of iatrogenic harm;

And to my wife and daughter, for their unwavering support.

Contents

PREFACE

On the morning of Wednesday, 13 December 2006, four-year-old Rebecca Riley died in her family's home in Hull, Massachusetts, after gasping her last on a pile of old magazines and newspapers just a few feet away from the bed where her parents slept. Later that morning Rebecca's mother Carolyn discovered the child's lifeless body, clad in only a pink pull-up diaper, her face and hair covered in frothing, foamy body fluids. She was already cold to the touch. Rebecca's father Michael was still slumbering abed, after repeatedly hitting the snooze alarm.

The autopsy revealed that Rebecca's death was caused by an overdose of clonidine, an antihypertensive drug she had been prescribed two years earlier for Attention-Deficit Hyperactivity Disorder, or ADHD. The pathologist also noted that Rebecca had signs of heart and lung damage, which she ascribed to the prolonged use of clonidine.

Kayoko Kifuji, the pediatrician at Tufts University Medical Center who had prescribed clonidine to Rebecca after a twenty-minute consultation, agreed to stop treating patients and was placed on paid administrative leave while the commonwealth investigated the case.[1] Dr. Kifuji received immunity from prosecution in return for testifying against Michael and Carolyn, both of whom were convicted in separate trials of the murder of their daughter. Tufts Medical Center affirmed that Kifuji provided "appropriate care" for Rebecca, and in the autumn of 2009 she was allowed to resume treating patients.[2]

Every day across this great land of ours, children are swallowing pills for something called "Attention-Deficit Hyperactivity Disorder." This is still largely an American obsession, by the way—the United States spends several times as much on ADHD meds than all the rest of the world put together—although the rest of the world is catching up with us. The idea that millions of children—mostly boys—are walking around with defective brains that require them to ingest powerful psychotropic drugs every day of their lives in order to be able to cope with the quotidian tasks of childhood has become received wisdom.

So what is the story? What are the harms caused by this mass drugging of children? What are the benefits? Who benefits? These questions form the basis of this book. In my quest for answers, I have examined the scientific literature, scrutinized news accounts, conversed with experts, and borne witness to the stories of those whose loved ones have been devastated by these drugs.

I will confess my bias at the outset: I believe our default preference should be not to drug kids for behavioral problems, and that the burden of proof rests on anyone who thinks this is a good idea.

In this book I do not discuss any quasi-medical interventions for ADHD. You won't find anything in here about biofeedback, special diets, acupuncture, Ayurvedic medicine, etc. For reasons I will make clear, I do not believe ADHD is even a coherent diagnostic category, so it is meaningless to talk about a "treatment" for this condition.

There is no credible evidence of any long-term benefits resulting from drugging children diagnosed with ADHD. However, the harms are indisputable. I contend that a perhaps even greater harm is inflicted by distracting us from having a meaningful conversation about the social, familial, and medical roots of children's problems.

There are literally hundreds of reasons why a given child might have problems with inattention or hyperactivity. Far better to identify the source of the child's problems and address that, rather than to attribute those problems to some mythical disease entity.

Once upon a time the mass drugging of children was the subject of spirited debate, but that controversy seems for the most part to have died down. My goal is to re-ignite that controversy.

I have not attempted to write a balanced book, because I believe that what is needed is a balanced debate. You already know everything the drug companies want you to know about the purported benefits of their wares. My task here is to present the other side of the story.

CHAPTER ONE

THE INVENTION OF A DISEASE

The Ebers papyrus is one of the oldest known medical texts, dating from some 1,500 years before the birth of Jesus of Nazareth.[3] In it, the unknown author or authors recommend dosing children with a mixture of opium and flyspecks to keep them from crying.[4]

So the idea of drugging recalcitrant children into submission is nothing new. But it is only within the space of a single lifetime that this idea has been applied with a ferocity unmatched in human history. How did we get here? How did bad behavior come to be regarded as a neurological disease, requiring treatment with brain-altering drugs?

Let's take a trip back in time, shall we? Let's examine the early history of the diagnostic category that came to be known as "ADHD," and see what lessons we can learn.

A Lack of Moral Control

Sir George Frederick Still, the founding father of British pediatric medicine, is credited with the first clinical accounts of children afflicted with what now would be called Attention Deficit Hyperactivity Disorder, or ADHD, in a series of lectures delivered to the Royal College of Physicians on March 4th, 6th, and 11th of 1902.[5] Dr. Still had collated information on twenty children (fifteen boys and five girls), all between the ages of four and thirteen, and all of whom exhibited normal intellectual development along with a lack of what he called "moral control."

In reading Dr. Still's account, one thing is for certain: this was a bunch of seriously disturbed kids, who lied, stole, destroyed property, viciously attacked other children and even adults, masturbated openly, touched other children sexually, smeared their feces, banged their heads, walked in their sleep, tortured animals, and set fires. These antisocial behaviors seemed completely resistant to punishment. In some cases, these behaviors appeared only after the child had exhibited some degree of moral development, while in others the development had never occurred at all.

Some of these children exhibited other odd compulsions—one went around to the other family members to say "goodnight" five times in one evening, while others consumed garbage or materials that weren't food at all—plaster, chalk, book covers, pieces of blanket.

Dr. Still also noted:

> *A notable feature in many of these cases of moral defect without general impairment of the intellect is a quite abnormal incapacity for sustained attention... As might be expected, the failure of attention was very noticeable at school, with the result that in some cases the child was backwards in school attainments, although in manner and ordinary conversation he appeared as bright and intelligent as any child could be.*[6]

What was the source of these children's problems? The family histories of these children were rife with tales of abandonment, drunkenness, illness, and insanity. In one case, the child's father had murdered his mother.

No consideration was given to the possibility that these children's difficulties may have had their origin in the children's maladaptive reactions to these adverse experiences. Rather, Dr. Still seems to regard all this as evidence that these children arose from inferior genetic stock. To buttress this argument, he notes that many of these children displayed what he called the "stigmata of degeneration":

> *In 15 cases head measurements were taken; in seven of these the maximum head circumference was decidedly below the average for the age... In four out of the 15 cases the frontal region was abnormally narrow. The palate showed some deformity in seven of these 15 cases; all seven were strikingly high and narrow and two of them formed a sharply pointed V anteriorly.[7]*

Dr. Still also noted that many of these children were the product of complicated deliveries and/or had suffered from seizures, and he placed the blame for their problems squarely on their own supposedly broken brains, not on their life circumstances.

What was the prognosis for these children? Dr. Still was pessimistic, but held out some hope:

> *The limit of possible improvement may be a very narrow one and, whether it be narrow or wide, there is probably little hope in this particular group that the child will ever acquire a normal degree of moral control; but during the earlier years of childhood it is hardly possible to foresee to what extent careful training and environment will improve these cases.[8]*

Organic Drivenness

In the years that followed, the view that these behavioral problems were the products of broken brains gained traction. During the years 1916 through 1924, an epidemic of encephalitis swept across the world.[9] More than one million were afflicted, many died, and the survivors were left with an often-dizzying variety of devastating neuropsychiatric sequelae.

Some of the survivors included children who exhibited behaviors similar to those described by Dr. Still: lying, theft, destruction of property, encopresis, hypersexuality, cruelty to animals, setting fires, and vicious attacks on other children. One ten-year-old encephalitis survivor snatched up his baby sister from her crib and swung her about by her heels.[10] Nevertheless, as one clinician noted, "The lack of restraint exhibited by these children does not necessarily imply any great degree of mental impairment."[11]

In 1934, two psychiatrists from the Yale University School of Medicine, Eugen Kahn and Louis M. Cohen, proposed the term "organic drivenness" for a syndrome found in some encephalitis survivors, encompassing the following symptoms:

> *1) A high degree of general hyperkinesis with either choreiform or tic-like (myoclonic) movements in the face, trunk, and extremities; 2) Outstanding difficulty approaching an almost complete inability in maintaining quiet attitudes (be it only for a few seconds); 3) Abruptness and clumsiness in the performance of movements, even of relatively simple ones; 4) An explosive motor release of all voluntarily inhibited activity.[12]*

Drs. Kahn and Cohen attributed the symptoms of "organic drivenness" experienced by encephalitis survivors to unspecified lesions in the brainstem. They went on to note that the syndrome could also be found in patients who had never suffered from encephalitis, and concluded, without a shred of corroborating evidence, that these children's problems must also be due to some kind of lesions in the brainstem as well.

Again, many of the same antisocial behaviors described by Dr. Still more than thirty years before were found in children described as suffering from "organic drivenness," including theft, violence, encopresis, and hypersexuality.[13] Drs. Kahn and Cohen never demonstrated that this grab-bag of complaints had a common underlying brain pathology. Rather, they proclaimed it to be so. And from here it was only a short step to regarding this condition (or these conditions) as a drug-treatable disease.

A Chemical Solution

Amphetamine was first synthesized in 1887 by the Romanian chemist Lazar Edeleanu, who dubbed the new compound phenylisopropylamine. This drug is structurally similar to epinephrine and norepinephrine, the chemical messengers that mediate the "fight-or-flight" response. The pharmacological properties of amphetamine went unrecognized for forty years, until the molecule was re-synthesized by the chemist Gordon Ailes, who found the drug acted as a central nervous system stimulant.

Known colloquially as "speed," amphetamine is classified by the DEA as a Schedule II controlled drug, with a high potential for abuse and dependence.[14] This substance exists in two molecular forms, called optical isomers, which are mirror-images of each other. The right-handed form, dextroamphetamine, is considered more effective than its left-handed twin, levoamphetamine. Benzedrine is the trade name for amphetamine sulfate, while Dexedrine and Dextrostat are trade names for dextroamphetamine sulfate. The ADHD drug Adderall is a mixture of four different amphetamine salts. (The term "Adderall" was coined by advertising executive Roger Griggs and is a contraction of "ADD for all.") Lisdexamfetamine, sold under the trade name Vyvanse, is a prodrug which is converted into dextroamphetamine in the body.

In 1937, pediatrician Charles Bradley became the first to report that amphetamine improved the behavior of difficult children. Dr. Bradley was Director of the Emma Pemberton Bradley Home, Rhode Island's first psychiatric hospital for children. The home had been founded by a bequest from George Bradley, a distant relative of Charles, in memory of his own daughter Emma, who had contracted encephalitis as a child and died from the disease at the age of twenty-seven.[15]

Every history of the diagnostic category which later became known as "ADHD" tells the story of Dr. Bradley and his work on the effects of amphetamine in troubled children. But what is usually glossed over or never mentioned at all is why he started giving the drug to kids in the first place.

At the time, Dr. Bradley was using the technique of pneumoencephalography in order to document any brain injury his patients might have sustained.[16] Pneumoencephalography is a now-obsolete procedure in which a needle is inserted into the spinal canal to withdraw a significant quantity of spinal fluid, which is replaced by air or some other gas, in order to make the brain and spinal cord show up better on an X-ray. The procedure required the child to be strapped into a chair and, after enduring a painful lumbar puncture, to be turned upside-down and rotated into different positions in a specified sequence, in order to allow the air to displace the cerebrospinal fluid in the spaces inside and outside the brain. The procedure was usually followed by severe headaches, neck stiffness, fever, elevated heartbeat, and high blood pressure, any or all of which could last for days. It could take weeks for the normal amount of cerebrospinal fluid to be regenerated.

A 1973 paper stated "The occurrence of a transient improvement in mental state after pneumoencephalography does not seem to have been documented."[17] No surprise there.

At any rate, Dr. Bradley did become concerned about the misery this practice was causing his young charges—although, evidently, not concerned enough to stop doing it. Instead, he tried administering Benzedrine to a group of thirty children after undergoing pneumoencephalography.[18] While the drug did nothing for their headaches, he found that fifteen of them became "distinctly subdued in their emotional responses," while fourteen exhibited improved academic performance. Oddly, there seemed to be no correlation between these two categories of effect. Only seven of the children improved in both areas.[19]

Nevertheless, encouraged by these results, Dr. Bradley began using both Benzedrine and Dexedrine much more widely. By 1950 some 350 children in his care had received one or both of these drugs. Overactive children became more subdued and easier to handle, while shy children became more outgoing, and academic performance improved. Most gratifying was the results obtained with children judged to be suffering from "psychopathic personality," a label corresponding more or less to Dr. Still's category of children lacking "moral control." Over eighty percent of these children were said to have improved on the drugs.[20]

Side effects, according to Dr. Bradley, were mostly minor and transient, and the effects of the drugs did not wear off with prolonged use. In other words, the children did not develop a tolerance for the drug.

And what about Dr. Bradley's pneumoencephalographic studies of the brains of his troubled young wards, which caused so much distress to these children? They yielded no findings that were of any benefit to medical science whatsoever.

Despite the amazing results reported by Dr. Bradley on the effects of amphetamine on troubled children, little attention was paid to these findings at the time. But all that was to change in a few years.

Bizarre Experiments

The same year Dr. Bradley published his results on 350 children given amphetamine for disordered behavior, a French neurologist, Henri Gastaut, presented some findings to the Annual Meeting of the International League Against Epilepsy.[21] Subjects were administered an intravenous infusion of Metrazol, a drug known to induce convulsions, and were then exposed to flashes of light of varying frequencies produced by a strobe lamp, a procedure that induced "a muscular jerk of general flexion but predominantly in the upper limbs." The gradual infusion of the drug enabled researchers to calculate precisely the "myoclonic threshold," or the amount of Metrazol per kilogram of body weight needed to induce these violent fits, which Dr. Gastaut called the "myoclonic response."

Now, at this point the reader might be forgiven for deciding that injecting human beings with neurotoxins and then assaulting their senses with strobe lamps in order to cause violent fits is not such a great idea, but that is not the conclusion Dr. Gastaut wanted us to draw. Rather, he proclaimed, this procedure is "a clinical neurophysiological test which provides a method for the exploration of certain sub-cortical structures among which the most important are those of the diencephalon and most especially of the thalamus."[22]

By this time Dr. Bradley has departed from the Bradley Institute and accepted a position at the University of Oregon Medical School, where he helped found the Department of Child Psychiatry.[23] But bizarre experiments on the brains of children at the Bradley Institute continued, under the aegis of Maurice Laufer, who had succeeded Bradley as Director.

In a 1957 paper,[24] Dr. Laufer and two of his colleagues described what they called the "hyperkinetic impulse disorder," characterized by hyperactivity, short attention span, poor powers of concentration, unpredictability, impulsivity, inability to delay gratification, irritability, explosiveness, low frustration tolerance, and poor schoolwork. Dr. Gastaut's "photo-Metrazol activation" had by this time come to the attention of Laufer, who along with his co-workers administered this procedure to fifty patients, including thirty-two who had been diagnosed with hyperkinetic impulse disorder.[25]

The results showed a significant difference in the myoclonic threshold between the children with the hyperkinetic syndrome and the controls, leading the authors to conclude that "underlying the hyperkinetic syndrome is a dysfunction of the diencephalon."[26]

However, examination of the data shows that there was considerable overlap between the experimental and control subjects.[27] The myoclonic threshold test was not diagnostic, in the way that, say, testing for elevated glucose levels is diagnostic for untreated diabetes. It is not clear what these experiments added to the clinical observations, other than lending the enterprise a veneer of scientific legitimacy.

Dr. Laufer and his co-authors noted that while many of the children diagnosed with the hyperkinetic syndrome had suffered brain traumas or infections, many of them had not. They chalked this up to "inaccurate or incomplete histories, a succession or combination of minor insults, none of which seem significant in themselves, minor infections during the mother's third trimester of pregnancy and minor infections in the baby in the first few months of life, and lastly the hazards of normal birth."[28]

At this point the existence of a biological cause for the hyperkinetic syndrome seems more like an article of faith than a testable hypothesis.

Dr. Laufer and his colleagues took a potshot at mothers "who themselves have had a strong drive toward masculinity and dominance" and who "seemed to derive great satisfaction from their hyperkinetic infants," and then followed this up with a discussion of the psychological difficulties involved in the syndrome:

> *In the crowded classrooms of today, the teacher often becomes hostile toward a child who, despite seemingly good intelligence, can not sit still, can not keep his mind on his work, hardly ever finished the assigned task and yet unpredictably may turn in a perfect paper.[29]*

Are these behaviors the product of a diseased brain? Or are they the perfectly understandable result of bright and energetic child being forced to sit through classes conducted at a pace far below his natural ability, and endure rote learning and unimaginative assignments at the hands of an overburdened schoolteacher who doesn't have the time or energy to provide him with something more stimulating? One might wonder if hiring more teachers, paying them more, and providing them with more resources might be a better solution than drugs.

Dr. Laufer and his co-authors cautioned readers:

> *It is also possible that symptomatic control of behavior and relief of anxiety by medication, by its 'magical' effect, may interfere with the course of psychotherapy and may also make the child feel that he has no responsibility for his conduct and no difficulties which need further work.[30]*

Unfortunately, these words of caution were all but forgotten in the years that were to follow.

Post-Encephalitic Behavior Disorder

Two years later, psychiatrist Sol Levy addressed the American Psychiatric Association on the subject of "post-encephalitic behavior disorder," a syndrome characterized by erratic behavior, hyperactivity, short attention span, impulsivity, and poor schoolwork.[31] Oddly enough, no evidence of the patient ever having suffered from encephalitis was required for this diagnosis to be rendered. Dr. Levy noted, correctly, that these behaviors are often seen in patients known to have sustained brain damage, and then jumps to the conclusion that all children with this ill-defined "syndrome" must also be suffering from brain damage—even if there are no measurable signs of such damage.

But all this violates a basic principle of science, not to mention common sense, that the burden of proof always rests on the person making a claim. Dr. Levy shifts this burden to anyone who disputes his claims.

Dr. Levy also heaps scorn on his benighted psychoanalytically-oriented colleagues who looked at the role of psychological factors in the genesis of these complaints:

> *Because of this attitude which has been prevalent during the past 20 or 30 years, post-encephalitic behavior disorder has become one of the forgotten entities, and furthermore, because of the emphasis on the so-called psychogenic origin of this type of behavior which was then treated only with psychological methods, a great deal of harm was done to the child suffering from such an illness, and to his family, since the real causation was not recognized and the proper treatment was not instituted.[32]*

As Dr. Levy makes clear, by "proper treatment" he means "drugs."

Dr. Levy's attack on his psychoanalytically-oriented colleagues is followed by a case history in which he seems to be preposterously undercutting his own argument. He tells us the story of B.T., a 13-year-old boy who came to the attention of the psychiatric profession for truancy, stealing, running away from home, theft (including seven automobiles), and violent attacks on both children and adults.[33]

We learn that B.T. had an alcoholic, violent father who committed suicide when the boy was eleven, leaving behind a wife who was unable to cope with their troubled son, who in the year and a half that followed underwent placement in no fewer than fifteen different foster homes. But all this takes a back seat to the fact that when B.T. was eighteen months of age, he suffered a bout of double pneumonia with a fever that reached a high of 107 degrees.[34]

Fortunately, with the help of fifteen milligrams of benzedrine sulfate daily, a seemingly miraculous change ensued:

> *His behavior improved markedly, restlessness and hyperactivity subsided, concentration span improved, and although he had been on probation in school, he was immediately taken off since the teacher reported very satisfactory adjustment at school with marked improvement in his grades, and better socialization with other children.*[35]

Minimal Brain Dysfunction

In 1962 psychologist Sam Clements and psychiatrist John Peters of the Child Study Center at the University of Arkansas Medical Center published a paper titled "Minimal Brain Dysfunction in the School-Age Child,"[36] in which they described a syndrome including specific learning deficits, perceptual-motor deficits, general coordination deficits, hyperkinesis, impulsivity, emotional lability, short attention span, neurological signs, and borderline abnormal or abnormal EEG. None of these signs or symptoms was either necessary or sufficient for a diagnosis of "minimal brain dysfunction," as the authors themselves made clear: "It is important to reemphasize that a given child may not have symptoms in all or even many of these areas; each child has his own particular cluster of symptoms."[37]

Indeed. Their description of this syndrome goes on for two pages, and includes everything from poor spelling to homicide.[38] It is not clear what is to be gained by regarding this grab-bag of widely disparate problems as manifestations of the same "syndrome."

It is also not clear why the authors included "borderline abnormal or abnormal EEG" in their description, since by their own admission there is no consensus among scientists as to the significance of EEG findings in this group of children.[39] It is hard to see why EEG's were mentioned at all, other than to lend the enterprise a veneer of scientific legitimacy.

The choice of the term "Minimal Brain Dysfunction" was significant. The term "brain dysfunction" places these problems squarely within the jurisdiction of the medical profession, while the modifying adjective "minimal" exempted these doctors from providing any evidence of any common neural substrate underlying these complaints.

Presumably, everything we think or feel or do involves the brain. So is every problem with human thoughts of feelings or behaviors properly regarded in terms of "brain dysfunction?" If not, then which ones are and which ones are not? The authors give us no guidance on this point.

The authors state that children with this (ill-defined) syndrome often respond well to a combination of drugs and "infrequent" counseling.[40] They also dismiss out of hand the idea that anything the parents do or fail to do could have any relation to their child's problems:

> *The prevailing climate of opinion in both professional and 'magazine' psychiatry is such as to create in these parents the conviction that they are somehow, by some magical aberration in their attitudes and behavior, to blame for the child's condition.*[41]

Thus we see both in this paper and in Dr. Levy's 1959 address to the APA the germs of the "drugs not hugs" school of thought which was to dominate the field in the years to come.

Minimal Brain Damage

A 1966 paper by Yale University neurologists J.H. Pincus and G.H. Glaser described a syndrome they called "minimal brain damage," marked by hyperactivity, inattention, impulsivity, and intellectual deficits of varying degrees.[42] The authors also included "listlessness and withdrawn, negativistic behavior" as one of many symptoms,[43] without explaining how they knew that both too much activity and too little are manifestations of the same syndrome. In addition, they acknowledged that "the distinction between a normally 'active' child and a hyperactive one is largely qualitative."[44]

Drs. Pincus and Glaser suggested a wide range of possible causes, including prenatal hemorrhage, toxemia, low birth weight, and neonatal asphyxia, although again, they noted that many children with this syndrome have not experienced any of these insults, and many normal children have. The authors also noted that there are no consistent anatomic, electrophysiologic, biochemical, or neurological correlates for a diagnosis of "minimal brain damage," and that children so labeled generally outgrew these symptoms by the age of eighteen.[45]

In short, the authors had created a diagnostic label for a "syndrome" with no common cause and no measurable signs, encompassing a wide range of complaints, some of them mutually exclusive, intergrading imperceptibly into normality, most of which were indistinguishable from youthful immaturity, and which they themselves acknowledged the child could be expected to outgrow as he got older.

The authors extolled the value of stimulant drugs in treating this syndrome, although in fairness they recommended a number of nondrug interventions as well, including a stable home environment, "consistent, firm, and fair discipline," hands-on learning, parental counseling, and psychotherapy.[46] The reader may be wondering what, if any, additional benefit drugs will bestow upon a child who is provided with all these other things.

Disturbing Behaviors

In 1969, psychologist C. Keith Conners of the Harvard Medical School and Massachusetts General Hospital introduced a rating scale to be used in drug studies of children judged to be "hyperactive" or suffering from other behavioral problems.[47] This scale, which came to be known as the Conners Comprehensive Behavior Rating Scale, is often used to screen children for ADHD.

The original questionnaire consisted of thirty-nine items and was to be completed by the child's teacher, with each item to be rated as follows: "Not at all," "Just a little," Quite a bit," and "Very much." Various other forms of the questionnaire have been employed, to be completed by teachers, parents, or the kids themselves.

Items include "Sits fiddling with small objects," "Sullen or sulky," "Tattles," "Acts 'smart.'" Didn't these things used to be called "behaving like a child?"

Any deviation from the norm is pathologized. "Submissive" is an item, as is "Defiant." "Excitable" is listed, as is "Inattentive." "Stubborn" made the cut, and so did "Overly eager to please."

Other items seem indicative of serious problems, including "Overly serious or sad," "Destructive," "Steals," "Lies," "Temper outbursts," "Fearful." If a child is presenting with any or all of these disturbing behaviors, wouldn't it be preferable to find out what is going on that child's world that is so disturbing, rather than drugging him into a state of temporary acquiescence?

Could a child's hyperactivity be due to a lack of outdoor free play time, or an undiagnosed medical condition? Could her inattention be due to the fact that she comes from a chaotic or abusive home environment, or even just that she can think of more interesting things to occupy her mind with than whatever her overworked teacher has in her lesson plan for the day? No consideration at all is given to the *context* of a child's behavior—an approach which places the source of the problem squarely within the child, and exempts the adults around him from doing anything, other than diagnosing and drugging the child.

Dr. Conners went on to become a major force in the ADHD industry and was one of the planners of the largest and longest study of drug treatment for ADHD, the MTA Study. Towards the end of his life he would express concern regarding the skyrocketing rates of diagnosis and drugging for that condition.

Little Monsters

January of 1973 saw the publication of *The Hyperactive Child* by Paul Wender,[48] a research psychiatrist at the National Institute of Mental Health and Assistant Professor of Pediatrics and Psychiatry at the Johns Hopkins Hospital.[49] This was the first book ever published on the subject intended for a lay audience, and it begins with Dr. Wender's description of hyperactive toddlers, whom he portrays literally as monsters:

> *The parents frequently report that after an active and restless infancy, the child stood and walked at an early age, and then like an infant King Kong, burst the bars of his crib and marched forth to destroy the house.*[50]

This passage is followed by his description of the "typical" hyperactive child.[51] "Hyperactivity" may be manifested by the child being too easily distracted, or by his relentless focus on a particular task ("Usually it is an activity they chose themselves," Dr. Wender adds, as if that were a bad thing). The hyperactive child may be too independent, or not independent enough. He may have problems in intellectual development and perception, or he may not. He may have difficulties in coordination, or he may be "well-coordinated" and "an excellent athlete." He may have difficulty making friends, or he may make friends easily. Indeed, the "hyperactive" child need not be hyperactive at all; according to Wender, one of the symptoms of "hyperactivity" is excessive sluggishness.

Dr. Wender notes that the annoying behaviors exhibited by these children often are held in abeyance when the child is interacting one-on-one with a responsive adult,[52] but he never considers that this "syndrome" may simply be another name for lack of adult attention. Finally, he notes that the "symptoms" of hyperactivity usually disappear around the time the child reaches puberty.[53] That used to be called "growing up."

Next comes a discussion of the medications commonly used to treat hyperactivity, beginning with this preamble:

> *The hyperactive child is in the same position as the child with diabetes, epilepsy, or rheumatic fever. Children with these disorders must take insulin, anti-epileptic drugs, or penicillin for the rest of their lives.*[54]

Dr. Wender also notes that some parents object to "medicating" their children for "hyperactivity" because they "fear that the medication is related to the substances currently feared as 'drugs.'" Reassuringly, Wender puts these irrational fears to rest:

> *They sometimes fear that, like the drug addict, the child will feel so good after taking the medication that he will become addicted to it. This is never true of the medications employed by physicians in the treatment of hyperactivity.*[55]

Dr. Wender subsequently moved his base of operations to the University of Utah Medical School, where he authored the "Utah Criteria" for the diagnosis of ADHD in adults. He later helped found the American Society for Clinical Psychopharmacology, and in 1995 he published the first monograph addressing adult ADHD. He even created an eponymous medical sign in his own honor, putting himself on the same level as giants like Jean-Pierre Charcot, William Osler, and Rudolf Virchow.

And what exactly is "Wender's sign?" It consists of—tapping your foot.[56]

When Dr. Wender died in 2016, his obituary in *Attention Deficit Hyperactivity Disorders* listed some of his numerous honors and awards and, after noting that "he did not always suffer fools gladly," eulogized him as "The Dean of ADHD."[57]

Magic Pills

A 1973 review paper by psychologist L. Alan Sroufe summarized the current state of affairs in the treatment of "minimal brain dysfunction."[58] By that time, according to Dr. Sroufe, 150,000 children with behavioral or learning problems were being treated with stimulant drugs. How was that working out?

One point seems beyond dispute: short-term studies have demonstrated that when children diagnosed with MBD take these pills, it improves their ability to concentrate on repetitious, boring tasks. In fact, some doctors had suggested that this response to stimulant drugs is a diagnostic feature of MBD.[59]

But these pills have the same effect on children without this diagnostic label, and on adults as well.[60] Does the entire human race suffer from MBD?

Dr. Sroufe noted that there was no evidence of organic brain damage in the vast majority of children diagnosed with MBD, no measurable neurological or biochemical signs of this condition, and no evidence of intercorrelation between any of the vast variety of symptoms postulated for this disorder.[61] In other words, the presence of any of these symptoms did not predict the presence of any other, which seems to counter the notion that MBD is even a coherent diagnostic category.

In addition, Dr. Sroufe pointed to the lack of attention given to the toxic effects of stimulants and their potential for abuse, as well as the lack of oversight regarding the prescribing of these drugs, with some children being put on medication without a single contact with a physician.[62]

Furthermore, the emphasis on drugging was a distraction from the real source of these children's problems: "The performance of poorly rested, malnourished children can probably be improved by stimulant drugs, just as occurs with hypoxic or overly fatigued adults."[63] Dr. Sroufe also raised concerns for the potential damage to a child's self-concept:

> *The child can conclude that he is not responsible for his behavior. 'I can't help being bad today. I haven't had my pill.' The child comes to believe not in the soundness of his own brain and body, not in his own growing ability to learn and control his behavior, but in 'my magic pills that make me into a good boy and make everybody like me.'*[64]

He also decried the mixed messages implicit in the drugging of problem children with stimulants:

> *In educational programs designed to counteract drug abuse young people are told that drugs are a 'chemical cop-out,' and that if they have personal difficulties, they should work on them rather than try to solve them with drugs. They also are warned not to experiment with drugs because of potential dangers from chronic use. On the other hand, the use of stimulants for children with learning and behavior problems is widely advocated as a quick and practical solution, even when the long-term use of such drugs has not been proven to be harmless.*[65]

Perhaps most important of all, Dr. Sroufe decried the lack of credible data showing that these drugs produced any meaningful long-term benefits in terms of the children's behavior and academic achievement—precisely the outcomes we would want to see improved by stimulant drugs.[66]

In the Eye of the Beholder

Three years later, a study by psychologist Herbert Rie and his colleagues attempted to fill this gap.[67] In Dr. Rie's study, twenty-eight underachieving children were referred from the Children's Hospital in Columbus, Ohio, as well as from neighboring schools. The study employed a double-blind, cross-over design: after the initial assessment, half of the children were randomly assigned to methylphenidate, a drug similar in its properties to amphetamine, and the other half to placebo. After twelve weeks, all subjects were assessed for a variety of outcome variables. Then, the children who had been given methylphenidate were given placebo, and those who had been given placebo were given methylphenidate, so that each child served as his own matched control. After another twelve weeks the children were assessed once again.[68]

Some of the more interesting results were obtained before the randomization phase even began. There was little or no correlation between children's activity levels or behavior problems and academic performance. There also was little or no correlation between hyperactivity as assessed by parents, by teachers, or by means of actometer.[69] Is "hyperactivity" in the eye of the beholder?

But the most interesting results were obtained at the end of the study. There was *no* drug-attributable improvement in five out of six indices of scholastic achievement: No improvement in vocabulary, reading, spelling, or either math subtest. Only in the area of word association was there a significant, drug-attributable improvement.[70]

Oddly enough, the parents' teachers' perceptions of the students' academic performance improved, even though the actual performance had not.[71]

So how did the drug affect the children? The words of Dr. Rie and his co-authors are worth quoting at some length here:

> *Children who were retrospectively confirmed to have been on active drug treatment appeared, at the times of evaluation, distinctly more bland or 'flat' emotionally, lacking both the age-typical variety and frequency of emotional expression. They responded less, exhibited little or no initiative or spontaneity, offered little or no indication of interest or aversion, showed virtually no curiosity, surprise, or pleasure, and seemed devoid of humor. Jocular comments and humorous situations passed unnoticed. In short, while on active drug treatment, the children were relatively affectless, humorless, and apathetic.[72]*

While such changes may be considered beneficial by harried schoolteachers and beleaguered parents, the rest of us may wish to step back and consider where all this is going.

Is There a True Syndrome of Hyperactivity?

On 27 October 1981, the book *Hyperactive Children: A Handbook for Diagnosis and Treatment* was published by clinical psychologist Russell Barkley of the Medical College of Wisconsin and the Milwaukee Children's Hospital.[73] In the first chapter Dr. Barkley writes:

> *Is there a true syndrome of hyperactivity in which the major symptoms covary, respond uniformly to treatment, and have a single etiology? The answer to this question seems to be "no."[74]*

Oddly enough, this did not deter Dr. Barkley from writing a 450-page book about the diagnosis and treatment of a syndrome which, according to Dr. Barkley, doesn't even exist.

In the chapter on "Drug Management of Hyperactivity" he notes:

*The important point to be made here is that some hyperactive children can develop tics or even Tourette syndrome in response to methylphenidate and perhaps to other stimulant drugs as well. In some of the 10 cases reported in the literature and two cases in my own clinic, hyperactive children with a prior history of tics developed Tourette syndrome after being treated for only a few weeks to a few months with methylphenidate. In these cases the Tourette syndrome did **not** disappear after withdrawal from the stimulant drug. The children are now being given haloperidol for symptom control.[75] (Emphasis in the original.)*

In tracing the early history of the diagnostic category which later came to be known as "ADHD," five themes are apparent: 1) The lumping together of widely diverse (and sometimes mutually exclusive) complaints under a single diagnostic label; 2) The general dismissal of the role of psychological and social factors in the genesis of these conditions; 3) The attribution, in the absence of any compelling evidence, of these complaints to some unspecified central nervous system lesion; 4) An uncritical acceptance of the usefulness of drugs in treating these conditions; and 5) The deployment of a lot of neuroscience jargon to camouflage what is really going on.

Despite all this, the diagnosing and drugging of children for ill-defined behavioral syndromes was to skyrocket in the decades that were to follow.

CHAPTER TWO

STIMULANTS BLAST OFF

A Grave Peril to Our National Security

When Maurice Laufer and his colleagues announced the results of their studies on the effects of amphetamine on troubled children, the world paid very little attention. But all this was soon to change, thanks to another much more famous event that took place later that same year—the launch of the world's first artificial satellite, Sputnik.

In his book *Hyperactive: The Controversial History of ADHD*,[76] historian Matthew Smith describes how Sputnik threw the nation into a panic, with far-reaching effects no one could have foreseen. Commentators warned that the Soviet Union, with its supposedly superior educational system, would achieve world dominance through the development of superior technology:

> *"The message which this little ball carries to all Americans if they would but stop and listen is that in the last half of the twentieth century—in this age of incredible technological change—nothing is as important as a trained and educated mind. This sphere tells us not of the desirability but of the URGENT NECESSITY of the highest quality and expanded dimensions of the educational*

effort. It states more dramatically than ever before that the future of the twentieth century lies in the hands of those who have placed education and its Siamese twin, research, in the position of first priority."[77]

"So now the humor is on us to enter into a frantic catching-up competition with Soviet technological education, a burning urge to create as fast as we can an imposing quantity of specialists. The alternative is grave peril to our national security."[78]

"The launching of Sputnik I shocked the public and the educational profession out of their complacent assumptions that in science, technology, and education America was, as a matter of course, ahead of the rest of the world, and that we had no reason to be seriously concerned about competition from the Soviet Union."[79]

"Our Republic today is living through the most critical period in its history. The underlying factor here is of course the passing of the great oceans which for centuries protected us as powerful bulwarks under whose protection free institutions developed. We are now exposed to every military, political, economic, or ideological storm that arises anywhere on the planet."[80]

"When Sputnik rose into orbit, it aroused more than incredulous amazement; it was a blow to American pride. It awakened and spurred us to rigorous self-examination of our total educational system."[81]

"Today a sense of crisis has been aggravated by the long cold war and the sudden revelation of the technological strength of a supposedly 'backward' rival."[82]

The reform of the American educational system was portrayed as a patriotic duty. A "We're-all-in-this-together" spirit pervaded these exhortations:

> *"If we succeed, our educational system will be truly a strength and bulwark of national security, both for ourselves and for those other nations which cherish freedom and human dignity. This is indeed a date with destiny—a time when teachers must rise to the challenge of the space age."*[83]

> *"And so there is a tremendous problem before American education in 1958. It is essentially a problem of the preservation of the integrity of freedom: (a) through the provision of adequate teaching and learning in science and technology (b) through the reestablishment upon a sounder basis of national competence, in all lines, to deal with the times, and (c) through the freedom to teach every American child up to his capacity to learn, in science or anything else."*[84]

> *"There any many other developments that might be mentioned add up to substantial progress in the first year of the space age. They do not, however, justify complacency. Much remains to be done along many lines; we are only well started on the job. The most basic need of all is that of developing and maintaining a sense of urgency on the part of the public, the profession, and the students."*[85]

> *"We must regard it, not only as a means of individual success and personal cultivation, but also as an indispensable means in the building of national health and strength on the foundations of freedom."*[86]

Along with this came an elevation of introverted, cerebral types, previously scorned as "eggheads," to the position of national saviors:

"It is popular fashion to ridicule and condemn what the Americans call the 'egghead,' the man who from boyhood up deliberately and consciously pursues intellectual pursuits… A country neglects its eggheads at its peril. For it is the egghead who is the greatest realist. It is the egghead who invents **Sputnik***, not the captain of football or the winner of the sword of honor, nor the president of the Junior Common Room. It is the egghead who discovers penicillin, who splits the atom, who thinks of the printed circuit, the electronic brain, the guided missile…"[87] (Emphasis in the original.)*

"The bitter, brutal fact is that, both in education and in the lay community, the human intellect has been held in contempt. 'Egghead' has become a scornful appraisal of the educated man."[88]

"There has been similar progress in less tangible matters. The word **egghead** *is much less popular than it was; the good student and the intellectual are regarded with growing respect."[89] (Emphasis in the original.)*

In addition, emphasis was placed on identifying "underachievers" and helping these boys achieve their full potential as scientists and engineers:

"Now the teacher is more and more to be charged with discovering the gifted child, and with doing something special for him."[90]

"Even more significant to the average family, however, is the amount of attention being given to smoking out and stimulating the effort of the underachievers."[91]

"We must increase our efforts to identify and educate more of the talent of our nation."[92]

"There is currently great concern about the use of talent in our society. Educators are troubled by the fact that a large proportion of the intellectually able students do not attend college, and officials

> *concerned with the national security and technological advance-*
> *ments of our society are worried about the increasing shortage of*
> *scientists being trained by the American educational system. It is*
> *evident that there is much wastage in this system, and steps must*
> *be taken to use our bright young secondary school students to full*
> *advantage.*"[93]

These concerns may seem quaint in an era in which wars are fought not with Polaris missiles but with improvised explosive devices and narwhal tusks. But they were very real at the time.

All this culminated on the passage of the National Defense Education Act on 22-23 August 1958. This bill, which was signed into law by President Eisenhower on 2 September of that year, authorized the establishment of testing programs to discover able students. It also authorized guidance and counseling programs for advising students to undertake the course of study best suited to their abilities, aptitudes, and skills; encouraging them to complete their secondary education; and preparing them for admission to colleges and universities of their choice.

A number of other measures were authorized as well, including loans for needy students and fellowships for graduate students; expansion of teacher training for colleges and universities; increased funding for vocational training and for the study of mathematics, science, and foreign languages; and the establishment of systems for the collection and disseminating of statistical data to enhance the effectiveness of program planning, administrative policy formation, and the provision of services.[94]

Since then the student loan program has metastasized into a monster which seems to exist solely for the purpose of saddling young people with a colossal burden of debt at the very beginning of their adult lives. But no doubt some good came out of some of the other measures in the bill. One unfortunate by-product, however, was the expansion of behaviors pathologized as "hyperactivity."

How did this come about? Concomitant with the elevation of the eggheads was a denigration of their more rambunctious peers—those boys who in another era might have been looked upon with benign indulgence, the young Tom Sawyers who might have been satisfied with leaving school and staying on the farm or getting a job at the local paper mill, but now were seen not just as a waste of potential but as a threat to national security:

> *"If present trends continue, professional workers will be in heavy demand. White collar jobs grow at a more rapid rate than blue-collar jobs, and it is quite clear that except in one area of employment there will be little demand for unskilled workers— the slow learners and high school dropouts who constitute a major problem in large city slums."*[95]

> *"There is no longer any **place** in our society for the school dropout."*[96] *(Emphasis in the original.)*

> *"We can no longer ignore the early school dropout on the excuse that we need a large labor force of uneducated muscle men."*[97]

So not only were more young people staying in school longer than ever before, but more and more was being demanded of them. Standards were raised, especially in the areas of science and mathematics, school days were lengthened, and teachers piled on more homework.[98] At the same time, disciplinary methods that had been taken for granted since time immemorial were increasingly frowned upon. Moreover, the post-war era saw large numbers of women, including teachers, depart from the salaried work force and start families, and the resulting Baby Boom meant more children needed to be educated than in any other time in history.

Overcrowded classrooms, teacher shortages, erosion of pedagogical authority, and more and more boys expected to attend school longer and study more advanced subjects than ever before—all this was a recipe for problems. Diagnostic labels like "minimal brain dysfunction" and "hyper-activity" provided a convenient explanation for these problems.

And the drug companies were all too willing to step in and help.

Shaping Life Styles

Methylphenidate was first synthesized in 1944 by the chemist Leandro Panizzon, who worked for the Swiss pharmaceutical firm Ciba. (In 1970, Ciba merged with Geigy to form Ciba-Geigy, which in 1996 merged with Sandoz to form industry behemoth Novartis.) This drug is sold under a variety of names, the best-known of which is Ritalin, a trademark patented by Ciba in 1954. The moniker "Ritaline" (later shortened to "Ritalin") was coined by Panizzon, supposedly after he administered the drug to his wife Rita and she found it improved her tennis game.[99]

Concerta, Metadate, and Adhansia XR are all long-acting forms of methylphenidate. Daytrana is methylphenidate in the form of a trans-dermal patch. Focalin consists of the right-handed, pharmacologically active form of methylphenidate.

Originally the drug was given mainly to patients in mental hospitals, including those diagnosed with major depression and schizophrenia as well as patients recovering from lobotomies. But as asylums were shuttered in the 1960's, Ciba had to look for a new market. This time they targeted elderly patients suffering from mild depression or anxiety. One advertise-ment for Ritalin depicted a lady of a certain age, seated at a kitchen table in front of a pile of potatoes, staring morosely into the distance. In the "after" photo she looks just as morose as ever, but at least this time she's peeling the potatoes.[100]

The first randomized controlled trial of methylphenidate for children with behavioral problems was published in 1963 by psychologist C. Keith Connors and psychiatrist Leon Eisenberg of the Johns Hopkins University School of Medicine.[101] These researchers conducted a ten-day trial on the effects of the drug on kids in two residential care settings and concluded that, at least in the short term, methylphenidate decreased the frequency of disruptive behaviors and increased children's ability to attend to mundane tasks—just as Drs. Bradley and Laufer had reported amphetamine did.

In other words, the drug produced changes in the children that an exhausted parent or a harried schoolteacher would likely regard as improvements. Since then, literally hundreds of studies have replicated these findings. Moreover, such protean categories as "Learning Disability" and "Minimal Brain Dysfunction" and "Hyperactivity" could be extended to include almost any kind of childish behaviors that adults found annoying—and they were.

Ciba was happy to underwrite symposia of "recognized authorities"—including the aforementioned Dr. Conners, along with Sam Clements and John Peters (the eminent doctors from the University of Arkansas Medical Center who invented the diagnostic category of Minimal Brain Dysfunction)—and to fund their research. They also sent teams consisting of a company salesman and a sympathetic doctor to meetings of parents to promote these new diagnostic categories and the company's chemical remedy.[102] In addition, they produced educational materials for parents such as the thirty-two-minute film, *The Hyperactive Child* [103] (available in two versions, one for lay audiences and one for physicians), as well as a booklet titled *The MBD Child*, which emphasized the shape-shifting nature of this diagnostic category:

> *MBD is never exactly the same in two children, and the precise cause is not known—so MBD is difficult to pin down to a simple definition.*[104]

Even retail pharmacies ran advertisements directed at parents of "restless, aggressive, and impulsive" children, advising "the earlier the problem is identified and helped, the better the social adjustment that will be made," adding "There are certain drugs available for therapy that can be of great help."[105]

Ciba targeted doctors as well, producing a booklet titled *Physician's Handbook: Screening for MBD*[106] authored by Drs. Peters and Clements. In the prologue they explain the importance of their work:

No concern should have a higher national priority than that of providing the fullest opportunity for physical and intellectual development of every child.[107]

On page five, they offer this helpful definition of Minimal Brain Dysfunction:

MBD is a broad entity based on the concept that there are brain abnormalities underlying and corresponding to the observed symptoms which constitute the entity.[108]

The authors soft-peddle the drugs, which they do not get around to mentioning until page seventy-eight, and without ever referring to Ritalin or any other specific nostrum by name. "Side effects rarely require discontinuation of the medication," they inform us, and instead attribute the youngsters' dislike of the drugs to "sibling or peer pressure."[109]

In addition, Ciba purchased advertisements in medical journals which entreated practitioners to "Help the MBD child achieve his full potential."[110] Company reps reached out to teacher training institutes, probation officers, PTA meetings, and any other community groups which they felt might be receptive to their message. In his sales report, a Ciba executive gushed about a doc who brought two hyperactive children to an in-service meeting of medical educational personnel "to use in a demonstration on the basic symptoms of Functional Behavior Problems," adding "That's getting involvement, folks."[111]

The memo did not record how the "two hyperactive children" felt about being put on display in this fashion.

Schools would contact parents of difficult children, helpfully referring them to doctors who all too often were quick with the diagnosis and casual about the follow-up. In one school district in the suburbs of San Francisco, the school psychologist always referred parents to one particular doctor who already had two thousand patients on Ritalin, Dexedrine, or some combination of drugs, and who described his function as "shaping the life styles of these children and their families."[112]

The efforts paid off—literally. By 1971, Ritalin accounted for fifteen percent of Ciba's annual profits.[113]

My Son Came Home Crying Hysterically

Not everyone was so sanguine about all this. Parents who did not readily acquiesce to drugging their kids might find themselves pressured to do so. One mother reported that the school had issued her an ultimatum: "Put the child on drugs or we will not be able to keep him in the school." Lacking the resources to send her child to private school, and not wishing to see him caught in the middle of an acrimonious struggle, reluctantly she gave in to the school's "unremitting" pressure.[114]

Daniel Young of Little Rock, Arkansas (home of the University of Arkansas Medical Center), described his family's experiences thusly:

> *We received almost daily notes from the children's teachers and calls from the school. We were told our children had completely quit trying and were failing every subject.*
>
> *My son (who was then eight years old) was not allowed to have recess with the other children because it was too stimulating. The final blow came when my son came home crying hysterically. After I calmed him down I found out the problem. He had been put into a cardboard box for two weeks. I went down to the school in a rage. The box was gone.*
>
> *They did not deny that the cardboard box had been used for him. He was easily distracted. I was told this way he could learn without distractions.*

> *Near the end of the school year I received the final and decisive*
> *call from the school principal [who said] that the school officials*
> *were seriously considering taking it out of our hands. When I found*
> *out how they hoped to accomplish this, I was panic-stricken.*
>
> *The school officials were contemplating using our children in a*
> *trial court case to see if the children could be put [on medication]*
> *without the parents' consent.[115]*

The Youngs picked up and moved and enrolled their children in another school in another state where, they reported, they had no further problems.

The mother of yet another boy prescribed Dexedrine for "hyperactivity" offered this account:

> *David would complain that he didn't like the feel of his body when*
> *he took the pills. It took his appetite away and he would cry a lot.*
> *His dreams got so bad he couldn't even talk about them. He would*
> *get up in the night and walk the floor for hours. His body would*
> *shake and he would quiver something terrible.[116]*

The boy's doctors kept increasing his dosage until it reached forty milligrams per day. Finally, one morning the boy collapsed and begged his mother to allow him to stop the pills. She called the school and informed them he would not be coming in. Later, school officials initiated action against the family for truancy.

While some parents chafed at having their children labeled and drugged, others seemed eager to find an external cause on which to assign blame for their progeny's bad behavior or disappointing academic performance. They formed organizations such as the California Association for Neurologically Handicapped Children, which provided information to medical and educational communities; sponsored films, in-service training, and conferences; and monitored and supported legislation affecting programs and funding for "learning disabled" children.[117]

One contemporary account described the movement's devotees thusly:

They appear to be totally trusting of the professionals and methods within the circle of enlightenment, ready to suspend all disbelief, and ready to make alliances with the drug companies where necessary. They talk in sycophantic superlatives about doctors who understand LD and have done so much for their children. They listen appreciatively when psychiatrist Camilla Anderson, keynoting at a symposium on learning disabilities, tells 1,500 suburban mothers that MBD causes everything from bad financial planning, violent crime and slums to unconventional sexual positions, and when she urges sterilization for all MBD victims, and they gratefully reprint Anderson's 164-item list of the most common (or worrisome) habits of children—all of them identified as manifestations of MBD: "perseverative masturbation," "gullible," "new generation psychology," "need for structure," "bossy," "demanding," "bed wetting," "running away."[118]

The authors went on to quote CANHC president Nancy Ramos who noted that while many learning-disabled children come from broken homes, "It's not the broken marriages that cause LD, it's that the learning-disabled child broke up the marriage in the first place."[119]

Even some of the True Believers began to have second thoughts. Caroline Rodriguez, another woman who served as CANHC president, was almost impeached after raising concerns about drugging kids for behavioral problems. Her own son fell down and broke his leg after being prescribed the anticonvulsant Dilantin, and he suffered liver damage after taking another drug, while a friend's son began having crying fits after starting on Ritalin:

I see lots of kids on Ritalin, and I'd hate to call that improvement. The kid is a bag of bones, but as long as he behaves and shuts up, nothing else is important. A lot of CANHC people are hyperactive parents whose logic is faulty.[120]

Irreparable Harm

An article in the *New York Times*[121] that ran 6 February 1968 was the first major story in the popular press on the salubrious effects of these new drugs. The piece covered the proceedings of the International Congress for Children with Learning Disabilities, held at the Sheraton-Boston and Statler-Hilton hotels, and featured these words from a pediatrician who plumed himself on his "practical gutsy approach of the doctor out in the boondocks who has to do something when the kids are brought to his office,"[122] adding:

> *I don't know what the drug will do in 20 years, but I have to try to do what we can do now to keep the kid from winding up in juvenile hall.*[123]

The author of the article concluded thusly:

> *One of the most promising though still highly experimental approaches to drug therapy is the stimulation of the manufacture of ribonucleic acid in the brain. Studies have concluded that this substance, known as RNA, may constitute the chemical basis of learning.*
>
> *If true, it is conceivable that memory and intelligence could some day be improved by RNA injections.*[124]

Since this article ran more than fifty years ago, no credible evidence has come to light showing that the administration of stimulant drugs results in reduced incarceration rates or any other meaningful long-term benefit. The promised injections of RNA to improve memory and intelligence have not been made available, either.

A major story in the *Washington Post*[125] that ran on 29 June 1970 took a more critical tone. The piece focused on Omaha, Nebraska, a city in which, it was claimed, between five and ten percent of school pupils had been prescribed Ritalin or other behavior-modification drugs. Bryon Oberst, a local pediatrician who was instrumental in introducing the behavior modification program to that city the year before, averred that the drugs made children "more successful" and "more self-confident," adding:

> *I see them every three to six months and we check their brain wave patterns yearly until they revert to normal.*[126]

The article acknowledged the role of the drug companies in promoting the use of their wares, citing an unnamed school official who noted:

> *Oh, they come around and address meetings on the subject, but it's always pretty much of a soft sell. They mention the products and the claims, but they don't push too hard.*[127]

The behavior modification program was not received with open arms by everyone. The black community in Omaha was especially skeptical. At a school board meeting, parents and community organizers charged that the city was trying to drug black children into submission.[128]

One mother stated that her son's teacher "badgered" her on the telephone every night for a month and a half to have the boy put on drugs. The mother finally relented and obtained a prescription for the child but never actually gave him the drugs, although she told the teacher she had. The teacher, for her part, noted with pleasure the improvement in the lad's academic performance.[129]

The article concluded with these remarks from Dr. Oberst:

> *They are definitely happier. One of my mothers came home from a meeting and found her child's homework finished on the table. And the child had written a note saying "Thank you mother, I feel much happier."*[130]

Despite these words of reassurance from the eminent doctor, this article marked the beginning of a period of critical scrutiny in the popular press, with articles in the *Saturday Review*,[131] *Evergreen Review*,[132] and the *Village Voice*[133] highlighting the lack of knowledge of the long-term harms or benefits of these drugs, both for the children involved and for society in general. *Newsweek*[134] and *US News and World Report*[135] were guardedly equivocal, while the *New Republic*[136] went on the counterattack:

> *On June 15, Miss Maryl Harris, a black militant student with an arrest record for sit-ins at an Omaha university, began building an election issue for Mr. Ernest W. Chambers, her candidate for the Nebraska legislature from Omaha's 11th District. She attended a school board meeting to charge, based on her experience with one student in an extracurricular class on black studies she was teaching, that school children from the ghetto were being drugged into conformity in the classroom. The boy had told her, when she remarked on his unusual behavior, that he had been placed on drugs because of his school conduct. From June 15 until June 29 when the story of the Omaha experiment broke on a national basis, Mr. Chambers, who had decided to use kids undergoing medical treatment as an issue, began developing the strategy which successfully carried him into the state legislature. But the Pandora's box he opened remains open, and irreparable harm has been done to children.*

The *Washington Post* piece also drew this finger-wagging admonition from *Good Housekeeping*:

> *Most everyone agrees that charges stemming from Omaha and inflammatory newspaper reports (that drugs are doled out as part of fascist, racist, government-financed or school-organized plots to "drug helpless children into submission") are just plain silly.*[137]

The rhetorical excesses were by no means limited to one side of this debate. Representative Cornelius Gallagher, a member of the New Jersey congressional delegation, took to the House floor to declaim:

> *On the basis of these considerations, Mr. Speaker, I am now commencing an investigation by my privacy subcommittee to determine if any federal funds whatsoever have been used in this monstrous project.*
>
> *Incidents such as the Omaha test may be exaggerated, but they seem to represent the most concerted attack on our basic humanity ever mounted in the history of the world.[138]*

That fall, Representative John Rarick of Louisiana introduced a bill to enjoin the Department of Health, Education, and Welfare from using government funds to "promote, subsidize, or propagandize the use or administration of any drug, narcotic, barbiturate, or sedatives to any child in the public school system."[139] The bill died in committee.

Rarick, for his part, was a virulent racist better known for his vitriolic attacks on Jewish people and black people than for his stance on stimulant medication.[140] As for Gallagher, his career came to an end two years later when he was imprisoned for tax evasion.[141]

The same year the *WaPo* piece ran, an article in the *Saturday Review* by Careth Ellington, author of *Shadow Children*, averred:

> *The prescription of d–amphetamines and methylphenidates (respectively Dexedrine and Ritalin) then, could be compared to the use of insulin by the diabetic…[142]*

Happy Pills

Less than a year later, a story in the *Los Angeles Times*[143] told the tale of one David Martin, M.D., described as "the leading proponent of public acceptance for the so-called 'Happy Pill,'" who traveled the length and breadth of the State of California, touting the benefits of Ciba-Geigy's blockbuster drug. The piece featured these words of wisdom from the general practitioner:

> *We gave [Ritalin] to one terrible little boy and a few minutes later the child was actually taking out the garbage for his mother.*
>
> *The diagnosis [of hyperactivity] can best be made by the parent or teacher. Why, my wife was even able to diagnose one of these kids simply on the basis of what his mother said on the golf course.*
>
> *Now I want you to understand we aren't curing these kids; we're just keeping them under control. It's just like we don't cure diabetics with insulin.*
>
> *Usually we'll start your 3- or 4-year-old with five milligrams three times a day, then up it to 15 milligrams by the time they are 8 or 9.*
>
> *We can go as high as 100 to 140 milligrams a day if we have to.*[144]

The Most Dangerous Psychoactive Drug

September 1975 saw the publication of *The Myth of the Hyperactive Child* by husband-and-wife reporting team Peter Schrag and Diane Divoky. The book was a scathing indictment not just of stimulant drugs for kids but of the cradle-to-grave surveillance state and the ever-growing apparatus of behavior modification coming to pervade every aspect of modern life. The authors issued this stark warning:

> *From a political and social perspective, the most dangerous psychoactive drug is precisely the one that is medically the safest and psychologically the most effective.*

> *What of the drug which, in fact or belief, has few negative medical side effects but which nonetheless makes the patient-student-prisoner-citizen more docile and manageable?*
>
> *The belief in "My magic pills make me into a good boy" is, after all, a political as well as personal statement in which institutional benevolence and the need for personal accommodation [to institutions] are taken for granted.*
>
> *It is the ideology of drugging, the idea that people can and should be chemically managed, that represents the most pervasive imposition on personal liberty and the most dangerous extension of authority.*[145]

Three years later, a survey of forty-eight physicians in Alameda and Contra Costa counties in California found that many of them agreed with this statement:

> *Depriving a hyperactive child of Ritalin is similar to depriving a diabetic of insulin.*[146]

These People Will Do Anything to Get Attention

Diane Montoya of Taft, California, never wanted to be a patient advocate, but she found herself forced into that role after she witnessed firsthand the devastating effects Ritalin had on two of her children.[147]

Diane's older son Frank was quiet and inattentive and did not fare well in his first year at kindergarten. After his IQ was measured at seventy-two, he was made to repeat kindergarten and at the end of his second year was placed on Ritalin.[148]

Frank was also placed in a class for the "Educable Mentally Retarded"—without his parents' consent, in blatant violation of state law. Every morning at 11:00, Frank and the other Ritalin children would be made to line up in the hallway to receive the daily dose. Other children taunted them and called them "retarded," and Frank would come home crying.[149]

After the boy suffered a grand mal seizure, Diane took him off Ritalin once more and sought help from specialists. After a year and a half on the drug, Frank's IQ was assessed again and was found to have dropped to fifty-two.[150]

Diane's younger son Joe was also placed on Ritalin, after his teacher caught him hiding a worm in his pocket. The boy became lethargic and cried easily and was made to repeat the first grade. When there was no apparent change in the boy's academic performance, his mother took him off the drug for two weeks, and then asked Joe's teacher how he was doing. When the teacher replied "fine," Diane revealed she had stopped giving him Ritalin. Subsequent to that admission she began receiving a torrent of complaints about the boy's classroom behavior, and she dutifully put him back on the drug.[151]

Diane explained that her decision to give the drug to her sons was based on her faith in the family's trusted pediatrician, Agnes Tarr:

> *When Dr. Tarr told me anything, it was like the Gospel. She'd been taking care of my kids since they were born, and I didn't think she would ever lead me wrong. So when she said this is what Frankie and Joe needed, I believed her. It was a whole new thing to me—some pill that wasn't going to cause me any harm but would help Frankie learn and Joe behave.[152]*

Juanita Morrison was another mother whose son had been put on Ritalin at the behest of school authorities. Her husband never saw first-hand the effects the drug had on the child until the family went on vacation and Juanita decided to give their son half a pill because he was "acting up." The boy's father recalled:

He just sat there and stared straight ahead for hours. I told my wife when we got home we were going to take those pills and dump them down the toilet.[153]

Juanita Morrison, Diane Montoya, and some other parents contacted the Youth Law Center, a federally funded organization offering free legal services to children. At first, they hoped to avoid having to go to court, asking just that the school district review its policy on psychoactive drugs and EMR classes, and to assure them that parents would be granted full information and choices of alternatives regarding the education of troubled children.[154]

At a raucous meeting of the Taft School Board, Juanita challenged the superintendent over some statements he made which she felt contradicted what he had told her earlier in private. In the middle of a heated exchange, Juanita collapsed on the floor with a heart attack. As she was being carried out, one audience member sneered "These people will do anything to get attention."[155]

The school board denied all the parents' requests. Diane Montoya and the other parents filed suit, asking for $425,000 in damages.[156] The board filed a counter-suit against the parents and the Youth Law Center, alleging they had "deliberately, intentionally, and maliciously abused the process of court by filing this action to embarrass, intimidate, and coerce" school officials to forgo the administration of Ritalin, "notwithstanding that such administration is lawful and proper in all respects." A year later Juanita suffered a second heart attack, and underwent open-heart surgery. She died a few days later.[157]

In 1980, the school district settled with the parents for $210,000, split between seventeen different families.[158] By then, the controversy about stimulant drugs for children had largely dropped off the radar. Few Americans seemed to care anymore.[159] And, by then, Skylab had fallen, and few Americans cared anymore about space exploration, either.

But by that time, the process of assembling a machine for giving as many drugs as possible to as many children as possible was nearly complete. Only one more component needed to be put into place to make the number of prescriptions for stimulant drugs for kids soar like—well, like a Saturn V rocket. And that component was a document which future historians may one day regard as influential as *The Communist Manifesto* or *Mein Kampf*—the third iteration of the *Diagnostic and Statistical Manual of Mental Disorders*, or the *DSM-III*.

CHAPTER THREE

HYPERACTIVITY BECOMES ADHD

The Re-Branding of Psychiatry

By the end of the 1970's, psychiatry was facing a crisis of identity that seemed to threaten its very existence. Then as now, psychiatry was the only medical specialty with its own anti- movement, sparked by tomes such as *The Myth of Mental Illness* by psychiatrist Thomas Szasz[160] and *The End of Psychiatry* by psychiatrist E. Fuller Torrey.[161] The Rosenhan experiment had convinced many that psychiatrists were unable to distinguish the insane from the sane.[162] The so-called minor tranquilizers, such as Valium, had been exposed as the dangerous and highly addictive drugs they were, while the major tranquilizers, such as Thorazine, were derided by patients forced to take them as instruments of torture. Other somatic interventions for mental illness, such as lobotomy and insulin coma, were as discredited as bloodletting. The tired old dogmas of Herr Doktor Freud seemed about as scientific as astrology or tarot reading.

About the only thing psychiatry had left to offer was talk therapy, and while no doubt many individual psychiatrists did some good in this capacity, there was a growing awareness among the public and the psychiatrists themselves that the conditions they were treating weren't really illnesses, and what the psychiatrists were doing wasn't really practicing medicine.[163] At the same time, psychiatrists practicing talk therapy were facing increasingly stiff competition from a growing army of lesser-paid professionals—psychologists, counselors, social workers, clergy, and lay therapists of various sorts. Medical school graduates were avoiding psychiatry in droves, and psychiatrists had the lowest salaries of any medical specialty.

Psychiatry was at a crossroads. Practicing psychiatrists could have concentrated their efforts on talk therapy, and accepted the salary of a clinical psychologist or a social worker. Medical schools could have begun shuttering residency programs in psychiatry, and the American Psychiatric Association could have merged with the other APA, the American Psychological Association.

In short, psychiatry could have begun the process of dismantling itself as a medical specialty.

Of course that didn't happen. Instead psychiatry embarked on a vigorous re-branding campaign, as documented by author Robert Whitaker in his blockbuster work of nonfiction, *Anatomy of an Epidemic,*[164] in order to convince the public (and themselves?) that psychiatrists were real doctors treating real diseases. A massive media campaign was fostered, in order to sell the public the idea that the biological bases of mental illness had been found, or at any rate would be found some time really soon, and that psychiatry had safe and effective medications for these conditions.

The 2 April 1979 issue of *Time* magazine featured a cover story heralding the new biological psychiatry. Titled "Psychiatry on the Couch: To Shake the Blues, Freud's Disciples Seek New Directions," the piece quoted one prominent psychiatrist as follows: "We will learn to think of ourselves, our personalities, as an orchestra of chemical voices in our head."[165]

The article went on to promise a new era in which:

> *It would become possible to diagnose mental illness from a simple blood, urine, or spinal fluid sample. Once imbalances in body chemistry are determined, doctors would be able to adjust them by administering the appropriate drugs.*[166]

Forty years later these promises remain entirely unfulfilled.

The linchpin of this enterprise was the APA's new version of the *Diagnostic and Statistical Manual of Mental Disorders*, or *DSM-III*, released in February 1980, amid promises that it would put the business of psychiatric diagnosis on a more scientific footing.[167]

This new edition of the *DSM* was impressive, certainly in terms of heft. Whereas the previous iteration, *DSM-II*, published in 1968, was a puny 134 A5-sized pages, the new rendition weighed in at a beefy 494 A4-sized pages. The 1968 category "Hyperkinetic Reaction of Childhood" was replaced with two new ones: Attention Deficit Disorder without Hyperactivity (ADD) and Attention Deficit Disorder with Hyperactivity (ADD-H).

A diagnosis of ADD required three symptoms of inattention from a checklist of five, plus three symptoms of impulsivity from a checklist of six. A diagnosis of ADD-H required all of the above plus two symptoms of hyperactivity from a checklist of six. The maximum age for onset of symptoms was set at seven years. Antisocial behaviors had been removed from the diagnostic checklist and placed under a separate label, "Conduct Disorder."

Seven years later *DSM-III* was replaced with the revised version, *DSM-IIIR*, which punched in at a beefier 567 pages. The twin categories of ADD and ADD-H were subsumed into a single one, Attention Deficit Hyperactivity Disorder, or ADHD. In order for a diagnosis to be rendered, a child needed to exhibit at least eight symptoms from a checklist of fourteen.

The increased emphasis on inattention, as opposed to hyperactivity, guaranteed that an increased number of girls would be diagnosed with this condition, although this would remain primarily a label applied to boys.

For many years, Ritalin was the treatment of choice for this diagnostic category, but consumption of that drug peaked in 2012. Meanwhile, the consumption of amphetamine has been increasing, and in 2016 went on to surpass that of Ritalin.[168] The use of lisdexamfetamine has been increasing as well. Other drugs which are occasionally prescribed for this condition include:

- Methamphetamine (Desoxyn), a chemical derivative of amphetamine

- Tricyclic antidepressants, notably amitriptyline (Elavil), nortriptyline, and imipramine

- Atomoxetine (Strattera), which inhibits the uptake of norepinephrine

- Antihypertensives, such as guanfacine (Intuniv, Tenex) and clonidine (Kapvay)

Pemoline (Cylert) used to be prescribed for ADHD but has since been withdrawn from the market after being linked to cases of liver toxicity.

In the years that followed the publication of *DSM-III*, the number of boys and girls diagnosed and drugged for a variety of conditions skyrocketed, with ADHD leading the way. And what did we get in return for this relentless drugging?

Unreliable Narrators

A study published in August of 1982 by Esther K. Sleator and her colleagues may have been the first indication in the scientific literature that something was amiss.[169] The authors interviewed fifty-two children who were currently or formerly taking medication for ADD, and checked the details garnered in the course of these interviews with information gleaned from conversations with parents and teachers. Three notable findings emerged.

The first was that nearly half of the children reported that they disliked or hated taking medication for ADD. Sample comments from these children included:

> *"It makes me sad."[170]*

> *"I wouldn't talk or smile or anything."[171]*

> *"It makes me feel strange."[172]*

> *"I don't know how to explain it, I just don't want to take it anymore."[173]*

The second was that many of the children who stated that they liked or felt indifferent to the medication were later found to be lying to the interviewers. These children employed a variety of strategies to avoid being drugged, ranging from deliberately failing to remind a parent to administer the medication, to cheeking the medication and then surreptitiously throwing it away, to outright refusal.[174]

A third finding was that the interviewers, including the treating physician, were almost totally incapable of discerning which children were telling the truth to them and which were lying. Of twenty-three interviews later found to be partially or totally unreliable after comparison to information from other sources, twenty-one had been coded by the study authors as having "good credibility." The authors themselves noted "Clearly most of the children whose interviews proved unreliable came across to the interviewers as sincere and believable."[175]

Dr. Sleator and her co-authors concluded that "The intensity of the dislike of many hyperactive children for taking stimulants is a troubling phenomenon."[176] No argument there. So did any of this cause them to re-assess whether drugging children for behavioral disorders is a good idea? Certainly not:

> *The problem is made more difficult by the fact that many of the most vigorous objectors, according to all observers, are greatly benefitted by medication in school achievement, in freedom from the open disapproval of elders at home and in school, and in improved peer and sibling relationships. Our observations that such improved behavior and functioning occur frequently are confirmed by an abundance of well-controlled published studies which support the view that there is an important role for stimulant drug treatment of hyperactive children.*[177]

The authors go on to ask "Is it justifiable to urge children to follow what is to them an aversive regimen whose benefits are perceived by associates but not by themselves?" and then proceed to answer their own question with a resounding Yes, likening the drugging of children for behavioral problems to childhood immunization and mandatory school attendance.[178]

Misperceptions

In 1994, the APA released the newest version of the *DSM*, *DSM-IV*, which clocked in at a ponderous 934 pages. The diagnostic category ADHD was split into three subtypes: Predominantly Inattentive Type, which required at least six symptoms from a checklist of nine; Predominantly Hyperactive Type, which required at least six symptoms from another checklist of nine; and Combined Type, which required at least six symptoms from each checklist. The maximum age for the onset of symptoms still was set at seven years.

Since there is no overlap in symptoms between the "Inattentive Type" and the "Hyperactive Type," it is not clear in what sense these conditions are "subtypes" of the same disease—other than because the authors of the *DSM-IV* said so.

The newly expanded criteria guaranteed that more children would be labeled as having this disorder. Two studies, one in the United States[179] and one in Germany,[180] screened children for ADHD using both the *DSM-IIIR* criteria and the *DSM-IV* criteria and found that sixty percent more kids were eligible for a diagnosis under the new criteria. The proportion of girls eligible for a diagnosis also increased.

A 1995 survey of 380 randomly selected members of the American Academy of Pediatrics listed several "misperceptions" that child patients and their parents were said to harbor regarding ADHD medication and ADHD itself.[181] Parental "misperceptions" included beliefs that children will outgrow ADHD, that medication makes their children drugged or zombielike, that ADHD drugs are addictive, and that the drugs inhibit growth. Child "misperceptions" included beliefs that ADHD drugs made them feel different, that ADHD medications are like illicit drugs and should not be ingested because they are taught in school to "just say no" to drugs, and that the drugs harm them.

It's interesting to note that the children's own reports of how the drugs affect them are labeled "misperceptions." The paper also stated that a large portion of parents believe ADHD is due to a chemical imbalance.[182] That belief was not labeled a "misperception."

An Overabundance of Drugs, a Paucity of Evidence

By 1998—more than fifty years after Dr. Bradley reported his results on the effects of amphetamine on difficult children at the Emma Pemberton Bradley Home—at least eleven major reviews had failed to find convincing evidence for any meaningful long-term benefits to stimulant medication for ADHD and related conditions. In a 1978 paper, clinical psychologist Russel Barkley declared "The major effect of stimulants appears to be an improvement in classroom manageability rather than academic performance."[183]

In the years that followed, this was a recurring theme in the scientific literature:

"Academic achievement and productivity are not appreciably improved by the drugs, despite the positive effects on classroom conduct."[184]

"While stimulants may increase academic productivity, (a) the effect on standardized test scores is not particularly robust; (b) individual reaction is quite variable, (c) the clinical implications for adult outcome appears to be minimal; and (d) some behavioral interventions are clearly superior."[185]

"Follow-up studies that exist presently suggest little long-term impact of sympathomimetic drugs on school achievement, peer relationships, or behavior problems in adolescence."[186]

"There is minimal evidence that extended stimulant treatment improves cognitive deficits or associated problems such as conduct disturbance, low self-esteem, poor peer relationships, or academic underachievement."[187]

"These long-term studies suggest that stimulants do not affect the clinical course or outcome of children with ADHD."[188]

"Stimulant pharmacotherapy does not typically correct academic or social deficits. These drugs do not improve learning, increase positive peer interactions, or enhance learning and achievement."[189]

*"Long-term efficacy of stimulant medication has not been demonstrated for **any** domain of childhood functioning."*[190] *(Emphasis in the original.)*

"Most of the studies are very brief, of not more than a few weeks' duration at most. Some studies were ultrashort, lasting only days. There is a dearth of evidence on long-term studies."[191]

"The dearth of extended treatment studies stands in marked contrast to any generalizations about long-term outcomes."[192]

"It is important to emphasize that pharmacotherapy alone, while highly effective for short-term symptomatic improvement, has not been shown to improve the long-term outcome for any domain of functioning."[193]

A 16 September 1997 article in the *New York Times* quoted ADHD researcher Judith Rapaport:

There's no controversy that drug treatment improves attention and behavior in the short term. The Holy Grail is to show whether stimulant drugs taken long term do anything.[194]

While Dr. Rapaport likened evidence of long-term benefits of these drugs to the Holy Grail, others might consider it an absolute minimum requirement that ought to have been fulfilled before these drugs were given to millions of children.

Confusing a Symptom with a Diagnosis

The year 1998 saw the publication of *The Hyperactivity Hoax* by Sidney Walker, a practicing neurologist and psychiatrist.[195] After acknowledging that the great majority of children labeled "hyperactive" are perfectly normal kids responding in a predictable manner to their circumstances, Dr. Walker emphasized a point that had been all too often ignored: hyperactivity can also be a symptom of a vast variety of serious and even life-threatening diseases, such as lead poisoning, mercury poisoning, manganese toxicity, head injuries, carbon monoxide poisoning, iron-deficiency anemia, vitamin deficiency, hyperthyroidism, temporal lobe seizures, subclinical diabetes, cardiac conditions, brain tumors… the list goes on and on.

Most of these can be cured or at least ameliorated if diagnosed and treated properly, and yet children suffering from any of these conditions may find themselves labeled "hyperactive" and lumped together with a whole lot of perfectly healthy children, and many of them will end up being prescribed Ritalin. Dr. Walker noted these practitioners are confusing a symptom with a diagnosis, and likened the process to that of a doctor who diagnoses every patient who coughs with "coughing disorder" and prescribes cough drops, without bothering to find out whether the cough is caused by strep throat, tuberculosis, or lung cancer. The treatment may mask the symptoms temporarily, but the underlying disorder remains.[196]

The NIH Consensus Development Conference

In November of 1998 NIH Consensus Development Conference on Diagnosis and Treatment of Attention Deficit Hyperactivity Disorder was held in Bethesda, Maryland. One of the featured speakers was psychiatrist Peter Breggin, who had already risen to national prominence with his books *Toxic Psychiatry*[197] and *Talking Back to Prozac*[198] (with Ginger Ross Breggin). Dr. Breggin's talk focused on the harms of stimulant drugs for ADHD[199]—and his findings were devastating.

Data culled largely from randomized, placebo-controlled trials included the following harms:

> *CENTRAL NERVOUS EFFECTS: Psychosis, hallucinations, convulsions, nightmares, nervousness, anxiety, irritability, crying jags, dysphoria, impaired cognition, dizziness, headache, tics, nervous habits, stereotyped activities or compulsions, decreased social interest, and constriction of affect and spontaneity ("zombie-like effect")[200]*

> *GASTROINTESTINAL: Anorexia, nausea, vomiting, stomach pain, cramps, dry mouth[201]*

> *ENDOCRINE/METABOLIC: Pituitary dysfunction, weight loss, growth suppression[202]*

CARDIOVASCULAR: Palpitations, tachycardia, hypertension, arrhythmias, cardiac arrest[203]

OTHER: Blurred vision, rashes, anemia, leukopenia[204]

WITHDRAWAL AND REBOUND: Insomnia, evening crash, depression, overactivity, and rebound of ADHD-like symptoms[205]

Had enough? It gets worse. Dr. Breggin pointed out that the FDA's own adverse drug event reporting system included fifty cases in the combined category of overdose, overdose (intentional), and suicide attempt.[206]

The FDA's adverse drug event reporting system is thought to capture between one and ten percent of all adverse events.

Dr. Breggin also mentioned a study that had shown brain atrophy in nearly half of children who had been treated with stimulants, adding "Brain scan studies that attempt to show a pathology of ADHD are almost certainly measuring pathology caused by psychostimulants."[207]

Dr. Breggin laid it on the line:

> *Spontaneous or self-generated activities—play, mastery, exploration, novelty seeking, curiosity, and zestful socialization—are central to the growth and development of animals and humans and necessary for the full elaboration of CNS synaptic connections.*[208]

> *Psychostimulants consistently cause two specific, related adverse drug effects in animals (and also humans).*[209]

> *First, stimulants suppress **normal** spontaneous or self-generated activity and socialization.*[210] *(Emphasis in the original)*

> *Second, stimulants promote **abnormal** stereotyped obsessive/ compulsive asocial behaviors that are repetitive and meaningless.*[211] *(Emphasis in the original)*

These drugs suppress normal spontaneous, self-generated behaviors and socialization; they promote abnormal compulsive, asocial, compliant behaviors deemed suitable to structured and often suppressive situations, such as many classrooms.[212]

This drug-induced suppression of behavior and mental function is independent of the child's mental state; it occurs in healthy animals and children.[213]

He wound up by noting that no study had demonstrated any positive long-term outcome that lasted beyond eighteen weeks, and that all the studies showing bad outcomes for patients with ADHD had been performed on children treated with stimulant drugs, concluding:

*"The use of psychostimulant drugs for the control of behaviors labeled ADHD in children **should be stopped**."*[214] *(Emphasis in the original.)*

The conference also featured a question-and-answer session with the media. Attendees were treated to the following exchange between NPR correspondent Joe Palca and pediatrician and panel member Mark Vonnegut:[215]

MODERATOR: "We have agreed that there is no consistent diagnostic test for ADHD. Our knowledge about the cause or causes of ADHD remain speculative. I would now like to open the forum to questions from the press."

JOE PALCA: "It sounds a little bit like you're saying that the definition is a little bit like the Supreme Court's definition of pornography, which is you know it when you see it." [Laughter]

MODERATOR: "We're gonna disagree. And I would like any member of the panel to describe a typical ADHD in terms of symptomatology. Mark, would you like to—? Since you see them in your practice."

MARK VONNEGUT: "There, there, uh, I mean—I think the panel has been frank in—you know, the difficulties here are immense in terms of, of, uh, um—these kids—I mean, um, uh—It is hard—It's very hard to know how to answer this question. These kids, um— In my experience, when you see these kids, um, they are, you know, several standard deviations different in terms of they cannot sit still, they cannot attend, they're, um, they cannot, you know, even when, um, uh, they are as if driven by a motor. There are some good clinical descriptions, um, of these kids…"

"Uh, uh, I do, I think part of the problem is the profession keeps changing the diagnosis. We have DSM-IV, the latest thing, but we have no, we have no guarantee that DSM-5 won't give us yet another diagnosis. But certainly I think we have the feeling, um, again, that's not very satisfying, uh, and I'm sure somebody else on this panel should have and could have done a better job with this question, so I'll stop talking now."

Highlights from the panel's consensus statement[216] include the following:

An independent diagnostic test for ADHD does not exist.[217]

There is no information on the long-term outcomes of medica-tion-treated ADHD individuals in terms of educational and occupational achievements, involvement with the police, or other areas of social functioning.[218]

Despite the improvement in core symptoms, there is little improve-ment in academic achievement or social skills.[219]

> *Effective treatments for ADHD have been evaluated primarily for the short term (approximately 3 months).*[220]

> *There is a paucity of data providing information on long-term treatment beyond 14 months.*[221]

Despite the admitted lack of evidence for any meaningful long-term benefits of stimulant drugs for children's behavioral problems, despite Dr. Breggin's warnings of the harms, and despite Dr. Vonnegut's stammering inability even to explain to his fellow conferees what ADHD is, the panel did not recommend against the continuing use of these drugs.

Little is Known

The years that followed were marked by a consistent failure to produce any credible data demonstrating any meaningful long-term benefit of stimulant medication for ADHD, a point that was repeatedly emphasized in the literature:

> *"Over the short term, the immediate effects on academic productivity do not translate into gains in achievement but over longer periods of treatment, small effects may emerge."*[222]

> *"Neither behavior management nor stimulant treatment can boast of measurable gains in **long-term** outcome studies."*[223] *(Emphasis in the original.)*

> *"Little is known, for example, about outcomes such as educational achievement, employment, or social functioning."*[224]

> *"Several controlled studies have investigated the short-term effects of methylphenidate given at dosages ranging from 2.5 to 20 mg. These trials show measurable efficacy but are clearly limited by small sample size, brief duration of treatment, and restricted range of efficacy and safety outcomes."*[225]

"We were unable to demonstrate that the methylphenidate effect is maintained beyond 4 weeks... The paucity of long-term trials is problematic, because children routinely receive methylphenidate in clinical contexts for much longer than was observed in the present collection of small trials."[226]

"Pharmacologic treatment and behavior management are associated with reduction of the core symptoms of ADHD and increased academic productivity, but not with improved standardized test scores or ultimate educational attainment."[227]

The MTA Study

The National Institute of Mental Health Multisite Multimodal Treatment Study was designed to close this gap in knowledge and to identify best practices for helping children diagnosed with ADHD.[228] The study population consisted of a total of 579 children, all between their seventh and tenth birthdays (average age was eight and a half), all diagnosed with ADHD (Combined Type). Each child was randomly assigned to one of four treatment arms: medication plus behavioral therapy, medication alone, behavioral therapy alone, and "usual community care."[229]

The study planners gave the drugs every chance to work. All of the children were started on Ritalin, and doses were carefully titrated to find the optimum for each child. Children who did not respond well to Ritalin were titrated on the following alternative medications, in this order: dextroamphetamine, pemoline, imipramine, and, if necessary, others approved by a cross-site panel. Children attended monthly half-hour medication maintenance visits (as opposed to the standard one or two brief visits per year) with a pharmacotherapist who provided support, encouragement, and practical advice, and who prescribed dose adjustments if necessary. The pharmacotherapist also kept in touch with the child's teacher by means of monthly telephone conversations. Parents were supplied with readings from an approved list in order to educate them about the importance of drug treatment for ADHD. Medication compliance was "facilitated" by monthly pill counts, saliva measurements of methylphenidate levels, and encouraging families to make up missed visits. The randomization phase of the study lasted fourteen months, at which point all children were released to usual community care.[230] The progress of these children was followed for a total of eight years.

And how did all this work out for the kids? At the end of the fourteen-month randomization phase, the researchers found the kids in the medication and the combined treatment arms, compared to the ones in the two unmedicated arms, exhibited superior results in terms of three outcome variables: parents and teacher's rating of inattention, and teachers' rating of hyperactivity.[231]

But the eight-year follow-up results of the MTA Study, published in May of 2009, were nothing short of astonishing. The good news was that kids in all four treatment arms tended to get better over time. That's not really very surprising—that used to be called "growing up." What was surprising was that the eight-year follow-up found no significant differences between any of the four treatment arms for any of twenty-four outcome variables.[232]

No effect on ADHD symptoms. No effect on oppositional behavior or antisocial behavior. No effect on anxiety or depression. No effect on reading skills, math skills, grade point averages, or grade retention. No effect on social functioning, psychiatric hospitalizations, traffic tickets, or auto accidents[233]—the list goes on and on.

In fairness, it should be pointed out that a substantial fraction of the children assigned to "usual community care" were also prescribed ADHD medication by their primary care providers. Could this have blurred the differences between the treatment groups? The researchers themselves nixed this idea, noting that their own analysis showed no correlation between initial or continuing severity of symptoms and the decision to start, continue, or stop medication.[234]

This was huge. Millions of children had been given powerful, brain-altering stimulants, in some cases for years and years, and now a large multiyear randomized controlled trial had failed to find *any* long-term benefits of these drugs.

In addition, at the three-year follow-up the researchers found the drugs stunted the children's growth. The largest difference (more than one-and-a-half inches) was between children assigned to one of the two medication arms who had been continuously medicated, with children who never received medication, either before or after randomization. Moreover, the researchers found no evidence of growth rebound in medicated children.[235]

Oddly enough, the researchers did not recommend against the use of these drugs in children. Indeed, in their "Executive Summary," they declared "It is important to express caution about interpretations based on the nonsignificance of statistical tests"[236]—as if the burden of proof is on anyone who questions whether giving powerful stimulant drugs to small children is a good idea.

Fleeting Benefits and Permanent Harms

Four years later, the APA released the newest version of the *DSM*, *DSM-5*, which by then had swollen to a gargantuan 1,521 pages. Seven out of the nine members of the ADHD and Disruptive Behavior Disorders Work Group had taken money from drug companies,[237] including Shire (the manufacturer of Adderall), Novartis (Ritalin), and Eli Lilly (Strattera).

The eighteen core symptoms for a diagnosis of ADHD remained unchanged, as did the three subtypes: Inattentive, Hyperactive, and Combined. The cutoff point for the onset of symptoms was increased from seven years to twelve. Moreover, for adolescents and adults, the number of symptoms from either checklist (hyperactive or inattentive) needed for a diagnosis was decreased from six to five, and the checklists included new examples (e.g., "often loses mobile telephones") making it easier to apply them to adults.

Upon inspection it becomes obvious that these "symptoms" are hopelessly subjective and context dependent. Every one of them is qualified by "often," raising the obvious question: How often is too often? It seems obvious that a diagnosis of ADHD will depend at least as much on the time and patience and energy a child's caregivers have, as on any intrinsic qualities of the child.

In fairness, it should be pointed out that the criteria specify the "symptoms" must manifest in at least two different contexts, which in practice almost always means school and home. But if a child's parents are being pressed by school authorities to have their child diagnosed as "ADHD," can we be sure the judgement of the parents is independent of that of the teacher?

Moreover, as we will see, the law has created a perverse set of incentives which may make obtaining a diagnosis of ADHD seem like an attractive option to some parents.[238]

Let's take a closer look at just one of the "symptoms" of ADHD, number 2-d: "Often unable to play or engage in leisure activities quietly." Guess what? Children do not play quietly. They chatter incessantly. They yell, and scream, and laugh. That's part of being a kid. One might wonder if the "experts" who came up with this symptom checklist ever had children—or ever were children. As educational psychologist Michael Corrigan points out in his book *Debunking ADHD*, *all* of these "symptoms" are exhibited by *all* children *often*.[239]

And if all else fails, there are the twin categories "Other Specified Attention-Deficit/Hyperactivity Disorder" and "Unspecified Attention-Deficit/Hyperactivity Disorder" which may be rendered for cases which do not meet even these minimal criteria. The upshot of all this, as Dr. Corrigan explains, is that if a clinician wants to give a child a diagnosis of ADHD, he can find reason to do so.[240]

In September of that year, a systematic review[241] noted that besides the MTA Study, no randomized controlled trial had ever assessed the effects of drug treatment for ADHD for any period longer than fifteen months, and concluded "There is little evidence to suggest that the effects observed over the relatively short-term are maintained throughout longer periods of impairment." The authors of the review did not recommend that doctors stop prescribing these drugs, but instead called for more studies.

March of the following year saw the publication of *The ADHD Explosion* by clinical psychologist Stephen P. Hinshaw and health economist Richard M. Scheffler. In Chapter Two, the authors state:

> *The large-scale Multimodal Treatment Study of Children with ADHD (MTA) study revealed major success for well-monitored medication in reducing ADHD symptoms.*[242]

As evidence, they cite the fourteen-month outcomes for the MTA Study, ignoring the eight-year follow-up which found no difference between treatment groups for any of twenty-four outcome variables. It seems unlikely the authors could have been unaware of the eight-year follow-up, which was published in 2009. The second author listed for that paper was Stephen P. Hinshaw.

That same month, an essay appeared in *Time* by behavioral neurologist Richard Saul titled "ADHD Does Not Exist." Dr. Saul noted that the diagnostic criteria in the latest edition of the *DSM* are so vague and subjective that the entire US population could potentially qualify, adding that there are over twenty medical conditions that can cause symptoms of ADHD including sleep disorders, undiagnosed vision and hearing problems, substance abuse, iron deficiency, allergies, and many others.

Dr. Saul summed up matters thusly:

> *In my view, there are two types of people who are diagnosed with ADHD: those who exhibit a normal level of distraction and*

> *impulsiveness, and those who have another condition or disorder that requires individual treatment.*
>
> *For my patients who are in the first category, I recommend that they eat right, exercise more often, get eight hours of quality sleep a night, minimize caffeine intake in the afternoon, monitor their cell-phone use while they're working and, most important, do something they're passionate about…*
>
> *For my second group of patients with severe attention issues, I require a full evaluation to find the source of the problem. Usually, once the original condition is found and treated, the ADHD symptoms go away.*[243]

In June of 2017, the young adult outcomes of the MTA study were made public. By that time, sixteen years had elapsed since the termination of the experimental phase of the study, and the subjects had reached an average age of twenty-five years. At this point there was no difference between the different treatment groups in terms of severity of ADHD symptoms. However, the "consistently medicated" subjects averaged nearly two inches shorter than those who received "negligible" treatment.[244]

In plain English, the short-term benefits, such as they are, of drugging kids fade away with time—but the growth suppression is permanent.

On 7 August of the following year, *Lancet Psychiatry* published a meta-analysis by psychiatrist Andrea Cipriani and his colleagues of 133 randomized controlled trials of ADHD drugs: methylphenidate, amphetamine (including lisdexamfetamine), and several others.[245] Primary endpoints were efficacy, as assessed by clinicians' and teachers' rating of symptoms, and tolerability, or proportion of subjects dropping out because of side effects. Secondary outcomes included acceptability, or the proportion of subjects dropping out for any reason, as well as changes in weight and blood pressure. These outcomes were assessed at twelve weeks, twenty-six weeks, and fifty-two weeks.

The researchers found that all the drugs were more effective than placebo at twelve weeks, and that methylphenidate was the most acceptable drug for children and adolescents, while amphetamine was most acceptable for adults. These drugs were also found to raise blood pressure and decrease weight, in both children and adults. There were not enough data for the twenty-six- or fifty-two-week endpoints. Dr. Cipriani and his co-authors concluded "Our results support methylphenidate in children and adolescents, and amphetamine in adults, as the first pharmacological treatment choice for ADHD."[246]

But we already knew that these drugs, in the short term, produce changes in children that overworked schoolteachers and exhausted parents may regard as improvements. No one has ever disputed that point. The question is: Does drugging children diagnosed with ADHD result in any long-term benefits that outweigh the harms? This study added absolutely nothing to our understanding of that question.

Moreover, as John B. Warren, Executive Editor of the *British Journal of Clinical Pharmacology*, pointed out in a letter to *Lancet Psychiatry*, choosing "tolerability" as a primary endpoint is setting the bar pretty low: "Tolerability to heroin does not confirm its safety, and tolerability to homeopathic remedies does not confirm their efficacy."[247]

Dr. Warren also argued that the study authors' assessment of risks and benefits of ADHD drugs was biased. He noted that "efficacy" is a composite endpoint of many symptoms grouped into score-based rating scales. Probably none of these symptoms by itself is powerful enough to enable a change to be detected. By contrast, there was no comparable composite endpoint for harms. Warren compared the researchers' approach to searching for benefits with a microscope while looking for harms with a passing glance.[248]

In November of 2018, a meta-analysis[249] re-confirmed something that had already been known for years—that the youngest half of children in a grade are more likely to be diagnosed with and drugged for ADHD than their older classmates in the same grade.[250] Clearly, many of the "symptoms" that fall under the diagnostic label "ADHD" are simply childish behaviors the kids could be expected to grow out of—and after all this time, there is still no convincing evidence that stimulant drugs aid this process in any meaningful way.

CHAPTER FOUR

THE PHARMACEUTICAL EMPIRE

The Most Profitable Organizations on the Planet

The same year that the Taft School District reached a settlement with angry parents whose kids had been harmed by stimulant drugs, and the same year the American Psychiatric Association released the final version of the *DSM-III*, another much more ballyhooed event occurred—the election of Ronald Wilson Reagan as the fortieth President of the United States of America.

Reagan's landslide victory had been preceded the year before by Margaret Thatcher's assumption of the office of Prime Minister of the United Kingdom. Both leaders had campaigned on a platform of deregulation—or in Reagan's memorable turn of phrase, "getting the government off the backs of the American people"—and both had been heavily influenced by the Nobel-Prize-winning economist Milton Friedman.

A point almost no one seems to remember now is this: when Friedman talked about deregulation, he really meant it. He wanted to *abolish* all government regulatory agencies. If people didn't like a particular product, they wouldn't buy it, and companies would stop making it. If people were hurt or killed by medications or any other commodity, they (or their loved ones) could file suit, and that would ensure product safety.

Whether or not that could have ever worked is a moot point, since it was never tried, not in the US or the UK nor anywhere else. What we got instead was a system which combined some of the worst aspects of capitalism and socialism—a chimera which has been variously termed late capitalism, neoliberalism, state capitalism, or corporate socialism, along with other names. Under this paradigm, the regulatory agencies were left largely intact, but they were transformed into the handmaidens of the industries they were purported to regulate—a well-documented process known as regulatory capture.

David Healy is a psychiatrist and a leading critic of the pharmaceutical industry. For most of his career he was Professor of Psychiatry at Bangor University in Wales, but just recently he switched his base of operations to the Department of Family Medicine at McMaster University in Ontario. In his recent books *The Decapitation of Care* and *Shipwreck of the Singular*, he notes that at the time Reagan assumed the office of the presidency, the pharmaceutical industry was facing increased competition from generic drugs, and had warned Congress that its share prices were about to collapse.[251] But the drugmakers were able to avoid this fate, by means of a variety of tactics.

The FDA, which is supposed to be an agent of the American people, increasingly came to be funded by the same companies it was supposed to be in an adversarial relationship with. Organizations such as the CDC and the WHO also were funded by Pharma.[252] Access to clinical trial data was increasingly restricted, and by 2000 there was no access to the data.[253] All this meant that new drugs could be brought on to the market on the basis of a statistical change in a marginal effect.[254]

A new player appeared on the scene: the pharmacy benefits management organization. The PBM's bought pharmacy chains and required patients to purchase drugs from those very same chains. Backroom deals were cut involving rebates and spread pricing. Drug prices soared, and the PBM's made billions.[255] And, within a few years, the drug companies themselves had become the most profitable organizations on the planet.

When I asked Dr. Healy if this was due to the invisible hand of the marketplace, he replied "No, this was due to the invisible hand of metrics."

Dr. Healy indicated that the roots of the current situation extend back farther than the dawn of neoliberalism and the Reagan-Thatcher era, and arise from modern society's obsession with numerical goals and targets—an obsession which cuts across ideological boundaries and which has transformed health care into health services, an enterprise which has lost all sight of the patient:

> *In the 1960's we began to get targets—we got targets for blood pressure, we got targets for blood sugar, we got targets for blood lipids—and we got rating scales. Increasingly across medicine by the 1980's we were treating the targets rather than the patient.*
>
> *DSM-III fits into all that, and that began before Reagan. Robert Spitzer was put in charge of the DSM committee in 1974 and right from the start he had an operational agenda. So I think it's the fault of the left to blame Thatcher-Reagan and to blame neoliberalism. My view is that what we've got is a technocratic agenda which follows metrics, and it's one the left had endorsed before Thatcher and Reagan and had done as much ultimately to impose as anyone on the right has done.*

Dr. Healy noted that the rating scales employed in psychiatry—such as the Hamilton Rating Scale for depression or the Conners Comprehensive Behavior Rating Scale for hyperactivity—originally were intended to function as a checklist, a reminder of things the treating clinician should touch upon in his interview with a patient. But that idea has been lost in the modern era of health services:

> *If you don't have a free-floating interview, if your view is that the rating scale is some kind of scientific instrument rather than it just being there to remind you about things you may want to ask at the interview, then the exchange between doctor and patient becomes much more standardized. And this is like a Big Mac hamburger. You know they're not in the business of producing the best possible hamburger ever—they want exactly the same hamburger every time.*
>
> *And whether you're Freudian or biological or whatever— once you check the thing and produce a number and once there's a pill that's going to make the numbers look a little bit better— supposedly—then there's tremendous pressure on the doctor, and the parent that brings the child, and the school system to make the numbers look better.*
>
> *It's not clear what ADHD is at all—I don't particularly think there is a condition that I would be happy to call ADHD—but you can make a checklist and you can show in a bunch of people that the stimulant group of drugs seem to produce some kind of benefit, and the logic of these days makes it close to impossible for any doctor to avoid giving you one of the stimulant drugs if you happen to mention at some point in the interview that you're not able to focus quite right.*

Dr. Healy explained that an improvement on a rating scale need not translate into any meaningful benefit in the life of the patient, citing the example of patients in antidepressant trials who may be judged to be "improving" every single day, right up to the day they kill themselves. He went on to note that the concept of risk management, a notion which first appeared in health care, has had effects there opposite to those it has had everywhere else:

> *See, in the mid to late 1980's it becomes an issue in the wider public domain, and we're being told we live in a world where the risks that people pose to each other may be greater than the risks that nature poses to us. And this led to the Green movement, the pushback against nuclear power, a concern about the chemicals that were in the environment, a wariness of the things that men were doing. But in health care it's led to just the opposite—it's led to the sense that we need to consume more chemicals and more devices.*

The upshot of all this, as Dr. Healy writes in *Shipwreck*, was that:

> *The experience of most Western physicians was like that of Rip van Winkle; they fell asleep in the 1970's in a Medical Republic and woke two decades later in a Pharmaceutical Empire.*[256]

How did all this work out for the rest of us?

Fed-Up Parents

On 5 May 1987, an article in the *New York Times* noted that the Drug Enforcement Administration announced that it had raised the production ceiling for Ritalin to twice what it had been just two years before. The same article informed readers "Ritalin is the best treatment for youngsters with a brain chemical abnormality known variously as hyperkinesis, hyperactivity, minimal brain dysfunction, and, most recently, attention deficit disorder."[257]

The attribution of ADD to a "brain chemical abnormality" seemed a bit odd, especially since a few paragraphs down the article stated "Medical authorities do not know exactly how [Ritalin] works on the brain or even what causes attention deficit disorder."[258]

As prescriptions for Ritalin for kids soared, fed-up parents began to push back. The same year the DEA raised the production ceiling for Ritalin, the first blow was struck in what would become the second round of the Ritalin wars. The plaintiff in *Lorenzo v. Yusin* claimed her son suffered headaches and depression after taking his prescribed Ritalin for three months, and that these toxic effects continued even after she stopped giving him the drug. The case never went to a verdict. On the fourth day, a mistrial was declared after the plaintiffs alleged racism on the part of school officials, after having been enjoined by the judge from doing do.[259]

That same year, a $125-million-dollar lawsuit was filed on behalf of Lavarne Parker, a mother from the suburbs of Atlanta, after her son Melvin reacted badly to the Ritalin he had been prescribed. The suit was filed by the law firm Coale, Cananack, and Murgatroyd with the aid of the Citizen's Commission on Human Rights, which, for the record, is an organization sponsored by the Church of Scientology. Lawyers for the plaintiff alleged that the boy had been stigmatized as mentally ill and threatened with suspension from school if he did not take the drug.[260] A December 1987 article in the *Los Angeles Times* stated that the boy had been kept in a dazed stupor, suffered severe brain damage and emotional distress, and remained depressed and suicidal even after stopping the drug.[261]

The same article quoted an Atlanta doctor as saying

> *Ritalin is the recommended treatment by experts throughout the country for attention deficit disorder, much as insulin is for diabetes.*[262]

The lawsuit was dismissed the following year, but there were more to come.

On 6 May 1988, an article appeared in *JAMA* with the sneering title "The Ritalin Controversy: What's Made This Drug's Opponents Hyperactive?"[263] The piece stated that by then eight Ritalin-related malpractice lawsuits had been filed. Five of these were in Massachusetts and had been filed by the Citizens Commission on Human Rights.[264] Parents claimed that the kids given these drugs experienced a variety of toxic effects including loss of sleep, appetite suppression, growth suppression, tics, depression, aggression, and psychosis.[265]

In addition, Ritalin had been blamed for the actions of fifteen-year-old Rod Matthews of Dedham, Massachusetts, who was charged with second-degree murder after he bashed in another boy's head with a baseball bat.[266] A month before the homicide, Rod wrote a note to his health teacher saying he had an urge to set houses on fire and that he was afraid that he was going to kill someone. The teacher took no action, other than to tell the boy that arson and murder were felonies.[267] Matthews was sentenced to life in prison.[268]

That October, another article in the *Los Angeles Times* mentioned that by then 750,000 children in the United States were taking Ritalin, and quoted a prominent pediatrician thusly:

> *If a child truly has attention deficit disorder, then he has a chemical problem and needs Ritalin as much as a diabetic needs insulin.*[269]

Saying No

In May of 1988, school officials in Derry, New Hampshire, informed Valerie and Mike Jesson that their eight-year-old son Casey would no longer be allowed to attend class unless they agreed to give the boy Ritalin. The Jessons just said No and filed suit against the school district.[270]

Casey had already tried Ritalin, and the experience had not been a happy one. In Kindergarten he had been diagnosed with hyperactivity and put on the drug. The toxic effects he experienced included mania, withdrawal from others, loss of appetite, sleep disturbances, and bedwetting. After twenty months, his parents took him off the drug and reported that his condition improved immediately.[271]

School officials felt otherwise and devised an "Individualized Education Program" (IEP) for the boy, which recommended special classes, counseling for both Casey and his parents, and Ritalin. The Jessons refused.[272]

The IEP also contained these insights:

Casey is only able to learn in a regular classroom when he is heavily invested in the activity. For most academic instruction he needs one-to-one or small-group instructions, clear behavioral limits, and frequent changes of activities. He also needs to be able to move around during the day to help burn off excess energy.[273]

In plain English: the kid needs engaging schoolwork, age-appropriate expectations, individual attention, clear boundaries, consistent discipline, and plenty of free playtime. But these are precisely the things every child needs to thrive. So is the lack of these things a drug-treatable brain disease?

The case was decided in favor of the Jessons, who were awarded compensatory damages. This was the only case in the second round of Ritalin lawsuits to end in victory for the plaintiffs.[274]

A Child in Distress

By 1994, all the other lawsuits filed in the second round of the Ritalin wars had failed, and the percentage of American children being drugged for ADHD, which had dipped slightly in the wake of the bad publicity, began to climb upwards once more.[275]

A study published two years later found that the number of children being drugged for ADHD had risen to 1.5 million. The vast majority of these kids were on Ritalin. The reasons for this increase included more children staying on these drugs into their teen years, more girls being given the drugs, increased drugging of children for symptoms of inattention without hyperactivity, and "a growing positive public image of medicating youths for ADHD."[276]

And it wasn't just the consumption of stimulant drugs by children that soared—the rate of polypharmacy did as well. For the period 1993-1994, just under five percent of pediatric office-based visits involved the prescription of a stimulant drug along with another type of psychotropic drug. By 1997-1998 that proportion had skyrocketed to twenty-five percent.[277]

On 15 November 1997, a special report in the *New York Times* illustrated the hollowness of the medical approach to human dysfunction. Titled "A Slide into Peril, with No One to Catch Her,"[278] the piece told the story of Sabrina Green, a child who had the deck stacked against her from the beginning. The story begins with this description of Sabrina, in the days before her death:

> *There was the sight of the dirty-haired child, in shoes two sizes too big, stumbling along to school last spring, apparently not taking the medication that stabilized her hyperactivity.*[279]

Born to a cocaine-addicted mother, Sabrina spent the very first days of her life suffering from the withdrawal effects of that drug. Meanwhile, her mother had abandoned her in the hospital, and didn't come back to claim her for two months. Child welfare workers looked into the case, and even though this was their third investigation of Sabrina's mother, they apparently saw no reason why she should not retain custody of the infant. Sabrina's father was addicted to drugs, just as her mother was, and doesn't seem to have played a meaningful part of her life.[280]

Sabrina was born into a cesspit of family dysfunction. One of her brothers was scalded to death as an infant during a visit with a family friend. Another was murdered. At the time the article was written, two more of her brothers were in prison—one for murder. Sabrina's mother was manifestly unfit to take care of a tot, and often left Sabrina in the care of her nine-year-old brother, who took on the responsibility of watching her and changing her diapers.[281]

When Sabrina was three years old, she watched her mother die from a drug overdose. At this point, she was placed in the care of a family friend, and seems to have thrived for the next six years. But then fate dealt Sabrina a cruel blow: the family friend died of cancer at the age of forty-nine.[282]

At this point, Sabrina was placed in the custody of her thirty-one-year-old half-sister Yvette, who already had ten children of her own and was living on welfare payments of $2189 a month. Yvette's common-law husband, and father of eight of her ten children, lived in the same household, in apparent defiance of welfare regulations. No mention is made of any contribution he may have made to the household finances. Yvette's own sister complained to authorities that Yvette's apartment was filthy, and that Yvette was unfit to care for eleven (!) children, but no action was taken.[283]

At school, Sabrina's unkempt appearance and poor hygiene caused her to be tormented by the other kids, who called her "Stinky Mouth." In May of 1997 Sabrina ran away from her home and sought refuge with a family friend, begging "Please don't send me back. I'll be good."[284]

In the Autumn of that year, Sabrina seems to have stopped attending school, although officials there still marked her "present." Her guardians kept her tied to the bed at night to prevent her from "stealing food." On 8 November of 1997, Sabrina Green was found dead of untreated burns, gangrene, and blows to the head. Her half-sister Yvette and Yvette's husband were charged with murder.[285]

Is the story of Sabrina Green typical of children who receive the label "hyperactive?" No, it is not. But is does highlight the perils of society which offers distressed children like Sabrina a label and a prescription, in lieu of meaningful help.

The Third Round of Ritalin Lawsuits Commences

By 1999, the line of children waiting outside the school nurse's office waiting for their mid-day dose of Ritalin had become a familiar sight in many elementary schools. In rural areas, some harried nurses had to cover five or six different elementary schools, and demands on their time had become so onerous that some states were discussing allowing clerical workers to hand out the daily meds.[286]

In May of the following year, a class-action lawsuit was filed in Texas against Novartis, the maker of Ritalin, as well as the American Psychiatric Association and the patient advocacy group known as CHADD, or Children and Adults with Attention-Deficit Hyperactivity Disorder.[287] Dr. Breggin, who had spoken about the harms of Ritalin at the 1998 NIH Consensus Development Conference, served as a consultant to the plaintiff's lawyers. The suit alleged that Novartis failed to disclose information about a wide variety of toxic effects of Ritalin, including cardiovascular and central nervous system effects. This was followed by similar class-action lawsuits filed in New Jersey, California, Florida, and Puerto Rico.[288]

In September of 2000, after the lawsuits were filed in California and New Jersey, Novartis issued a statement:

> *Any charge that Novartis somehow "conspired" with nationally prominent professional and/or patient third-party groups is unfounded and preposterous. Furthermore, any charge that ADHD is not a medically valid disorder is contrary to medical evidence and psychiatric consensus.[289]*

The APA branded the allegations "totally ludicrous and false" while CHADD likened them to accusing the American Diabetes Association of conspiring with the manufacturers of insulin to invent diabetes.[290]

Expert Reports

The Pharmaceutical Empire and its allies fought back on other fronts as well. In November of 2001, a special advertising feature in *Family Circle* magazine produced by an organization identified as "EXPERT REPORTS"[291] began with an introduction authored by APA President Richard K. Harding. Some of Dr. Harding's comments follow:

> *We now know that mental illnesses—such as depression or schizophrenia—are not "moral weaknesses" or "imagined" but real diseases caused by abnormalities of brain structure and imbalances of chemicals in the brain.*

> *Nobody still believes that epilepsy is caused by possession by demonic forces, for which the victim should be blamed. Likewise, we are coming out of a dark ages [sic] of fear and shame regarding psychiatric illnesses.*
>
> *Just 20% of children needing care for a psychiatric impairment receive it. Women, especially, can lead the way in identifying mental diseases in their families, friends, and loved ones—and in themselves.[292]*

The article also featured a commentary from Harvard psychiatrist Timothy J. Wilens. After acknowledging that "There are no blood tests, brain tests, computer, or neuropsychological tests used to diagnose ADHD,"[293] he goes on to inform readers:

> *Contrary to what most parents think, medication is one of the most important treatments for ADHD and is essential for the long-term success of these kids.*
>
> *Stimulants have been extensively researched and are very safe and effective.[294]*

The supplement also mentioned that "EXPERT REPORTS creates advertising supplements that contribute to public understanding of important social issues." The funding source for EXPERT REPORTS was not identified.

The Third Round of Ritalin Lawsuits Fails

By March 2002, all five class action suits filed in the third round of Ritalin lawsuits had been withdrawn or dismissed. Novartis Chief Counsel Dorothy Watson stated:

> *We are extremely pleased.*
>
> *The fact that all five of the class action lawsuits have been dismissed sends a strong message that the decision of how to treat*

ADHD is between the parent, patient, and physician, and has no place in the courts.[295]

Please Mom Make it Stop

That August, a series of articles in the *New York Post* by reporter Douglas Montero told of parents who had claimed they had been coerced by school officials into having their children drugged for ADHD. Patricia Weathers of Dutchess County claimed she had been told that her son Michael Mozer, then in the First Grade, would be transferred to special education classes unless he began taking the drugs. School officials referred them to a pediatrician who prescribed Ritalin after spending just a few minutes reviewing the boy's file.[296]

By the time he entered the Third Grade, Michael suffered from insomnia, lack of appetite, and antisocial behavior. He began chewing on his own shirt sleeves, collar, and pencils, and once started gnawing on a test sheet.[297]

School officials then allegedly informed Patricia her son was bipolar and suffered from "social anxiety." His doctor prescribed Dextrostat and Paxil. In Patricia's words, the drugs turned him into a "zombie." Michael became psychotic and told his mother "Please Mom make it stop—there's a person inside my head telling me to do bad things."[298]

In December of 1999, Patricia stopped the drugs. The school district originally agreed to provide homebound instruction for Michael, but reneged on their promise after deciding that absence from school for "psychiatric reasons" did not constitute a "medical reason." Patricia found herself the object of a child abuse investigation for not drugging her son.[299]

She was cleared of all charges after Child and Family Services concluded that Michael's problems were a direct result of the drugs he had been prescribed. Six months later, the boy was diagnosed with a heart murmur.[300]

Another story in the *Post* reported that Brooklyn assemblyman Felix Ortiz was sponsoring a bill to prevent school officials from coercing parents to have their kids drugged. Ortiz also stated that since the original article had run, his office had received calls from at least forty-five parents who claimed to have been threatened by school officials in such a manner. The same article quoted Jill Chaifetz, executive director of Advocates for Children, as follows: "We hear about this every week on a regular basis."[301]

The Story of Gretchen LeFever

The story of Gretchen LeFever is a cautionary tale for the era of the Pharmaceutical Empire.[302]

Dr. LeFever was a clinical psychologist at the Center for Pediatric Research of Eastern Virginia Medical School. In the mid-nineties, she and her colleagues founded the School Health Initiative for Education (SHINE), a partnership between providers, parents, policy makers, and community members. The coalition carried out an extensive community needs assessment, identifying four major gaps in ADHD care: 1) Systematic behavior management; 2) School-provider communication; 3) Teacher training and education; and 4) Parent training and support. LeFever obtained federal, state, and local funding to carry out interventions for each of these gaps and to evaluate the effectiveness of these interventions.[303]

Dr. LeFever and her colleagues created a school-wide positive discipline program that resulted in a decrease in ADHD symptoms and a rise in scores in every subject area of standardized tests administered to the children. The coalition also successfully lobbied for the passage of a bill that would prevent teachers from making ADHD recommendations to parents. The rate of ADHD diagnoses in southeastern Virginia dropped by one-third.[304]

It was Dr. LeFever's research on the rate of ADHD diagnosis in southeastern Virginia that led to the undoing of her career at EVMS. In a

September 1999 paper in the *American Journal of Public Health*,[305] LeFever and her colleagues reported that the proportion of children in grades Two through Five in two Virginia cities receiving medication for ADHD during school hours was a staggering eight to ten percent. The highest rate was found among white boys, with an even more staggering one out of five being drugged for this condition.

Three years later, Dr. LeFever and her colleagues once again assessed the proportion of children diagnosed with ADHD in a Virginia school district, this time by means of parental surveys.[306] This time they found the proportion was one out of six, including a jaw-dropping one out of three white boys. Eighty-four percent of these children were being given stimulant drugs. They also found no difference between medicated and unmedicated children in the rates of suspensions, expulsions, or grade retention.

The attacks on Dr. LeFever's research began almost immediately.

In January of 2002, a "Consensus Statement" signed by clinical psychologist Russel Barkley and a "consortium of international scientists" appeared in *Clinical Child and Family Psychology Review*.[307] Dr. Barkley and eighty-four co-authors declared "Among scientists who have devoted years, if not entire careers, to the study of this disorder there is no controversy about its continuing existence." No argument there. They went on to proclaim that "hundreds of studies" had demonstrated "the effectiveness of medication," adding that "ADHD is not a benign disorder" and that it can cause "devastating problems" in sufferers, who are more likely than "normal people" to drop out of school, to have few or no friends, to underperform at work, to engage in antisocial activities, to use tobacco or illicit drugs, to experience teen pregnancy and sexually transmitted diseases, to speed excessively and have multiple car accidents, to experience depression and personality disorders as adults, and "in hundreds of other ways mismanage and endanger their lives."

The authors didn't even try to argue that drugging children for ADHD reduces the likelihood of any of these outcomes.

Dr. Barkley and his co-authors wrapped things up by smearing their opponents as know-nothings, likening their views to "declaring the earth flat, the laws of gravity debatable, and the periodic table in chemistry a fraud."[308]

Two years later, a critique of the Consensus Statement authored by psychiatrist Sammi Timimi and thirty-two of his colleagues appeared in the March 2004 issue of the same journal.[309] The authors began by noting:

> *History teaches us again and again one generation's most cherished ideas and practices, especially when applied on the powerless, are repudiated by the next, but not without leaving countless victims in their wake.*[310]

They went on to mention that each revision of the *DSM* for the past thirty years had increased the number of children eligible for a diagnosis. They also pointed out that while Dr. Barkley and his co-authors had claimed that "less than half" of those with the disorder are receiving treatment, Dr. LeFever's work had shown that one out of six white boys in two Virginia school districts were being drugged for ADHD (a figure later revised upward to one out of three).[311]

In the same issue, Dr. Barkley and twenty co-endorsers fired back,[312] stating that a subsequent study just completed for the same region was unable to replicate the results of Dr. LeFever and her colleagues, finding a prescribing prevalence closer to three percent, adding ominously "The reasons for such a gross disparity of results deserve investigation."[313]

In fact, the study Dr. Barkley and his co-authors referred to was a Ph.D. dissertation which was to remain unpublished a decade later. Barkley had been a member of the author's dissertation committee—a fact that he and his co-endorsers left unmentioned.[314]

Nevertheless, the requested "investigation" followed posthaste. An anonymous accuser alleged that Dr. LeFever had intentionally inflated the rates of ADHD diagnosis in order to push an anti-medication agenda, and that her research had been conducted without obtaining proper consent.[315]

In fact, Dr. LeFever was not anti-med, and had referred many children for medication evaluations. All of her research had been cleared by the EVMS Internal Review Board.[316]

Nevertheless, in April of 2004 EVMS decided to launch an investigation. Against their own policy and common protocol for investigations of scientific misconduct, they notified the media that LeFever was under investigation.[317] They also prematurely terminated her research and seized her computers.[318]

Thirty-nine psychiatrists and psychologists signed a petition stating that the school's actions were "an egregious violation of academic freedom."[319]

The investigation found no evidence of scientific misconduct on Dr. LeFever's part, although they did find a typographical error in the appendix of one of her publications, regarding the wording of one of the survey questions used by LeFever and her colleagues. Here is the survey question as reported in the 2002 paper in *Psychology in the Schools*:

> *Has your child been diagnosed with attention or hyperactivity problems known as ADD or ADHD?*

The actual wording of the question used by the researchers was:

> *Does your child have attention problems or hyperactivity problems known as ADD or ADHD?*

In July of 2004, Dr. LeFever was cleared of all charges of misconduct. She asked the editor of *Psychology in the Schools* to publish a correction regarding the typo in her 2002 paper. The editor first replied that the error was too trivial even to warrant a correction, but later relented. The one-paragraph erratum was published in February of 2005.[320]

Meanwhile, on 9 December 2004 a local school district official complained to EVMS that Dr. LeFever had misled her about the procedures used to obtain parental consent for the epidemiological study. The allegation was completely untrue. Nevertheless, as she would later recall, "Very weird things started happening."[321]

> *Suddenly, my university travel account was frozen. Everybody around me was getting nervous. People were shutting their doors at work.*[322]

Dr. LeFever met with her supervisor and another university official who warned her, ominously, "Well, your staff may be supportive of you—*for now.* That won't last."[323]

Dr. LeFever's research was terminated, she was placed on administrative leave, and EVMS assured public school officials that the study data would never be used. LeFever left the university the following June and accepted a position at Regent University. More than a decade of work in the epidemiology and treatment of ADHD lay in ruins.[324]

Today Gretchen LeFever is known as Gretchen LeFever Watson and serves as President of SLS, a consulting firm for organizational and professional development. I asked Dr. Watson if she believed this episode had any wider implications beyond the career of one researcher. This was her reply:

> *The Hampton Roads community was unique in that it was proactively tackling the problem of how we were handling child mental health or behavioral problems in school. They were being proactive, they were being creative, they were involving wide and varied inputs, and we were working at the research center and with people in the community to design responsive interventions, and layering research onto those interventions so we could see what was effective and what was not, and we were keeping the community informed the whole time. So it was a very dynamic, very intense,*

broad-based approach—community-driven solutions to children struggling to meet the demands placed on them in the educational environment and home environments. And things were working.

And now?

Children's Hospital, which is where my office was, is now launching a $224 million psychiatric facility for children. So instead of developing community responses, we are now developing a psychiatric hospital. And the reason for this hospital—it's been reported in the newspaper—was that we have so many children and adolescents in our region showing up in the emergency department with psychiatric problems. We don't know what to do with them. And we can't manage them with our current facility.

Of course, these children aren't showing up unmedicated for the first time—they're showing up already medicated. And nobody seems to be connecting the fact that probably all these medications that they're on is part of the reason why they're showing up in the emergency room.

I wonder—had we been able to continue down the path that we were, if we would have this need for this facility that's getting built right now?

Letting Everyone off the Hook Except Kids

By 2011, the number of kids being drugged for ADHD reached 3.5 million.[325] In January of the following year, psychologist L. Alan Sroufe, who nearly forty years previously had been one of the first to warn of the possible adverse effects of stimulant drugs, both to the kids and to society at large, authored an op-ed essay in the *New York Times* on the MTA Study.[326] Here are some of Dr. Sroufe's comments:

The large-scale medication of children feeds into a societal view that all of life's problems can be solved with a pill, and gives millions of children the impression that there is something inherently defective in them.

The illusion that children's behavior problems can be cured with drugs prevents us from seeking the more complex solutions that will be necessary.

Drugs get everyone—politicians, scientists, teachers, and parents—off the hook. Everyone except the children, that is.

Indeed. On 7 December 2015, the FDA approved Pfizer's Quilli-Chew, or methylphenidate in chewable cherry-flavored tablet form, for use in children as young as six.[327] Not to be outdone, barely a month later the pharmaceutical firm Neos Therapeutics announced it had obtained FDA approval for Adzenys XR-ODT, or amphetamine in a yummy orange-flavored pill, for kids the same age.[328]

Three years later, a review published in *PLoS* reported that total health care spending on ADHD for the year 2016 in the United States topped twenty billion dollars. For that kind of outlay, we could pay the mid-career salaries of an extra 365,000 teachers, or 827,000 teachers' aides.[329]

In tracing the history of the diagnostic category "ADHD" from its first appearance in the *DSM-IIIR* in 1987 to the present day, six themes are apparent: 1) The increasing expansion of the number of children eligible for a diagnosis; 2) The increasing amount of time children spend on drugs; 3) The increasing rates of polypharmacy involving stimulant drugs along with other types of psychoactive substances; 4) The failure of psychiatry to produce credible evidence for any long-term benefits of ADHD drugs; 5) A staggering lack of curiosity regarding the potential harms of these drugs; and 6) The shifting of the burden of proof to anyone who raises concerns about the lack of efficacy and the long-term harms of these drugs.

Anxiety over the Space Race was the spark that lit this fire. Drug company money was the accelerant that enabled the flames to spread. Successive iterations of the *DSM*, each one defining ADHD more broadly than the last, stoked the fire to a red-hot intensity.

Meanwhile, the post-Sputnik world, with its obsessive concern for training the next generation of scientists and engineers for the Space Race, seems almost as far gone as the lost world of Troy. But a new factor has entered this equation.

The rise of globalization means that young people who graduate from university today find themselves saddled with crushing student loan debt while having to compete for jobs against skilled workers on six continents The gig economy means the job security their grandparents took for granted isn't even a pipe dream for most of them. The Cold War ethos of "We're all in this together" seems to have been replaced by "Every man (and woman and boy and girl) for himself (or herself)." Is it any wonder that some seek to gain a competitive edge, for themselves or their children, by means of a label and a pill?

Whether or not these pills provide that competitive edge is another question entirely. But that scarcely matters anymore in the era of the modern Pharmaceutical Empire, in which many of us have more value to our rulers as consumers of drugs than as workers. To paraphrase a great thinker, the end object of drugging people is drugging people.

And when people take the drugs, in good faith, as directed, and suffer adverse reactions which are well-known toxic effects of these drugs, all too often instead of being taken off the drugs they find themselves the recipients of new diagnoses, more drugs, stronger drugs, and higher doses, until someone who began with no more than the problems of living ends up as a career mental patient, or dead.

We will take a look at how this process operates in the next three chapters.

CHAPTER FIVE

ADHD MEDS AND BIPOLAR DISORDER

A Manufactured Epidemic

An epidemic is stalking the land, a crippling, possibly lifelong, potentially fatal condition called childhood bipolar disorder.

The term "bipolar disorder" refers to episodes of mania alternating with depression. The first clinical descriptions of this condition were published within a few days of each other, early in 1854, by two French psychiatrists, Jules Baillarger and Jean Pierre Fairet. This was followed by an acrimonious conflict over which of these eminent doctors had priority, a dispute that lasted as long as both men lived.[330]

Emil Kraepelin, widely regarded as the founding father of modern psychiatric nosology, divided all mental illnesses into two broad categories. One of these was "dementia praecox," corresponding more or less to the modern-day notion of schizophrenia, with "general paresis of the insane," or syphilitic dementia, thrown in for good measure. The other was "manic-depressive insanity," corresponding more or less to the modern-day category of affective disorders. The latter he divided into three subcategories: depression, simple mania, and "periodic and circular insanity," or depression alternating with mania. This latter subcategory became known as "manic-depressive illness," and in 1966 the Swedish psychiatrist Carlo Perris coined the term "bipolar disorder" for this condition.

Whatever it was called, it was exceedingly rare, and virtually unknown in children. In 1931, psychiatrist Jacob Kasanin of Boston Psychopathic Hospital (now known as the Massachusetts Mental Health Center) reported that out of approximately 1,900 admissions per year, only two or three were for children suffering from affective disorders. This was all affective disorders, not just manic-depressive illness.[331]

But, as author Robert Whitaker points out in his blockbuster work of nonfiction *Anatomy of an Epidemic*, all this began to change after the initiation of the modern psychopharmaceutical era, with large numbers of children being dosed with stimulants and antidepressants.[332]

An April 1976 paper in the *American Journal of Diseases of Childhood* related what may be the first case histories of children suffering from mania after being given these drugs.[333] In reading these accounts, the most striking thing is the doctors' utter lack of curiosity regarding the circumstances that may have contributed to the distress that brought these children to the attention of the psychiatric profession in the first place.

A young boy in separate episodes fractured both forearms as well as several ribs and toes and amputated the distal joint of his left index finger, in addition to having to have his stomach pumped after several "accidental" drug overdoses. At the age of six an examination revealed "many scattered bruises and small, well-healed lacerations all over his body." The authors describe the boy as "accident-prone."[334]

The parents and teachers of this "accident-prone" boy described him as "hard to control," and so he was prescribed Ritalin. At first, he seemed to do well on the drug, but after a year and a half he became irritable and uncooperative, suffering from frequent crying spells, distractibility, insomnia, and hyperphagia. His doctors tried amitriptyline in addition to the Ritalin. When that didn't help, they added thioridazine, and then chlorpromazine, which caused the boy to suffer from cholestatic jaundice.[335]

The boy complained of being unloved and persecuted, and accused his doctors of poisoning him.[336] All this was interpreted by the authors as evidence of the boy's mental illness.

In the years to come the number of children diagnosed and drugged for bipolar disorder soared, and no one has done more to promote this than psychiatrist Joseph Biederman and his colleagues at Harvard Medical School and Massachusetts General Hospital. A 1996 paper by Dr. Biederman and several co-authors described the results of a study performed at the Pediatric Psychopharmacology Unit at Mass General.[337] The researchers screened 140 children referred for ADHD and found that eleven percent of them met the criteria for bipolar disorder as well. At the four-year follow-up, an additional twelve percent also qualified for the same diagnosis, indicating that something like twenty-three percent of children treated for ADHD will go on to develop bipolar disorder.

Three years later, the link between ADHD meds and childhood bipolar disorder was confirmed in a letter to the editor of the *Journal of the American Academy of Child and Adolescent Psychiatry* from Martha Hellander, Acting Executive Director of the Child and Adolescent Bipolar Foundation:

> *Most of our children initially received the ADHD diagnosis, received stimulants and/or antidepressants, and either did not respond or suffered symptoms of mania such as rages, insomnia, agitation, pressured speech, and the like. In lay language, parents call this 'bouncing off the wall.' First hospitalizations occurred often among our children during manic or mixed episodes (including suicidal gestures or attempts) triggered or exacerbated by treatment with stimulants, tricyclics, or selective serotonin reuptake inhibitors.[338]*

That same year saw the release of the first edition of *The Bipolar Child* by psychiatrist Demitri Papolos and his daughter Janice Papolos.[339] In the preface, the authors lay it on the line:

> *Many of the children were initially diagnosed as having atten-tion-deficit disorder with hyperactivity and put on stimulant medications; or they were first seen in the throes of depression with little or no consideration of the opposite pole of a mood disorder. As a result, a shocking number of them were thrown into manic and psychotic states, became paranoid and violent, and ended up in a hospital—unstable, suicidal, and in worse shape than before the treatment began.[340]*

The solution recommended by the Papoloses is not to refrain from giving children powerful, brain-altering drugs, but to make sure they get the right drugs:

> *Mood-stabilizing drugs such as lithium, Depakote, or Tegretol should be considered as a first-line treatment—early on—before episodes [of mania] become more frequent, and the illness warps the psychological development of a child and destroys the life of a family.[341]*

As the number of children being drugged with stimulants and antidepressants skyrocketed, so did the number of them afflicted with bipolar disorder. Between 1994-1995 and 2002-2003, the number of youth office visits for this condition rose a staggering forty-fold—from twenty-five per 100,000 youths to one thousand per 100,000.[342] Accompanying this increase was an explosion of angry, out-of-control adolescents admitted to hospital emergency rooms.[343]

Where is all this going? We have already noted that 3.5 million children currently are being treated with stimulant drugs for ADHD. Using the Biederman group's figure of twenty-three percent of ADHD kids going on to develop bipolar disorder, that works out to 800,000 cases of childhood bipolar disorder in the making—and that's not even counting the antidepressant-induced ones.

Early-onset bipolar disorder is a particularly pernicious form of this condition, characterized by increased vulnerability to substance abuse, psychotic symptoms, anxiety, panic, violence, arrests, and suicide attempts. In addition, patients with the early-onset form of this condition are more likely to present with rapid cycling, switching back and forth between depression and mania multiple times in a day—or worse, something called "ultra-rapid" cycling, in which the switching back and forth is essentially continuous.[344]

Desperate Remedies

Treatments for bipolar disorder include lithium salts; anticonvulsants such as Depakote, Tegretol, and Trileptal (often called "mood stabilizers"); as well as so-called "antipsychotic" drugs. All of these treatments come with serious toxic effects.

Lithium, the lightest metal on earth, was discovered in 1817 by the Swedish chemist Johan August Arfwedson. The word lithium literally means "rock stuff"—not a terribly informative name, but there you are.

The antimanic properties of lithium were discovered, more or less by accident, by the Australian psychiatrist John Cade while pursuing some half-baked theories on the supposed biochemical basis of schizophrenia. Working literally on his kitchen table at home, he injected guinea pigs with lithium urate and found it made the animals so listless and apathetic that they didn't even bother righting themselves when placed on their backs. Apparently he decided this was a good thing, and tried the drug out on ten of his patients suffering from mania. One of them died of acute lithium toxicity, a fact Dr. Cade never got around to mentioning in his published reports.[345]

The toxic effects of lithium include insatiable thirst and polyuria—both obviously the body's attempts to get rid of this poison. Other effects include abdominal cramps, nausea, vomiting, diarrhea, tremor, fatigue, ataxia, slurred speech, cognitive impairment, skin eruptions, weight gain, hypothyroidism, sky-high blood pressure, and irreversible kidney damage.

The toxic effects of Tegretol include vertigo, tremor, slurred speech, diplopia, headaches, and a drop in white blood cell count. Those of Depakote include androgenizing effects in females as well as liver toxicity, while Trileptal is known to cause dizziness, somnolence, ataxia, double vision, nausea, vomiting, headache, tremors, and abnormal gait. All three of these drugs have been linked to cases of spina bifida after being taken by pregnant women.[346] In 2008, the FDA issued a warning that all drugs of this class might increase the risk of suicidality and completed suicides.

The permanent damage to the central nervous system by antipsychotic drugs is by now well known. The most visible is tardive dyskinesia, a disfiguring, dehumanizing condition characterized among other phenomena by lip-smacking, grimacing, bizarre postures, and uncontrollable movements of the tongue. Even the names of these phenomena are dehumanizing: rabbit syndrome, fly tongue, worm tongue, and so forth.

Other toxic effects include dysphagia, hypersalivation, massive weight gain, gynecomastia, diabetes, seizures, atrophy of the brain, blood clots, stroke, and sudden cardiac death.

Yet another toxic effect is akathisia, or feelings of unbearable restlessness and distress. "Akathisia feels like you're being tortured from the inside out," psychiatrist Peter Breggin once told me. "People can't find the words to describe how it feels." Patients suffering from this drug-induced disorder may be driven to suicide.

David Healy, now a professor of Family Medicine at McMaster University in Ontario and the author of *Mania: A Short History of Bipolar Disorder*,[347] analyzed RCT data for the antipsychotics Risperdal, Zyprexa, Seroquel, Serdolect, and Geodon. He found the rate of suicidal acts in the treatment arm was almost four times that of the placebo arm. There were no suicides out of 1,351 patients given placebo, whereas the 12,817 patients in the treatment arm included 33 completed suicides.[348]

Or as Dr. Healy put it, graphically and succinctly:

> *When it comes to dead bodies in current psychotropic trials, there are a greater number of them in the active treatment groups than in the placebo groups. This is quite different from what happens in penicillin trials or trials of drugs that really work.*[349]

The Gateway Diagnosis

Something like sixty percent of patients diagnosed with early-onset bipolar disorder present with "co-morbid" ADHD.[350] In one study performed by Dr. Biederman and his colleagues, the rate was ninety-four percent.[351]

For the most part, the experts have studiously ignored the role of stimulants and antidepressants in creating this epidemic. Instead, they have maintained the ADHD is a "prodromal manifestation" of early-onset bipolar disorder.[352] But in fact this condition was unheard-of before we began dosing large numbers of children with stimulants and antidepressants.

Dr. Healy once told me that much as drugs such as marijuana and cocaine are said, rightly or wrongly, to serve as the gateway to more dangerous drugs, ADHD functions as a "gateway diagnosis," leading to more serious diagnoses and harmful treatments.

Dr. Breggin said much the same thing to me. A diagnosis of ADHD, he proclaimed, "is the start of a career as a mental patient, with the original diagnosis leading to more drugs, and more drugs, and eventually to childhood bipolar diagnosis, and multiple drugs including antipsychotic drugs, and hence this horrible outcome."

Indeed. As the incidence of childhood bipolar disorder skyrocketed, so did the consumption of antipsychotic drugs. Between 1993 and 2002, prescriptions for antipsychotic drugs in the United States for youths under the age of twenty-one increased by an astonishing six-fold—from 200,000 per year to over 1.2 million.[353]

And what are we getting in return for all this relentless drugging? Dr. Healy, at the time a Clinical Professor of Psychiatry at Bangor University in Wales, wanted to find out.

Dr. Healy and his colleagues analyzed asylum records in north-west Wales and compared them to records from the 1990's.[354] North-west Wales was almost ideal for this sort of comparison. Between the 1890's and the 1990's the population had changed almost not at all in terms of size, age structure, poverty, ethnicity, or rurality. Moreover, for both the 1890's and the 1990's, there was effectively one point of access for mental health services in north-west Wales: Denbigh Asylum in the 1890's, and the Hergest Unit in the 1990's. This was about as close to a controlled experiment as it is possible to get with this sort of thing.

Dr. Healy and his co-workers found that, in comparison to the 1890's, the total number of patients admitted for what would now be called bipolar disorder had risen by fifty percent. The average length of stay for this condition in the 1890's was longer, but by the 1990's the total number of hospital stays had almost quadrupled, so the aggregate time spent in hospital had increased as well.[355] They concluded:

> *These data are incompatible with simple claims that mood stabilizing drugs 'work.'*
>
> *If medical treatments are fully effective, then the index condition should disappear, as general paralysis of the insane disappeared after the introduction of penicillin.*
>
> *Modern treatments appear to offer few benefits compared with treatment 100 years ago.*

A 2007 review paper[356] by psychiatrists Nancy Huxley and Ross J. Baldessarini confirmed all this:

> *The previously accepted clinical and popular conception of the course of BPD is that it is marked by time-limited acute episodes of mania and major depression with recovery to euthymia and*

a favorable functional adaptation between episodes, and with a marked decrease of acute morbidity with effective mood stabilizing treatment.

In contrast, the emerging picture of the course of BPD is quite different, and includes slow or incomplete recovery from acute episodes, continuing risk of recurrences, and sustained morbidity over time even with continuous long-term use of modern treatments.[357]

The authors go on to drive this point home. Studies show that anywhere between nineteen percent and fifty-eight percent of adult bipolar patients were not living independently, with most of those residing with family members. Unemployment rates among bipolar patients had skyrocketed from fifteen percent in the 1970's to sixty percent or even higher. Only half of those who were working were employed at their pre-morbid level of functioning.[358]

In the abstract, the authors highlight their own adroitness at ignoring the possibility that treatments for bipolar disorder are making patients worse rather than better:

Disability and poor outcomes were prevalent, despite major therapeutic advances.[359]

Going Through the Roof

A 17 June 2000 article in the *Fort Worth Star-Telegram* profiled several area families each of which had a child afflicted with early-onset bipolar disorder.[360]

At the age of eighteen months, Heather Norris banged her head against a tray table in the course of a temper tantrum. A short time later, she became enraged in the course of a ride in the family car and banged her head against the windshield so hard she broke it. Heather was diagnosed with attention deficit disorder and prescribed Ritalin, which, in the words of the article, "sent her through the roof."[361]

Heather's mother obtained a copy of *The Bipolar Child*, and after showing that book to a psychiatrist obtained a diagnosis of bipolar disorder for her daughter, making Heather Norris the youngest child in the county with such a label. The article goes on to assure us "she is now taking medication and receiving therapy to help her control her outbursts."[362]

At the age of three Bryan Thompson was diagnosed with bipolar disorder "after he began taking Ritalin and his behavior grew worse." Now, at the age of five, he frequently threatens to kill his mother, who explains "I know it will be like this for the rest of my life."[363]

The article also quotes a local expert as saying "The earlier a problem is treated, the better chance a child has of living a healthy productive life."[364] Not a shred of evidence is adduced in support of this assertion.

Elephants in the Room

The year 2008 saw the publication of *Is Your Child Bipolar?*[365] by psychiatric nurse Mary Ann McDonnell and child psychiatrist Janet Wozniak, who begin with this acknowledgement:

> *We are forever indebted to our mentor Dr. Joseph Biederman, chief of pediatric psychopharmacology research at Massachusetts General Hospital.*[366]

Nurse McDonnell and Dr. Wozniak describe parents of bipolar children as "walking on eggshells" and refer to the condition as "the elephant in the room,"[367] then proceed to tiptoe around the real elephants in the room—the role of stimulants and antidepressants in causing bipolar disorder in the first place, and the abundant evidence that treatment makes these kids worse, rather than better.

According to the authors, fifty percent of children treated for bipolar disorder "have" ADHD. For children diagnosed as bipolar before the age of seven, the figure rises to a staggering ninety percent.[368] Elsewhere they acknowledge that fifty percent of children treated for depression also go on to develop this condition,[369] and yet they never put two and two together and consider the role of stimulant drugs and antidepressants in creating this epidemic.

These two experts inform us that "As many as 18% of untreated children die by suicide before their eighteenth birthdays."[370] Not a shred of evidence is adduced for this astonishing proposition. Nor do they cite any evidence showing that "treatment" reduces the rate of suicide in this group. Instead, they go on to kick over a straw man, asking rhetorically "If your child had a chronic physical illness—diabetes or cerebral palsy or cancer for example, would you withhold or delay treatment for her?"[371]

So how does "treatment" work out for these kids? The authors provide us with some actual case histories from their files, which are eye-opening, to say the least.

Tara was diagnosed and drugged for ADHD at the age of four years, first with Concerta, then Ritalin, then Strattera, then Wellbutrin, and then Adderall. She suffered from explosive rages that could last for up to two hours, sleep disorders, anxiety, and hallucinations of ghosts.[372]

Nurse McDonnell and Dr. Wozniak diagnosed Tara with bipolar disorder and started her on Abilify, Trileptal, and lithium. Her moods stabilized, and then Adderall XR was added to the mix, but the drug made her condition worse, so the two experts decided to taper her off it and try non-medical approaches to treat her ADHD.[373] The reader could be forgiven for wondering why her doctors didn't do that in the first place.

Tashina had been described by her preschool teacher as a "spirited kid" who "had more energy than she knew what to do with." This "spirited kid" was diagnosed with ADHD at the age of eight years and prescribed Ritalin and then Concerta. She suffered from crying jags and was switched to Adderall. Later her doctor added Paxil to the mix.[374]

After Tashina's doctor increased her dose of Adderall and Paxil in order to eliminate "residual symptoms," the child suffered from rage storms lasting half an hour or more, every single day. Her parents brought her to see Nurse McDonnell and Dr. Wozniak who diagnosed her as bipolar and prescribed Risperdal, which caused the child to gain weight and made her lethargic. Her grades dropped.[375]

The two clinicians lowered the dose of Risperdal and added Strattera to the mix. Her grades improved and she no longer is physically aggressive, although she can be "mean-spirited." Her weight is stable, but she has sleep problems, so Seroquel has been added to the mix. It would be interesting to see how this story turns out.[376]

We do know how things turned out for Lonnie. This child had been diagnosed with ADHD and prescribed Tegretol, which caused a rash. She was switched first to Tenex, which made her irritable, then to Ritalin, which caused tics, and then to clonidine and Dexedrine. She was brought to Nurse McDonnell and Dr. Wozniak at the age of ten.[377]

The two experts rendered a diagnosis of bipolar disorder, continued the child on Dexedrine, tapered her off the clonidine, and added lithium and Risperdal to the mix. They later added Paxil but this caused wild mood swings, so they discontinued the Paxil and added the tricyclic antidepressant nortriptyline in its place.[378]

Lonnie became suicidal and refused to go to school. The lithium was discontinued after causing extreme thirst and bloating. The two clinicians added Zoloft to the mix along with the benzodiazepine tranquilizer Klonopin, increased the dose of Risperdal, and switched her to a different form of Dexedrine.[379]

Lonnie's condition became worse. She began drinking, smoking marijuana, and sneaking out of the house to consort with older teenage boys. She also experienced wild mood swings, flights of grandiosity alternating with suicidal despair.[380]

She did succeed in getting accepted to college but she did not fare well there, failing to adapt, doing poorly in her classes, and abusing cocaine. She downed an entire bottle of Tylenol in an attempt to end her life and suffered serious liver failure. For a time it looked as if she would survive only with a transplant.[381]

Lonnie did not receive a liver transplant, but her medication doses had to be reduced. Shortly after that her fiancé ended his relationship with her, and at the age of twenty she committed suicide.[382]

They've Got Issues

In her 2010 book *We've Got Issues: Children and Parents in the Age of Medication,*[383] author Judith Warner tells the story of a five-year-old boy "who had always been in trouble"—disruptive, hyperemotional, and aggressive:

> *The boy's pediatrician, without any formal evaluation, suggested a trial of ADHD meds. The medication made the boy all but psychotic. At age five, he was talking about suicide.*
>
> *The mother stopped the drugs and took the boy to a child psychiatrist. The psychiatrist diagnosed him as bipolar on the spot—based on his reaction to the ADHD meds. (Many children end up being diagnosed as bipolar—and end up on bipolar meds—after becoming manic or violent or psychotic or otherwise out of control on stimulant medication or SSRI antidepressants.)[384]*

It would be hard to find a more clear-cut example of drug-induced toxicity than this one. Other such examples are cited, but none of this stops the author from demanding even more kids be put on these drugs.

Page 45 of her book contains this statement:

> *It wasn't until the late 1980s and early 1990s that psychiatrists started prescribing antidepressants widely to children and teens...[385]*

The opening sentence of the very next paragraph reads as follows:

> *Bipolar disorder wasn't considered a possibility for kids until the 1990s...*[386]

Seven pages later she tells the reader:

> *There weren't any bipolar kids until psychiatrists in the mid-1990s, influenced chiefly by the work of Harvard University's Joseph Biederman at Massachusetts General Hospital, began saying there were.*[387]

Warner in effect acknowledges there was no epidemic of childhood bipolar disorder until psychiatrists began dosing large numbers of children with antidepressants and stimulants, but rather than put two and two together, she attempts to explain this epidemic by means of some wild speculation about the harmful effects of "assortative mating"[388]—a proposition for which she adduces no data whatsoever.

Mental Health Services

A documentary aired on 17 March 2015 by the CBC news magazine *Fifth Estate* illustrates how adept the media have become at ignoring the twin elephants in the room. Titled "Chazz Petrella: The Boy Who Should Have Lived,"[389] the program told the tale of a young boy who committed suicide after years of entanglement with the mental health system.

"From the time he was out of the womb, Chazz Petrella was a boy on the go." So we are told, as we are shown images of Chazz leaping off a roof, jumping into a pool, and rolling down a hill and colliding with another boy. The presenter then intones ominously "Mental illness was something the Petrellas, like most families, didn't understand."

Chazz Petrella was the youngest of five children. His father owned a hairdressing salon, his mother was a sales manager, and in addition the two of them operated a hobby farm.

The presenter describes Chazz as "a boy in perpetual motion, a kid on the go," and so he was.

"Chazz was always full of energy, always ready to try anything," his mother recalls. "He loved to play. He loved life. He loved everything. He really, really did."

None of this sounds like a problem, and indeed there was no problem until the boy began his formal education. "Chazz couldn't seem to focus," the presenter proclaims. "And when he got frustrated, he got aggressive." They tried changing schools, but it didn't help. Chazz was tested for learning disabilities, but that didn't seem to be the problem. Chazz's pediatrician diagnosed him with ADHD and, we are told, "like thousands of children in this country, he was put on medication"—as if this were an incidental detail.

The medication didn't help. Chazz couldn't sleep, and he told his mother it felt as if he couldn't turn his brain off. He began acting out and smoking marijuana at the tender age of nine. He would sneak out of the window of his home and wander around for hours. He would go into rages, after which he would feel overwhelmed with remorse.

All this sounds suspiciously like stimulant-induced mania, or maybe even just a boy crying out for clear boundaries and consistent discipline, but no one inquires into this possibility.

The last straw came when Chazz threw a rope over a basement water pipe and left a chair nearby—clearly a threat of suicide. At the age of ten the boy was sent to a residential care facility, and six months later he returned home, seemingly much improved—for a time.

"They'd adjusted his medications," the presenter tells us—note her use of the plural—but she doesn't bother telling us what "medications" he was taking, as if this was a matter of no import.

Chazz's behavior soon took a turn for the worse again. He continued to have trouble sleeping, and went back to his old habits of sneaking out at night. When his parents installed window alarms, he cut the wires. He was hanging out with much older youths, in their late teens or even early twenties.

When school resumed, on the second day he went into a rage, overturning his desk and trashing the classroom. He was sent home, and his mother and pregnant older sister transported him to the mental health crisis center half an hour away. In the course of the journey, Chazz grabbed his sister by the hair and pulled her head backward—while she was driving the car. She managed to pull over to the side of the road and they succeeded in restraining him, and they resumed the journey. Again Chazz attacked his sister in exactly the same way. Chazz's mother called the police, and they transported him to the center in handcuffs.

Ultimately, nine separate agencies were involved in Chazz's case. Chazz was sent to another residential group home, then another, and yet another—his fourth. It was here that Chazz finally seemed to be getting better.

But he had been admitted on an emergency basis, and his parents were told that in order for him to return the following year, they would have to pay $21,000 in tuition—money they didn't have. Then they were told that the government would pay the full price, on one condition—that they relinquish custody of their boy to the state. The Petrellas refused.

That summer, late one night, the Petrellas made a video recording of their son, shrieking in agony. When his father urges him to go to sleep he screams "I can't do it! I can't! I need something to help me sleep!" When the elder Petrella reminds his son that he has already had his sleep meds, the boy screams "They don't do anything! I hate this so fucking much!"

"He had no control," his mother recalled. "He couldn't sleep. It's almost like he's crawling in his skin."

Two days later Chazz Petrella hanged himself in the back yard. He was twelve years old.

The pain felt by the Petrellas and everyone else who loved Chazz is not to be belittled. These are obviously good, decent people, whose lives have been shattered by forces seemingly beyond their comprehension.

But the producers missed a golden opportunity. We are never told which drugs Chazz was prescribed. The possibility that his worst problems may have been pharmacologically induced is not even considered, even though mania is an extraordinarily well-documented toxic effect of stimulant drugs, and his mother's description of her son's anguish— "It's almost like he's crawling in his skin"—is almost the textbook definition of akathisia.

Even more importantly, there is no discussion of a society which has failed miserably in accommodating the natural energy and exuberance of young boys, and which at the same time has sadly undermined parental authority and substituted in its place an alphabet soup of government agencies and a cornucopia of neurotoxic drugs. Instead the producers offer an improbable tale of a boy whose brain inexplicably went haywire for no apparent reason, and then wrap things up with some platitudes about the need for better mental health services.

Driving Kids Crazy

The following December, a paper in the *Journal of Clinical Psychopharmacology* examined the relationship between stimulant prescriptions for young people and hospitalization for psychosis or mania.[390] Researchers looked at all Ontario social assistance recipients aged twenty-five or younger for the period between 1 October 1999 and 31 March 2013 who were hospitalized for psychosis or mania within 180 days after receiving a prescription for stimulants. There were a total of 183 cases that met these criteria. Ninety percent of the stimulant prescriptions were for Ritalin.

The authors found that young people were almost twice as likely to be hospitalized for psychosis or mania within sixty days after receiving a prescription as they were within the control period, defined as 120-180 days after prescription.[391]

So are the drugs the cause of these young people's distress? More than fifty years ago, noted epidemiologist Sir Austin Bradford Hill set forth the guiding principles for establishing cause and effect in this field.[392] The *JCP* study satisfies most of the Bradford criteria:

1) Strength of association: The risk of being hospitalized for psychosis or mania in the first sixty days was nearly double during the risk interval—a huge increase.

2) Temporality of association: The hospitalization always followed the stimulant prescription, rather than preceding it.

3) Consistency of association: Numerous clinical case histories had already reported an association between stimulant prescriptions and psychosis or mania.

4) Theoretical plausibility: Stimulant drugs by definition result in increased levels of arousal and activity—the very essence of mania.

5) Coherence: The association between stimulant drugs and mania or psychosis is coherent, meaning it does not contradict other knowledge, and there are no competing or rival theories to explain the association.

6) Specificity of association: This one admittedly is lacking, as other classes of drugs are also known to cause mania and/or psychotic symptoms

7) Biological gradient: Again, this one is lacking, as the researchers did not look for evidence of a dose-response relationship

8) Experimental evidence: The evidence was of high quality, coming as it did from a large population-wide sample with each subject serving as his own matched control.

9) Analogy: We already knew that other psychotropic drugs can have a wide variety of harmful effects, including psychosis and mania.

The evidence is clear. In plain English, these drugs are driving kids crazy.

Perhaps even more disturbing was the revelation that sixty-two of these cases received another prescription after being discharged from the hospital, and of those, twenty-eight, or forty-five percent, were readmitted for psychosis or mania shortly thereafter.[393]

The Bipolar Bandwagon

The bipolar bandwagon keeps rolling. Once upon a time, children were raised on religious and national myths that placed their lives in a larger context of meaning, as well as stories that taught the importance of hard work (*The Little Red Hen*), preparation (*The Three Little Pigs*), and perseverance (*The Little Engine That Could*). They read about the young Abe Lincoln walking miles to return books he had borrowed, and the young Teddy Roosevelt overcoming his childhood asthma through strenuous exercise. Today, tomes such as *Turbo Max*, *Brandon and the Bipolar Bear*, and *My Bipolar Roller Coaster Feelings Book* teach the wee ones the importance of psychotropic medication compliance.

Dr. Papolos, first author of *The Bipolar Child*, is now the Director of Research at the Juvenile Bipolar Research Foundation, which bills itself as "the first and only nonprofit research foundation dedicated solely to promoting research to identifying the source of early-onset bipolar disorder." The organization's website features the Child Bipolar Questionnaire, "a reliable and sensitive diagnostic indicator for early-onset bipolar disorder."[394] Sample items from the questionnaire include "craves sweet-tasting foods," "attempts to avoid homework assignments," "has elated or silly, goofy, giddy mood states," and "fidgets with hands or feet."

The website coyly acknowledges the organization's "Pioneer Sponsors" but a comprehensive list of benefactors is nowhere to be found, and repeated emails to the foundation inquiring as to their source of funding went unanswered.

CHAPTER SIX

REBECCA
RILEY

The short unhappy life of Rebecca Riley is a parable for our times. Her diagnosis of Attention Deficit Hyperactivity Disorder at the age of two was followed by a downward slide which doctors, nurses, teachers, social workers, parents, and other family members seemed powerless to halt.

Born into a troubled family, Rebecca had the odds stacked against her from the beginning. Her father, Michael, had been forbidden to live in public housing with the rest of his family due to an alleged sexual assault against his wife's thirteen-year-old daughter from her first marriage. Michael denied the allegations, and no charges were ever filed in the case. He once attacked his own eleven-year-old son, banging the boy's head against the rear window of a pickup truck. His wife Carolyn filed a restraining order against him, although the order subsequently was allowed to lapse.

At the tender of age of twenty-eight months, Rebecca came under the care of Kayoko Kifuji, a board-certified pediatrician at the Tufts-New England Medical Center. (Sometime after she began treating Rebecca, Dr. Kifuji became board-certified in psychiatry as well.) Kifuji was a devotee of Joseph Biederman and his followers at Harvard Medical School and Mass General.

"They are by far the leading lights in providing leadership in the treatment of children who have disorders such as bipolar," her lawyer would later tell reporters. "Dr. Kifuji subscribes to the views of the Mass General Team."[395]

Indeed. After a twenty-minute initial consultation, Dr. Kifuji diagnosed Rebecca with ADHD and prescribed the antihypertensive drug clonidine.

The toxic effects of clonidine include a severe drop in blood pressure, which may be fatal, as well as rebound hypertension which can be lethal as well.

At the age of three Dr. Kifuji diagnosed Rebecca with bipolar disorder, and prescribed Depakote and Zyprexa in addition to the clonidine. Later the Zyprexa was replaced with Seroquel. At the time, none of these drugs had been approved for use in children.

Rebecca lived in public housing with her mother and two older siblings. Rebecca's older brother and sister had also been diagnosed with ADHD and bipolar disorder by Dr. Kifuji, and were taking the same drugs, and the family was receiving SSI disability payments for both children. They applied for disability payments for Rebecca as well, although this was never approved by the authorities. The children's mother, Carolyn, was taking Paxil for depression and anxiety. Michael identified himself as suffering from Intermittent Rage Disorder, although he was not taking any medication for this condition.

On one occasion Carolyn claimed to have lost an entire bottle of clonidine. Dr. Kifuji wrote another prescription for her. Ten days later Carolyn reported that water had gotten into the bottle of clonidine, ruining the contents, and Kifuji dutifully wrote yet another prescription for her, but only for a ten-day supply, to avoid the possibility of "losing" yet another entire month's supply. This did not end the problem, and investigators reviewing prescription records for the autumn of 2006 would later note an alarming pattern of Rebecca's supply of clonidine running out before it should have, again and again.

Running out of clonidine was not the only problem this family faced. A social worker visiting the Riley home in May of 2006 noticed a puddle of urine on the floor. Carolyn thoughtfully advised her to step around it but made no attempt to clean it up until the social worker told her to do so. Carolyn herself appeared heavily drugged and unable to respond to the needs of her children.

The social worker also expressed concern over the amount and types of medication Rebecca was taking, later telling investigators that she saw no evidence of mental illness in the child. Rebecca and her sister often were asleep when the social worker visited, and Carolyn herself fell asleep during one of these visits. Carolyn also declined to take advantage of child-care and parenting programs offered by Social Services. The social worker filed two reports with her superiors, but no action was ever taken, and after missing numerous appointments Carolyn terminated the agency's contact with the family.

In her notes from her first visit with Rebecca, Dr. Kifuji described Rebecca as a happy child with "bright affect." However, all this would soon change.[396]

Rebecca often slept through her appointments with Dr. Kifuji, and Carolyn herself fell asleep during one of these visits as well. Rebecca's preschool teacher and school nurse expressed concern over the tot, noting that most of the time she appeared lethargic and too weak to play with the other children. The child was barely able to walk up a flight of steps without help, and when the nurse held Rebecca in her lap she felt "like a floppy doll."

The nurse also noted that Rebecca had never exhibited any kind of aggressive behavior toward the other children, nor any other behavior that would support a diagnosis of either bipolar disorder or ADHD.

There were other concerns. Rebecca exhibited a need to urinate repeatedly during the day, another toxic effect of the drugs she was given. An aide noted that the child would void only a small amount of urine at a time, and afterward she often was so weak she was unable to pull up or fasten her pants.

Rebecca often arrived at preschool without a snack, attired in inappropriate clothing or wearing shoes that were obviously too big for her. The driver who transported Rebecca to preschool also conveyed her older brother to another school, and she would later tell investigators that the boy smelled so badly she had to open all the windows while he was in the vehicle.

On Tuesday 14 November 2006, Carolyn and the children moved out of public housing and into a home located at 70 Lynn Avenue in Hull, Massachusetts, which they shared with Carolyn's half-brother Jim, a tow-truck driver, and Jim's fiancée Kelly. Sometime around the beginning of December 2006, Michael moved in to join the rest of the family.

On Thursday 7 December, Carolyn filled an order for thirty-five clonidine tablets, or a ten-day supply. Based on past prescriptions, Rebecca should have had enough of the drug to last her until 7 January 2007. Unfortunately, Rebecca herself would not last that long.

On Saturday 9 December, Rebecca woke up at two o'clock in the afternoon and came into the kitchen and fiddled with a bowl of cereal for a while. Carolyn's sister-in-law Kelly gave the child some Sunny D juice to drink. That night Kelly and her husband Jim heard the child coughing and making whooping sounds.

The next day, Sunday 10 December, Rebecca climbed up into Kelly's lap. The child was extremely hot, her hair was damp with sweat and her clothing was soaked. Kelly and Jim observed Carolyn as she offered Rebecca some red liquid cough syrup in a coffee cup. Kelly would later tell investigators that there had been at least an inch of syrup in the cup.

The child took one sip and spat it out, so Carolyn gave her some Tylenol instead. Throughout the day Kelly and Jim repeatedly urged Carolyn and Michael to take the child to the doctor, and they promised to do so.

The day that followed, Monday 11 December, Rebecca woke in the morning still feverish, and so Carolyn gave her three children's chewable Tylenol. The family had an appointment with Social Services and arrived at 9:00 AM. Rebecca vomited in the lobby, and so Carolyn re-scheduled the appointment and they all left. Rebecca vomited again while in the car, and Michael would later recall seeing Depakote sprinkles in the vomit.

When they arrived at home, Michael screamed at Carolyn, "Your daughter fucking threw up in my car!" Kelly and Jim again urged Carolyn and Michael to take the child to the doctor. Rebecca vomited repeatedly that afternoon.

On the afternoon of the next day, Tuesday 12 December, Kelly and Jim noticed that Rebecca was acting strangely, appearing incoherent and not responding when people called her name. Michael retreated to his room and began working on models at his desk. Jim stormed into the room and grabbed Michael by the shirt collar and told him "If you won't bring her to the hospital, then I'll beat you so the ambulance will come and take you both!" Michael assured Jim that they had scheduled a doctor's appointment for Rebecca the next day.

No such appointment was ever made.

That evening, while Carolyn and Michael were out on an errand, Kelly and Jim became concerned for Rebecca. She would come out of bedroom, crying out for her mommy. Kelly told the child repeatedly where her mother had gone, but she did not seem to understand. Kelly picked up Rebecca and carried her into the bedroom. Normally, Rebecca would wrap her legs around Kelly like a monkey whenever she picked her up, but this time, Kelly later would recall, the child's body felt stiff as a board.

When Carolyn and Michael returned, Kelly begged them to take Rebecca to the doctor, and they promised to do so. That night Rebecca got up repeatedly and went into her parents' room, crying out for her mommy. Michael would scream at the child, often using profanity, and order her to "Get back in your room!"

Just past midnight, Jim was awakened by a page from the Hull Police Department requesting a tow. He arose and heard gurgling sounds coming from Rebecca's bedroom. After entering the child's room and wiping some vomit off her face, he then ran to Michael and Carolyn's room and kicked the door open and demanded they do something immediately. Carolyn got up and took Rebecca into the bedroom she shared with Michael. Meanwhile the requested tow was canceled, and Jim went back to bed believing the Rileys finally were going to take care of their child.

Sometime in the wee hours of the morning, Rebecca Riley died.

Based on the amount of clonidine Rebecca had been prescribed, she should have had seventy-five tablets left if she had been taking them as directed. Investigators found seven.

Both of Rebecca's surviving siblings were immediately taken away and placed in foster care, and both Carolyn and Michael were arrested and charged with first-degree murder.[397] News photos of Carolyn taken during her trial show her looking obese and bewildered. She was convicted of second-degree murder and sentenced to life in prison with the possibility of parole after fifteen years. Michael was convicted of first-degree murder and sentenced to life in prison without parole.[398]

On 25 January 2011, lawyers for the estate of Rebecca Riley announced that they had settled a malpractice lawsuit against Dr. Kifuji for $2.5 million, to be distributed to Rebecca's surviving brother and sister. Tufts said it agreed to the settlement in order to spare the siblings more heartache.[399]

CHAPTER SEVEN

A DEVASTATION BEYOND BELIEF

A Beautiful Child

He was a beautiful child.

That is how Anne, a nurse by trade, remembers her older son, William.

"He laughed a lot," she recalls. "He liked to have fun. He played the piano beautifully." He was fascinated by fire engines, and Anne used to take the boy to the local fire house for visits. The fire captain told Anne "Your son can roll up the fire hose better than some of my firemen."

He also was high energy. When he was five years old, he received a pair of roller blades for Christmas, and he put them on and went outside and practiced until the sun went down. "He was a fantastic roller-blader before the day was over," Anne says.

Night after night, the boy would run around the house in circles to burn off some of that excess energy. But when Anne's mother witnessed this behavior, she became concerned for her grandson. "He has anxiety," Anne's mother told her. "You need to take him to the doctor."

Anne protested "Mom, all they're going to do is give him medication," and her mother replied, "Well, then that's what they need to do. You need to have him evaluated."

Anne consulted with both her son's teacher and the school headmaster, both of whom agreed that there was nothing wrong with the boy. "But I was very eager to please my mother," Anne says ruefully. She took her son to a clinical social worker who told Anne the child had ADHD. Over the next five years, William was prescribed a variety of medications, including Ritalin, Adderall, and Dexedrine, along with the antidepressant Elavil, and for a short time, Zoloft.

The results were disastrous. Her son would appear perfectly normal all day long, Anne recalls, but when she picked him up at school his behavior would change instantly. "He would just explode. He would start pointing his finger at me and yelling at me. I would just be so dumbfounded that a little boy in a five- and six-year-old body could be attacking me."

Anne never connected the change in her son's behavior with the drugs. "I medicated the heck out of him," she recalls. "The poor child. I mean I look back and just go, 'What were we doing?'"

> *You're so frightened your child is going to misbehave that you're just feeding them these pills just as fast and as hard as you can and you don't want the time to get away from you because you're afraid they're going to blow up and explode. Well, they do, because it's just like a heroin addict without their heroin. They do explode. You don't give them what their body's been getting, and they have a reaction.*

When her son was ten, Anne read the book *The Bipolar Child* by Demetri Papolos, M.D., and his daughter Janice Papolos. "They described my child to a T. I just remember highlighting so many things in that book and crying and thinking 'Oh my gosh—my son has bipolar!'"

Anne took her son to a clinic and asked the doctor to prescribe Depakote for the boy. "I've got a book now telling me what to do and how to go to my doctor and say 'This is what I need,' and I was insistent." After a fifteen-minute consultation, the prescription for Depakote was dispensed, as requested. At the same time, all his other medications were discontinued.

"It was horrible," Anne recalls. "He became a zombie." Other times, the boy would undergo meltdowns, screaming and crying at the smallest provocation.

But the worst was yet to come.

A Day-Dreamer

He had a wonderful, creative, imaginative way of living.

That is how Michelle describes her older son Trevor—before he was diagnosed and drugged for ADHD.

"He was a day-dreamer," she recalls. "He had always been very artistic, creative, imaginative."

Michelle looks back with fondness on her days as a stay-at-home mother of two young boys. "I had a wonderful life I had carved out for myself," she remembers. "I had other mothers that were grateful to be stay-at-home moms and were very supportive. We had play groups together. I was active in my church. My husband was working in a family-owned business, and finances were not an issue." In her spare time, she played tennis and golf, and won trophies for mountain biking.

Michelle's tale of iatrogenic harm begins not with her son's diagnosis but with her own. A dark secret from her childhood came to light, and meanwhile her husband was facing work- and family-related stressors of his own. Their marriage began to crack under all this strain, leaving Michelle feeling depressed and anxious. She was prescribed Prozac and Klonopin, and after taking the drugs she suffered a breakdown which led her to be confined to a hospital psychiatric ward, where her husband served her divorce papers.

Michelle and her now-ex-husband shared custody of their two children. He was off working most of the time, Michelle recalls, and when the boys were staying with him they were raised mainly by nannies. Michelle offered to take the boys full-time, but her ex-husband refused.

Michelle says that when her older boy, Trevor, was in the second grade at a tony private school, he was well-liked but had problems keeping up with the other children academically—problems Michele attributes to not having a parent available to assist him with his homework when he came home to his father's house after school.

Michelle recalls feeling ganged-up on when she met with school authorities regarding her son's difficulties. "They're telling me if we don't medicate him he's not going to be asked back."

Trevor was evaluated by a pediatrician who diagnosed him with ADHD and prescribed Adderall. The boy reacted badly to the drug—depression, agitation, and mania—and he was switched to Ritalin. Michelle was concerned and filed a motion to gain full custody of her son, who by then had become volatile and was losing control of his emotions.

Meanwhile Trevor's pediatrician switched him to Metadate—the long-acting form of Ritalin—and the boy's condition deteriorated. He became upset, withdrawn, depressed, obsessed with death, and was sent home from Boy Scout camp for bizarre behavior.

Michelle's bid for full-time custody did not go well. The judge fined her $3,500 for wasting the court's time, which she had to pay on top of her attorney's fees. Meanwhile her son's condition continued to get worse. He suffered from nightmares and cut himself with a razor while staying with his father. A child psychiatrist diagnosed Trevor with an anxiety disorder and prescribed Celexa and Klonopin.

After the first dose of Celexa, Trevor suffered a psychotic break. He experienced hallucinations, tried to jump out of a moving car, threatened to leap out of a second story window, broke glass, expressed a desire to cut himself, and lay on the floor moaning like a wounded animal. The boy was hospitalized but then released at the demand of Michelle's ex-husband, who took Trevor to another psychiatrist who diagnosed him with bipolar disorder.

Soon after, Trevor was hospitalized and diagnosed with Substance Induced Mood Disorder, which the attending physician attributed to Klonopin. How he knew it was the Klonopin and not any of the other drugs the boy had been given was never made clear.

While staying with his father and his new nanny (the third one in three months), Trevor locked himself in the bathroom and refused to go to school. Desperate for answers, Michelle began searching bookstores and found the Papoloses' book, *The Bipolar Child*. After reading it, Michelle accepted that her child had a mental illness which would require treatment for the rest of his life. She even gave presentations to her son's class, "educating" them on the reality of the "brain disease" her boy had to cope with.

Trevor was subsequently prescribed a veritable cornucopia of psychiatric drugs—Depakote, Risperdal, Neurontin, Wellbutrin, Trileptal, Zyprexa, and Cogentin. Michelle says there are pages missing from her son's medical files, so there may have been other drugs prescribed as well. The boy was hospitalized again and Michelle begged the doctors to taper him off all the drugs, but they refused.

By this time Michelle was feeling exhausted and overwhelmed. She says she asked her ex-husband, who she says was making in excess of $200,000 a year, for more child support payments than the $1,000 a month he was paying, but he refused. At this point she was hospitalized for suicidal depression, and her ex assumed full custody of their two sons.

Michelle's tribulations continued. She lost a court battle over her mother's estate to a family member she says sexually abused her as a child. Then her boyfriend, a medical doctor, was diagnosed with an aggressive inoperable cancer and died six months later. The medications she was taking led to akathisia, which drove her to the brink of suicide. Her doctor told her she was bipolar, like her son, and that both of them suffered from a faulty genetic inheritance. Meanwhile, Trevor was struggling academically, skipping school, clashing with his father, and cutting himself.

With great anguish, Michelle moved out of state and began to put her life back together. Amazingly, just two months later, her ex-husband gave up custody of their son and allowed him to move in with her. She helped him taper off all his meds and he resumed his schooling—in regular classrooms, without an IEP, just like the other kids.

Aftermath

Today Michelle's oldest son is a grown man and doing beautifully. After graduating with a BA in business communications from a top university, he is now living abroad and pursuing a successful career, married, with a little boy of his own. Her other son did not fare as well. He escaped the turmoil surrounding his formative years by sinking into a morass of video game addiction. She describes him as a shut-in, living alone, obese, paranoid, unable to work, still supported by his father, and dependent on monthly depot injections of the antipsychotic drug Invega.

Meanwhile, Michelle went back to university and became a counselor. Today she works to help other families deal with their problems—without toxic brain-disabling drugs.

Anne and her son William did not fare well, either. About a year after stopping the ADHD drugs and beginning Depakote, the boy's condition finally seemed to be stabilizing. For the first time in years, he was genuinely smiling and laughing. But tests revealed he had elevated levels of liver enzymes. The Depakote was stopped abruptly, and a few months later he scribbled out a suicide note and shot himself dead.

There is a bizarre postscript to this story. Seven years later, Anne's younger son Warren was in middle school and doing beautifully. "He had lots of friends," Anne recalls. "The girls loved him." He was a rock climber, the SGA president, and the emcee for the school television show. He was not taking any psychotropic medication, although he was taking Claritin for his allergies.

One day Warren suffered abdominal pains and was rushed to the hospital, where he was prescribed an over-the-counter laxative, Miralax.

Claritin is a dibenzazepine, a chemical cousin to Elavil, which Warren's late brother William had been taking. Miralax consists of polyethylene glycol, also used by the chemical industry as a plasticizer, a sealant, a dispersant, an anti-foaming agent, and a wood preservative. In 2011, the FDA warned of a potential risk of neuropsychiatric effects associated with the use of polyethylene glycol, although it later decided that no further action was necessary.

Six days after Warren started taking Miralax, his mother left to go to the PTA meeting. Warren and his father were watching television together when the boy left the room and then came back with a gun and shot his father dead. Before this he had never shown any sign of violent behavior. The following year, he pled guilty to second-degree murder and was sentenced to twenty years and six months in state prison.

"Losing a child is a devastation beyond belief," Anne says. She goes on to relate an incident that occurred almost seven years after her older son committed suicide. "I remember putting my hands on my husband's face. I looked at my husband with great love and I said 'We are going to make it. We're going to be okay.'"

"As I said that to my husband, our little boy—I'll never forget—he came down the hall and said 'Hey Dad, my favorite program is beginning to start. Would you fix me some ice cream?'"

Three weeks later her husband was dead.

CHAPTER EIGHT

DIVERSION, MISUSE, AND ABUSE OF ADHD MEDS

We have already noted that the generic term for Adderall is "mixed amphetamine salts." Amphetamine, Ritalin, and cocaine all are central nervous system stimulants. The addictive properties of amphetamine, and its potential for abuse, have been well-known for at least the past sixty years,[400] and those of cocaine for longer than that.[401] Ritalin and cocaine both act on the same parts of the brain,[402] and rats trained to self-administer cocaine will enthusiastically accept amphetamine or Ritalin as a substitute—although they will not do so with wide variety of other drugs, or a saline solution.[403]

The toxic effects of cocaine include confusion, delirium, hallucinations, and psychosis. The same is true for amphetamine and Ritalin. It would seem naive to assume these noxious attributes vanish just because someone gives these substances catchy names and calls them "medicines."

Before we go any further, let's define our terms. According to the FDA,[404] "Diversion" means any intentional act that results in transferring a drug product from lawful to unlawful distribution or possession. "Misuse" is any intentional therapeutic use of a drug product in an inappropriate way—such as popping your dorm-mate's Adderall to help get you through final exams. "Abuse" is any intentional nontherapeutic use of a drug for the purpose of achieving a desirable psychological or physiological effect—or in plain English, to get "high."

Sweden's experience with the abuse of stimulant drugs is instructive. In that country, amphetamine was strictly controlled, but Ritalin and another stimulant, phenmetrazine, were widely available on the street. Concern over rising rates of hepatitis, septicemia, and psychotic reactions among abusers led authorities in that country to ban both drugs.[405]

In December of 1996, in response to concerns sparked by skyrocketing rates of prescriptions for Ritalin, the United States Drug Enforcement Agency held a conference to discuss the misuse and abuse of that drug. Highlights from the closing statement by DEA administrator Gene Haslip include the following:[406]

> *Since 1990, prescriptions for methylphenidate have increased by 500 percent, while prescriptions for amphetamine have increased 400 percent.*
>
> *The data shows that there has been a 1,000 percent increase in drug abuse injury reports involving methylphenidate for children in the 10 to 14 age group.*
>
> *Parents need to understand we are talking about very potent, addictive, and abusable substances.*
>
> *We have become the only country in the world where children are prescribed such a vast quantity of stimulants that share virtually the same properties as cocaine.*

The following March the International Narcotics Control Board issued a warning about the about the abuse potential of Ritalin, along with a stern rebuke to American prescribers:[407]

> *About 90 percent of global consumption [of Ritalin] is in the United States.*
>
> *A black market in the drug has emerged in recent years, with adolescents and even adults buying tablets from children under*

treatment or tablets stolen from school medical wards, in addition to the diversion of methylphenidate from pharmacies by theft or forged prescriptions.

Since the drug is touted as 'accepted medication' for children, abusers are unaware of its health hazards, which include addiction and a range of stimulant-abuse symptoms.

In August of that year, a police sergeant in Cedar Rapids, Iowa, told USA Today "We have Ritalin junkies. They'd rather do Ritalin than morphine or cocaine."[408] Abusers would often combine Ritalin with the opioid pentazocine, dubbing the concoction "Kibbles and Bits." A doctor quoted in the same article referred to the mixture as "the poor man's speedball."

The misuse and abuse of ADHD meds has been particularly well-studied on American college campuses. A 2002 study at a small competitive private college found that one out of three undergraduate students had taken a stimulant medication that had not been prescribed to him or her.[409] A 2010 study at a large public research university reported an almost identical figure.[410] For fraternity and sorority members, the figure was more than one out of two.

Almost none of these students purchased these substances from strangers or professional drug dealers. Instead, they obtained the pills from friends, either gratis or for a small fee (usually about three to ten dollars per pill).[411] Most of them had not been diagnosed with ADHD as children, and did not start taking the drugs until they entered college.[412]

Students' motivations for ingesting these drugs fell into two broad categories: academic and recreational.[413] Those who took stimulants for academic reasons reported the drugs enabled them to stay awake longer, increased their concentration, productivity, learning, and memory, and also made the subject matter more interesting. Students who took stimulants for recreational purposes often crushed the drug into a powder and snorted it, flooding the brain and enabling an instant high some abusers compared to the euphoria produced by cocaine.[414]

Students who abused ADHD meds often did so in conjunction with alcohol. They claimed the drugs helped them stay awake longer, and in addition made them more sociable and talkative. They further reported that stimulants helped them get drunk quicker, or to drink longer, or sometimes both. As one young man explained to researchers, with admirable brevity, "You get fucked up faster and you can keep going without passing out."[415]

Some of the female students also reported these drugs suppressed their appetites, enabling them to lose weight in a hurry before spring break or a major social event.[416]

It's not all fun and games. Between 1998 and 2005, prescriptions for young people aged thirteen through nineteen increased 133 percent for amphetamine and fifty-two percent for Ritalin. During the same period, the number of calls to poison control centers related to the ingestion of these drugs increased by seventy-six percent. Forty-two percent of these cases were "clinically significant," meaning they resulted in moderate effects, major effects, or even death.[417]

During the period 2005 through 2011, emergency room visits for adults involving ADHD medications more than tripled. The fastest increase was seen in the eighteen through twenty-five-year-old demographic. Half of these visits were for "nonmedical" uses of stimulants, and at least thirty percent of those involved alcohol.[418]

Sometimes abuse of ADHD medications becomes deadly, as the following examples illustrate:

- On 21 May 2010, after a night of heavy drinking with his hometown friends, Kyle Craig, twenty-one, stepped in front of a passenger train and ended his life. He had begun using Adderall as both a study drug and a party drug while at Vanderbilt University, at first obtaining the drug casually from friends and later faking symptoms of ADHD in order to acquire prescriptions.

The February before his death, while spending a semester abroad in Barcelona, he had abruptly discontinued the drug, apparently without any medical supervision.[419]

- On 20 December 2012, George Washington University law student John Hronrich died in his New Jersey home from an overdose of heroin and Adderall. John had already graduated from Rutgers University with a 3.93 grade point average and had one semester left before completing law school.[420]

- In the early morning hours of 20 July 2014, Josh Levine, a twenty-two-year-old recent graduate from the University of Michigan, was rushed to the hospital after being found lying unresponsive on the sidewalk in front of his apartment building after a night of partying. Josh was declared brain-dead upon arrival and taken off life support hours afterward. The cause of death was listed as cardiac arrest brought on by acute alcohol poisoning. Post-mortem analysis revealed both alcohol and Adderall in his system.[421]

- On the night of 26 August 2018, Texas A&M University freshman Joseph Little suffered prolonged uncontrollable seizures which lasted over half an hour. He was rushed to the College Station Medical Center where he died two days later. It was later revealed that Joseph had been snorting Adderall in order to help him stay awake while attending social events during fraternity rush week. He had no previous history of seizures.[422]

Of course, since time immemorial young people have done foolish things, and most of them survive. But does misusing ADHD meds lead to improved academic performance? The answer to that question is a big fat No. Three separate studies conducted at three different universities have found that misusing these drugs results in lower grade point averages.[423]

And why would anyone have thought otherwise? After more than forty years of research, not a single study has shown that taking ADHD medication as directed results in improved long-term academic outcomes.[424]

In the light of all this, the hand-wringing concerns raised by some experts who liken these drugs to "academic steroids" and worry that students may be exaggerating symptoms of ADHD in order to obtain prescriptions for stimulants and supposedly gaining an unfair advantage over their classmates seem misplaced.[425] Perhaps a more pertinent question is this: Why did anyone think that a substitute for learning self-discipline could be found in the form of a pill? And what are the long-term consequences to society of telling young people that there is?

CHAPTER NINE

TWO FAMILIES

The Typical All-American Kid

He was the typical all-American kid.

That's how Rick Fee of Virginia Beach remember his son Richard.

> *He was very outgoing. He had lots of friends of various backgrounds. He was an athlete. He was a very good student, and he associated with just about everybody. Usually with the cliques and the groups in the schools, the athletes stay with the athletes and the smart kids stay with the smart kids and all that kind of stuff. But Richard bridged all those different groups. He was very popular, well-liked, did extremely well academically, and personally we had a great relationship.*

Richard graduated from high school with honors in 2004 and won a full scholarship to Greensboro College in North Carolina, where he was an honors program student in biology and also found time to play on the varsity baseball team. It was during this period that he began using Adderall as a study aid, having obtained the drug from one of his teammates.

Richard mentioned his use of Adderall to his father. "That immediately set red flags off in front of me," his father recollects.

> *We had the discussion right then and there that the Adderall had not been prescribed to him, that it was a dangerous drug, that he did not need to be taking it, and he just should stay away from it. I was totally against his taking it because it wasn't his, it wasn't prescribed to him, he didn't need it.*

The subject never came up again, and the elder Fee thought the matter was closed. Unbeknownst to him, his son continued his surreptitious use of Adderall while away at college.

Richard graduated from the honors program and remained in Greensboro to study for the Medical College Admission Test (MCAT). He had big dreams, and planned to enlist in the Navy in order to finance his medical education—dreams which never came to fruition.

While staying in Greensboro, Richard obtained a prescription for Vyvanse from a local nurse practitioner. He took the MCAT at the end of 2009, but he did not pass. Like many a young person whose dreams had stalled, Richard moved back home with his parents.

In February of 2010, Richard visited Dominion Psychiatric Associates of Virginia Beach and met with psychiatrist Waldo Ellison, who wrote a prescription for Adderall for the young man. His parents knew nothing about this.

The winter segued into spring which in turn segued into summer. Richard seemed to be losing focus. He wasn't interested in studying for the MCAT anymore or even in finding a job. He told his father he had given up on the idea of medical school, substituting instead some vague plans for writing a book.

"His whole mindset and train of thought was just a little off," his father recalls.

The elder Fee decided to hire his son to work in the family business, and it was only then—after Richard had been put on the company insurance plan—that he found out about his son's prescription for Adderall.

"I told him 'You don't have ADHD. You don't need this medication.'" After that confrontation, Rick's relationship with his son began to deteriorate.

> *We started butting heads, and having arguments about the least little things. It got very loud and vocal and aggressive on his part.*

Rick decided to take the bull by the horns, and visited Dr. Ellison in his office. He remembers the encounter as "surreal." Ellison refused to come out from behind the glass partition in the receptionists' area. He also refused to discuss Richard's case, citing health information privacy laws, adding that he was the foremost expert in ADHD in the state of Virginia and that he prescribed more Adderall than anyone else.

Rick felt he had hit a brick wall with Dr. Ellison and exited. His parting words to Ellison were "You keep giving Adderall to my son, you're going to kill him."

Richard's condition continued to deteriorate. He began disappearing for days at a time, and he suffered from insomnia, hallucinations, and fevers which could be assuaged only by plunging into a pool of cold water—in the middle of winter. He became more aggressive and began threatening violence against his father. Rick and his wife began locking their bedroom door before retiring at night.

"This wasn't who he was before Adderall," Rick notes.

Ellison did agree to schedule a joint meeting with Richard and his parents, which was held in February of 2011. "Dr. Ellison was so arrogant," Rick recalls. Virginia's "foremost expert in ADHD" told the other man that he knew Richard better than the young man's own father did—on the basis of one forty-five-minute initial consultation and a few subsequent five-to-seven-minute med checks.

Rick told Dr. Ellison "If Richard continues to get Adderall from you, he can't live in our house."

Dr. Ellison then told Richard "I can't have you become homeless over this." He abruptly discontinued the Adderall, without offering any advice for tapering off the drug, and prescribed Seroquel and Abilify instead. (Rick says he does not believe his son ever took either drug).

Richard "flipped out," the elder Fee recalls. The young man's mother had already departed in her own vehicle, and while they were out in the parking lot Richard tried to run his father over with his car.

The office was just a few blocks from Dominion Psychiatric Associates. Rick ran home and found his son had spiraled into a rage—swinging baseball bats against the walls of the garage and then bringing out cans of gasoline and threatening to burn the house down.

"It was a horrible situation," the elder Fee recalls.

Rick managed to get his son calmed down. Richard returned to Greensboro for a time, then moved back in with his parents. For a time his condition seemed to be improving, but unbeknownst to Rick, his son returned to Dr. Ellison. He told the psychiatrist that he now had a job and was living on his own—neither of which was true. Without bothering to verify any part of the young man's story, Ellison wrote another prescription for Adderall.

Richard's condition took a turn for the worst, and one night he turned violent and assaulted his father. Richard was six feet three inches tall and weighed nearly 200 pounds—"all muscle," his father recalls—and the older man called the police. By the time they arrived, Rick had changed his mind, but the officers told him they had to take his son into custody. Richard was released that same night.

Richard went to stay with a friend for a time, and then returned home yet again. One afternoon father and son had a heart-to-heart talk. "I really have a problem," the younger man explained tearfully. "I want help."

Rick took his son to the emergency room, thinking that there he could find the help he needed. But after waiting for hours, Richard's willingness to get help seemed to be waning. "The longer he waited, the antsier he got," his father remembers.

At last Richard's turn came. He refused to allow his father to go with him into the back office, but he did assent to having his mother accompany him. They were referred to Richard Parker, a psychiatrist with the hospital's "Rapid Response Team."

Richard's mother took him to his appointment with Dr. Parker, and carefully explained to a therapist working in the office that her son was there because of his Adderall addiction. Then Richard met with Parker—and walked out with a prescription for Adderall. (He was also prescribed clonidine and venlafaxine, but Rick says his son never took either of those drugs.)

"I was absolutely livid," Rick recalls. "I was shocked. I remember telling my wife, 'We just can't catch a break here. This system is going to end up killing this kid.'"

Rick told his son the only way he could keep living under his roof would be for Rick to retain custody of the Adderall, doling out the pills one day at a time. Richard agreed, but that arrangement didn't last. The young man began ransacking the house, trying to find where his father had hidden the Adderall.

One night in July of 2011 Richard became violent, throwing things and shoving his father, and then, astonishingly, the younger man called the police and demanded they make his father hand over his Adderall. The police told Rick that his son was an adult and that he had to turn the drug over to him. Rick replied that if they made him do that, his son could no longer stay under his roof. He handed back the Adderall and then the police ordered Richard to leave the house.

Richard returned later that night, manic and violent. This time his mother called the police, and he ran off. Later he telephoned his mother and threatened to stab himself in the head with a hunting knife. He was subsequently taken into custody, handcuffed, and placed in the back seat of the patrol car, at which point he proceeded to try to kick out the windows. He was remanded to the Virginia Beach Psychiatric Institute.

Richard's mother called the therapist at Dr. Parker's office and explained her son's situation. "Parker said 'No more Adderall' and washed his hands of Richard," the elder Fee recalls. Parker never saw Richard again.

Richard was released from the Virginia Beach Psychiatric Institute after just five days. His family was not even notified. Richard went to stay with a friend for a time.

Rick reached out to his son and offered to rent an apartment for him. The younger man was able to obtain a job supervising crews cleaning up debris from a recent hurricane. He was off the Adderall, making good money, and he would stop by and visit his parents from time to time. At last, he seemed to be getting better.

But, again unbeknownst to his parents, Richard returned to Dr. Ellison who, incredibly, wrote yet another prescription for Adderall for him.

"He called me one day," Rick recalls, "And I forget exactly what he said, but I could just tell by the tone of his voice something was different." His speech was rapid-fire, and he seemed manic. Rick asked his wife to call their insurance company and check. They learned that Dr. Ellison had written three prescriptions for Adderall for their son, each one for a month's supply—one for August, one for September, and one for October.

"I called Ellison," Rick recalls. "I just lit him up. I was furious." When Rick told the other man his son had been remanded to the Virginia Beach Psychiatric Institute, Dr. Ellison claimed to know nothing about it. Rick threatened legal action if Ellison prescribed any more Adderall for his son.

Richard did receive one more prescription from Dr. Ellison, that October, for Eli Lilly's blockbuster drug Strattera. Rick says his son would not take the drug.

"He may have taken one or two," Rick allows. "But they didn't give him the high that the Adderall did. So he wouldn't take it."

On 7 of November, Richard called his parents and left a message for them. His mother called back that night and left a message for him, asking him to call. When he failed to respond, Rick and his wife went to his apartment and knocked at the door. When nobody answered, Rick climbed in through an open window and then let his wife in.

It was a sight he would never forget.

The Perfect Son

He was the perfect son.

That's how David Schopp of North Lauderdale, Florida, remembers his son Dylan.

Known to his friends as "Sunshine," both for his golden locks and his eternally cheerful disposition, Dylan Schopp seemed destined for great things. An active lad, he loved wrestling and ultimate Frisbee, along with cycling, snowboarding, jet skiing, and sky-diving. Renowned for his wise-cracking sense of humor, he was voted "Class Clown" by his schoolmates. Academically he did well enough—"Solid B's, some A's," his father notes.

"He was always wanting to make people smile and laugh," his older sister Dara recalls. As a senior in high school, she found herself, improbably enough, overshadowed by her younger brother, then a freshman. Upon meeting her, people would exclaim, "Oh, you're Dylan Schopp's sister?"

In the fall of 2012, Dylan enrolled in Florida State University in Tallahassee to study business, and was immediately caught up in the hard-partying lifestyle. He pledged a fraternity and was subjected to a grueling program of hazing—sleep deprivation, bullying, and who knows what else. Dylan was falling asleep in his classes, and in order to cope with it all he began taking illegally diverted Adderall, along with other drugs, in a wide range of formulations and doses.

"Sometimes you buy Adderall, sometimes you buy Ritalin," his sister explains. "Extended release or not extended release—whatever is available." At times, weed, cocaine, and Ecstasy were added to this mix. His grades suffered, and he failed a required course in financial accounting.

Dylan survived the hazing and the following semester returned to campus a full-fledged member of his frat, but his troubles were just beginning. He continued the abuse of Adderall, and his grades continued to suffer as well. On one occasion, after staying up all night studying with the aid of the drug, he was so impaired it took him seven minutes just to enter his ID number for an online exam.

In February, one member of his freshman pledge class informed university authorities about the abusive hazing practices in his fraternity. Dylan became obsessed with the idea that everybody would think he was the one responsible—the first signs of a paranoid mentality which would eventually become his undoing.

"He couldn't get that thought out of his head," his father recalls. "That was the beginning of the end."

In March of that year Dylan had a heart-to-heart talk with his family. "He sat us down on the patio," Dara remembers, "And he was telling us 'Something's not right in my head. I'm having weird thoughts. My brain is not right.'" A campus psychiatrist prescribed Zoloft, and Dylan's mother Debbie actually moved to Tallahassee, staying in a nearby motel, to help her son get through the semester.

That summer, back home from FSU, Dylan seemed to be thriving. He began working out again, he was eating well and sleeping well, and he appeared to have returned to his old self. That fall he returned to FSU.

"That semester," his mother recalls, "Was an absolute shit show."

Dylan plunged right back into the same hard-partying atmosphere. He rented an apartment with four of his friends and obtained a part-time job, but he soon got fired. He discontinued the Zoloft without any taper, and the paranoia returned. He became convinced people were talking about him behind his back. Seemingly anything could trigger the same repetitious loop of paranoid thoughts—an Instagram post, a song on the radio, the sight of an FSU T-shirt. Again his grades suffered, and again he failed the required course in financial accounting.

He went to the campus health center where a doctor prescribed the antipsychotic drug Abilify. The drug, in his mother's words, made him "wacky"—hallucinations, jerky movements, uncontrollable blinking.

Around Thanksgiving, another doctor discontinued Abilify and prescribed the antipsychotic Risperdal. Dylan's father recalls his son's agitated state and rapid-fire speech while on the drug: "I wanna go fishing, I wanna do this, I wanna do that, dat dat dat dat dat dat dat." Towards the end of the semester one of Dylan's friends telephoned David and Debbie, expressing concern that their son might be suffering from schizophrenia.

After that semester ended, Dylan discontinued the Risperdal. His mother suggested he stay at home and try to recuperate, and he agreed. He enrolled at Florida Atlantic University—a forty-minute drive each way—switching his major from business to public relations. He was back on the Zoloft, with yet another antipsychotic drug, Geodon, added to the mix.

The drugs caused sedation and weight gain, and made him "foggy," according to his mother. His eyes were bloodshot, and he was afraid of falling asleep at the wheel in the course of his long daily commute to FAU. Later he was switched to Klonopin, a so-called "antianxiety" drug.

Dylan's adherence to his medication regimen was sporadic, exposing him to both the toxic effects of the drugs and effects of withdrawal as well—seemingly the worst of both worlds. Every time he would stop the drugs and then start again, his condition seemed to get worse. Nevertheless, he managed to finish the semester with a 3.5 grade point average in his new major.

That summer Dylan began working in a restaurant, and once again he seemed to be thriving. He would come home after his shift with $500 worth of tips in his pockets—and, often, the phone numbers of young women who had taken an interest in him.

"Everybody loved him," his father recalls.

That fall Dylan resumed his studies at FAU, and once more his condition took a turn for the worse. He became obsessed with conspiracy theories, dark forebodings about the malevolent forces arrayed against society—ISIS, the Illuminati, and God knows what else.

Dylan decided to join the Army. His family supported his decision in principle, but they urged him to hold off until he got healthy and finished his degree and would be able to enlist as an officer. But Dylan decided his new dream could not wait.

He abruptly discontinued all of his medications, and on Monday 9 February 2015 was sworn into the United States Army. He proudly announced this step on his Facebook page, but an innocuous expression of congratulations from one of his friends brought his paranoid obsessions swirling into the forefront once more.

Dylan texted his sister to express his outrage, convinced that a sinister message lay behind his well-wisher's innocent words. They texted back and forth, until finally she wrote "Let's agree to disagree. I love you."

Dylan replied "I love you."

Those were his last words to her.

Aftermath

On the evening of 7 November 2011, Richard Fee hanged himself.

"Not a day goes by that I don't think about that," Rick told me.

When I asked Rick what lessons he wanted people to take away from this, he didn't hesitate before replying:

I am of the firm belief that ADHD is not a real disease, and that Adderall is one of the most dangerous prescription drugs in the marketplace. It's extremely powerful, and nobody really realizes the long-term effects of this. It's extremely powerful. Doctors that are prescribing it do not have their patients' best interests at heart.

Phony diagnoses, pushing pills, is not the way to go. If people are having issues, there are much better alternatives.

Richard's argument always was that a doctor would not prescribe him something that was going to hurt him. Obviously, that's not true.

People need to be their own advocate, and just not take for granted that what a doctor is telling them is always going to be one hundred percent accurate. Trust your instincts and trust your gut, especially when it comes to your kids.

And what about Dylan Schopp?

In fairness, it ought to be pointed out that Adderall was only one of many toxic influences in Dylan's young life, along with sleep deprivation and what sounds like a virtual cornucopia of other drugs. Nevertheless, it is obvious that Adderall was the gateway drug which led to polypharmacy and his one-way slide to his eventual demise. Five years on, Dylan's sister offers this assessment: "The abuse of Adderall was the spark that lit the fire."

Indeed. But what if things had been handled differently? The human brain is a wonderfully plastic organ, with prodigious power to heal itself. When this gifted but troubled young man first began suffering from Adderall-induced paranoia, what if, instead of being offered new diagnoses and new prescriptions, he had been given all the time he needed to recover, and then resumed his studies, steering clear of all drugs, legal and illegal?

We will never know. In the early morning hours of Thursday, 12 February 2015, in a park in the nearby town of Sunrise, Dylan Schopp ended his life. He was twenty-one years old.

CHAPTER TEN

ADHD MEDS AND SUBSTANCE USE DISORDER

We have seen that ADHD medications can easily be misused or abused, by either the prescription holder or someone else, often with devastating effects. But another question remains: does drugging kids for ADHD make them more vulnerable to becoming dependent on other substances later in life?

In 1998, psychologists Nadine M. Lambert and Carolyn S. Hartsough published the results of a long-term study begun in 1974 of 492 children diagnosed with hyperactivity, in kindergarten through the fifth grade, drawn from 191 public, private and parochial school classrooms in the San Francisco Bay area.[426] Eighty-one percent of these subjects were available for follow-up some twenty years later.

Drs. Lambert and Hartsough found that rates of dependence on tobacco, cocaine, and stimulants was greater among the hyperactive subjects than in a set of matched controls.[427] That's not really very surprising. No one get the label "hyperactive" unless his behavior is deemed a problem by somebody, and it doesn't come as a surprise that troubled kids sometimes grow up to be troubled adults.

What was surprising, to some, was when the researchers looked at the hyperactive subjects, the rates of tobacco and cocaine dependence were significantly higher among those who had been medicated than those who had not. Rates were highest of all for those who had been medicated for a year or more.[428] The rate of cocaine dependence in this group was almost twice that of the never-medicated subjects.

Why might that be? Anyone who knows anything about life as it is lived knows that the body adapts to the presence of any drug taken on a regular basis. This happens by means of a well-known process known as "down-regulation." When the body is flooded with a chemical substance that mimics the action of a given neurotransmitter, it responds by cutting down the amount of neurotransmitter released by the pre-synaptic neuron, and also by cutting down on the number of receptor sites on the post-synaptic neuron. This is why when you ingest any psychoactive drug repeatedly, you often end up needing more and more of it to achieve the same effect.

There could be other factors at work here as well. In *Talking Back to Ritalin*,[429] Dr. Breggin suggests that children who take stimulants—whether in the form of Ritalin, tobacco, or street drugs—get in the habit of using substances to deal with painful feelings, instead of learning constructive ways of coping with the difficult emotions that we all experience. And finally, children diagnosed with ADHD are often told they have a chemical imbalance which requires them to take prescription drugs to correct that imbalance. How big a step is it from there to using tobacco or street drugs in an effort to accomplish the same goal?

The year after Drs. Lambert and Hartsough published their results, a study by Joseph Biederman and Steven Faraone and some of their colleagues appeared to contradict these findings.[430] The Biederman group compared the rates of substance use disorder among three groups: medicated subjects with ADHD, unmedicated subjects with ADHD, and unmedicated controls. The researchers reported that the rate of substance use disorder was a staggering eighty-five percent lower in medicated subjects than in their unmedicated counterparts.

That may seem like an impressive finding, but several points need to be kept in mind. First, compared to the sample size used in the Lambert study, that of the Biederman group study was tiny—fifty-six medicated ADHD subjects and just nineteen unmedicated ones.[431] Second, the medicated and unmedicated ADHD groups were not comparable. Seven out of nineteen unmedicated subjects had a substance use disorder at baseline, whereas none of the medicated ones did.[432]

Finally, the impressive odds ratio of more than six to one reported by the Biederman group was achieved only after "adjusting" for co-morbid conduct disorder,[433] which is an acknowledged risk factor for substance use disorder.[434] Estimates of the proportion of ADHD kids with co-morbid conduct disorder range from thirty-five percent to sixty percent.[435]

A 2003 meta-analysis by the Biederman group also concluded that medicating kids for ADHD reduced the risk of substance use disorder, although this time the odds ratio was two to one, not six to one.[436] Moreover, when we look at the six studies included in the meta-analysis, the largest odds ratio by far was that reported by the Biederman group's 1999 study. The second-largest was that of the MTA study at the fourteen-month follow-up—and that study later found no long-term effect of medication on the rate of substance use disorder (vide infra).

What about the remaining four studies? Two of them, including the Lambert study, reported negative results—i.e., that medicated subjects had higher rates of substance use disorder than medicated ones. One found a small protective effect of medication, with an odds ratio of 1.1. And the remaining one was not a peer-reviewed paper but rather a poster presented at the Ninth Annual European Congress of Psychiatry.[437]

Meanwhile, like Gretchen LeFever, Dr. Lambert found herself a pariah in the scientific community. The National Institute of Drug Abuse refused to fund her efforts either to perform further follow-up studies or to conduct a more thorough analysis of the data she already had collected.

No major journal would publish either her new results or a re-analysis of her old research in order to enable her to reply to her critics.[438]

Unlike Dr. Watson, Dr. Lambert never had the chance to get her career back on track. On 26 April 2006, at the age of seventy-nine, she was killed in a car crash.[439]

The following year the data from the thirty-six-month follow-up from the MTA study were published. Unlike the Biederman group study, this study had not excluded children with co-morbidities such as conduct disorder—and the results showed no effect of initial treatment group assignment on subsequent substance use disorder.[440]

The year after that, the Biederman group published the ten-year follow-up results of their study of the effect of stimulant medication on substance use disorder.[441] In contrast to the promising results they reported more than a decade before, this time they found no effect of stimulant medication on the development of substance use disorder.

Dr. Biederman and his co-authors concluded:

> *The results in the present study converge with previous studies toward helping alleviate concerns among clinicians about future substance use disorder problems when prescribing stimulants to children with ADHD.*[442]

But not finding an effect is setting the bar pretty low. Isn't the whole point of giving these drugs to kids to make them better?

And even these unimpressive findings were achieved only after "correcting" for conduct disorder. So what Biederman and his colleagues were saying, in effect, was that drugging kids with stimulants has no effect on the likelihood of their subsequently developing a substance use disorder—provided you don't look at the kids who are most at risk for substance use disorder.

In fairness, it ought to be pointed out that the Lambert study was a naturalistic study, not a randomized controlled trial—but then again, neither were most of the others. The MTA study was, but that one was confounded by the fact that some of the children in the two medication-free arms were prescribed ADHD meds after the randomization phase ended. Would a closer analysis, comparing continuously-medicated subjects with never-medicated ones, have found a relationship between ADHD meds and substance use disorder? The study authors don't seem interested in finding out.

So let's get back to the original question: does drugging kids diagnosed with ADHD increase the likelihood of subsequent substance use disorder? Common sense, which deserves deference until the facts prove otherwise, tell us that plying children with dangerous and highly addictive drugs might increase the likelihood of drug addiction in some of them. Certainly Dr. Lambert's expansive long-term study showed that it did, and no one has ever debunked her methods or data, even though the ADHD industry would seem to have an enormous vested interested in doing so. The strongest evidence to the contrary comes from Dr. Biederman and his colleagues, many of whom have received massive infusions of cash from the manufacturers of these dangerous and highly addictive drugs[443]—and remember they stacked the deck by excluding kids with a concurrent diagnosis of conduct disorder from their analysis. Finally, no one who is in a position to do so seems interested in performing the definitive study—and that in and of itself may tell us something.

CHAPTER ELEVEN

IS ADHD A DISEASE?

Is ADHD a disease?

That all depends on what we mean by the word "disease." The *Oxford English Dictionary* offers this definition:

> *A condition of the body, or of some part or organ of the body, in which its functions are disturbed or deranged; a morbid physical condition; a departure from the state of health, especially when caused by structural change.*

The essential part of this definition is "a condition of the body," which implies something that can be measured, such as blood glucose levels in the case of diabetes—a point tacitly acknowledged by psychiatrists and other medical professionals when they compare (as we have repeatedly seen) ADHD meds to insulin.

But no one is claiming that ADHD is caused by a deficiency of Adderall. Have scientists demonstrated any kind of measurable biological lesion that causes ADHD? They certainly have tried. There are two categories of relevant studies here: neuroimaging studies and genetics studies.

Let's take a look at each of these in turn.

Neuroimaging Studies

Surprising Findings

In 1978, a group of Swedish researchers used the newly developed technology of computerized tomography to scan the brains of forty-six children referred to a clinic for suspected "minimal brain damage."[444] Fifteen of these children exhibited measurable brain anomalies of one form or another.

There was no control group, so we have no way of knowing the proportion of typically-developing children who have similar anomalies. Furthermore, for two-thirds of the MBD children, the researchers were not able to find any brain abnormality at all. Nevertheless, the authors concluded "It may be of some comfort to the parents and others to know that brain damage is the primary cause of the disturbance and not, for example, social or environmental factors."[445]

They never considered the possibility that attributing these children's problems to "brain damage" (despite the complete lack of evidence of brain damage in the majority of cases) might be a preposterous distraction from focusing on the social and environmental roots of these children's problems —which unlike brain damage, can be undone or mitigated.

Since then a mountain of data has failed to demonstrate any anomaly of brain structure or function that reliably distinguishes patients diagnosed with ADHD from those who are not—a point that has been repeatedly emphasized in the scientific literature:

> *"Computed tomography of the brain does not appear to be a necessary screening procedure in the evaluation of the child with minimal brain damage and learning disabilities. Most children evaluated with computed tomography can be expected to have normal scans."[446]*

"If anatomic abnormalities are present in ADD, they are not discernible using present-day CT technology."[447]

"No evidence of structural damage in the brains of children with hyperactivity has yet appeared."[448]

"There is no evidence at present to support psychological testing, laboratory measures of attention, electroencephalography, or neuroimaging studies in the clinical assessment of attention deficit hyperactivity disorders."[449]

"No specific abnormality in brain structure or function has been convincingly demonstrated by neuroimaging studies."[450]

"MRI is not currently diagnostically useful in the routine assessment or management of ADHD."[451]

That last quote was from a 2001 review article by psychiatrist F.X. Castellanos and his colleagues at the National Institute of Mental Health on neuroimaging studies of ADHD. The studies reviewed had reported a dizzying variety of anomalies of brain structure and function said to correlate with a diagnosis of ADHD, but most of the sample sizes were small—which is especially problematic given the high degree of variability in brain structure even in typically-developing subjects. Moreover, all of these differences were quantitative rather than qualitative—that is to say, no abnormality of brain structure and function had ever been shown to distinguish children with a diagnosis of ADHD from those who had no such label.

Even if such an abnormality ever be discovered, it would be an open question as to whether that anomaly was the cause of ADHD. We know that experience changes the brain—indeed, that is the whole point of having a brain. Any commonalities between the brains of children labeled ADHD might reflect common experiences associated with that label.

Moreover, as Dr. Castellanos and his co-authors themselves pointed out, most of the studies have not adequately controlled for drug effects[452]—even though, again, there is overwhelming evidence that psychotropic drugs cause measurable structural and/or functional changes in the brain. How could it be otherwise? If a drug did not have an effect on the brain, it would not be considered "psychotropic."

In order to fill this gap in knowledge, Dr. Castellanos and his co-workers published a paper in the October 2002 issue of *JAMA* describing the results of a ten-year study conducted at the NIMH of 152 children diagnosed with ADHD, including forty-nine never-medicated kids and 139 controls.[453] The researchers found that the brains of children diagnosed with ADHD were smaller than those of typically-developing kids. But perhaps the most surprising finding was that the unmedicated children had significantly smaller white matter volumes compared to both the controls and the medicated ADHD subjects.

None of these differences was diagnostic, and there was considerable overlap between the data sets. Nevertheless, these findings were greeted enthusiastically by the popular media. The headline in the *New York Times* proclaimed "Brain Size Tied to Attention Deficit Hyperactivity Disorder."[454] *Education Week* informed readers "ADHD Drugs Unrelated to Smaller Brain Sizes,"[455] while the *Detroit News* gushed "Ritalin is safe—and it works: Research dispels fears that drug hurts kids, and finds that it actually helps brains grow."[456]

There was just one problem: the unmedicated ADHD kids in the NIMH study were on average more than two years younger than the medicated ones,[457] and presumably shorter and lighter. Both brain size and white matter volume are known to correlate with age, so it's not surprising that both of these were smaller in the undrugged kids.

Dr. Castellanos and his colleagues claim to have controlled for that confounder by means of a secondary analysis of twenty-four unmedicated patients with ADHD, fifty medicated patients, and fifty-four unmedicated controls, and they reported that "all measures remained essentially unchanged."[458] But since the authors don't give us any details about this secondary analysis, we just have to take their word for it.

The following year, the Castellanos paper was the subject of a withering review[459] by psychiatrist Jonathan Leo and David Cohen, a Professor of Social Work at Florida Atlantic University, who asked:

> *Why is the control group two years older, taller, and heavier than the group of unmedicated patients? It seems odd that, given ten years and the resources of the NIMH, these experienced researchers could not have found a more appropriate control group.[460]*

Drs. Leo and Cohen also re-reviewed the brain imaging studies cited in the 2001 review paper by the Castellanos group. Of thirty-three studies, twelve did not report the medication history of the subjects. Of the remaining ones, in eleven of them all of the subjects had a prior history of ADHD medication treatment, while in seven more a majority of them had. Only two of the studies had been conducted on undrugged patients.[461]

A 2013 review paper[462] by Dr. Castellanos and a colleague concluded:

> *Based primarily on lesion studies in animals and humans, the imaging community initially embraced a prefrontal-striatal model of ADHD which expanded to include cerebellar involvement… This model has been largely supported by an ever-increasing number of structural and functional imaging studies.[463]*

The paper made no mention of the potential confounding role of drug effects.

Big Data

Meanwhile, a group of scientists, including Dr. Castellanos, formed the ADHD-200 Consortium to coordinate efforts to find the still-elusive biomarkers for ADHD. On 1 March 2011, they released a large-scale database consisting of 776 fMRI scans collected at eight independent imaging sites, along with phenotypic information including ADHD diagnostic status, ADHD symptom measures, age, sex, IQ, handedness, and medication history. They held a competition, inviting researchers to use the data from brain scans along with the phenotypic data to construct an algorithm that could be used to distinguish kids diagnosed with ADHD with typically-developing kids. This algorithm would then be tested against an additional 197 datasets which were released without providing ADHD diagnostic status.[464]

The winners were a team from the Johns Hopkins Medical Institutions, who devised an algorithm which was accurate sixty percent of the time.[465] For calibration, they could have achieved fifty-five percent accuracy by just guessing "typically-developing" one hundred percent of the time.[466] Moreover, the algorithm correctly diagnosed only twenty-one percent of the ADHD kids.[467]

Another team from the University of Alberta ignored the brain scan data entirely and formulated an algorithm using only the phenotypic data. While this was inconsistent with contest rules, the algorithm they submitted had an accuracy rate of sixty-two percent—surpassing that of the one created by the Hopkins team.[468] This suggests that any commonalities in brain activity of the ADHD kids may be just correlates of the phenotypic variables—age, sex, and so forth—which are known to correlate with ADHD, rather than manifestations of some disease process.

But rather than conclude that this is not a profitable line of inquiry, the ADHD-200 Consortium researchers wound up by calling for more funding for even larger studies.[469]

Bigger Data

On 15 February 2017 *Lancet Psychiatry* published the results of a "mega-analysis" conducted by the ENIGMA ADHD Working Group of brain scans of 3,242 individuals, including 1,713 persons diagnosed with ADHD and 1,529 controls.[470] This was the largest such analysis ever conducted, and the researchers found that overall brain volume, as well as the volume of several specific brain regions, was smaller in subjects diagnosed with ADHD than those who were not.

The paper's eighty-two authors concluded:

> *Data from our highly powered analysis confirms that patients with ADHD do have altered brains and that ADHD is a disorder of the brain. This message is clear for clinicians to convey to parents and to patients, which can help to reduce the stigma that ADHD is just a label for difficult children and caused by incompetent parenting.*[471]

This message was dutifully picked up by the mainstream media. *Newsweek* told its readers "Study Finds Brains of ADHD Sufferers Are Smaller."[472] CNN reported "People diagnosed with attention deficit hyperactivity disorder have smaller brain volume than those without the disorder."[473] Other outlets quickly followed suit:

> *"ADHD is a brain disorder, not a label for poor parenting."*[474]

> *"Children with ADHD have some smaller brain regions, study shows."*[475]

> *"These findings revealed that those with ADHD had smaller brain volume compared to people without ADHD."*[476]

The *Lancet Psychiatry* study was the target of a withering broadside by author Robert Whitaker in his Mad in America blog, co-authored by educational psychologist Michael Corrigan.[477] Whitaker and Dr. Corrigan noted the differences between the ADHD subjects and controls were not categorical differences, but rather were average differences—and tiny ones, at that. There was a more than ninety-two percent overlap in brain size between the ADHD subjects and the controls.

In plain English, nearly half the ADHD subjects had larger-than-average brain sizes. Nearly half of the control subjects had smaller-than-average brain sizes. And this relationship was true not just for overall brain size, but for every one of the brain structures the researchers looked at. The study produced no findings that could be used to distinguish the brain of a person diagnosed with ADHD from that of someone who was not.

In fairness, the CNN article did acknowledge this point—although that admission was buried in paragraph number thirty-seven. None of the other laudatory news stories mentioned the matter at all. Indeed, the article in *Newsweek* featured an impressive color photograph of sections of plastinated brains on display at the Plastinarium in Guben, Germany. The article never actually said that doctors can diagnose ADHD by looking at a patient's brain, but it's hard to imagine why they included that particular picture if they did not wish to leave their readers with that impression. This kind of mendacity is quite common in news stories about ADHD and other "mental illnesses."

The authors of the *Lancet Psychiatry* paper found no clinically significant differences whatsoever between the brains of subjects diagnosed with ADHD and those who were not, although they did find some statistically significant differences. What could be the cause of those differences? Could it be a drug effect? The researchers themselves flatly ruled out that possibility, stating "The brain differences we have reported are not caused by medication effects."[478]

The researchers did not find proof of a drug effect—but they don't seem to have looked very hard. All they did was compare those who had taken ADHD meds for at least four weeks with those who had never taken them. In other words, people who took the drugs for just four weeks were lumped in with those who had taken them for years and years—a tactic guaranteed to blur any drug effect. Would a more fine-grained level of analysis, looking for a dose-dependent relationship, have found something? The study authors don't seem interested in finding out.

Whitaker and Dr. Corrigan started a petition demanding that the paper be retracted. The petition garnered over 800 signatures, but to this day *Lancet Psychiatry* has refused to do so.

A Distributed Network-Based Pathology

On 18 February 2019, the journal *Neuroscience and Biobehavioral Reviews* published a meta-analysis titled "Brain Alterations in Children/Adolescents with ADHD Revisited: A Neuroimaging Meta-Analysis of 96 Structural and Functional Studies." The authors of the meta-analysis concluded:

> *To the best of our knowledge, this study is the largest meta-analysis of structural and functional neuroimaging experiments in children/adolescents with ADHD. We found **no significant convergence** across structural and functional regional alterations in ADHD, which might be attributable to clinical heterogeneity, experimental and analytical flexibility and positive publication bias, but could also point towards a more distributed, network-based pathology lacking a consistent expression at any particular location. (Emphasis added.)*

The possibility that "ADHD" is not even a coherent diagnostic category was not considered. At this point, the existence of an underlying brain pathology seems more an article of faith than a testable hypothesis.[479]

Genetics Studies

Nobody's Fault

Is ADHD genetic?

Perhaps a better question would be "What difference would it make if it were?" If it ever be demonstrated unequivocally that ADHD was a genetically-based condition, it still would not follow logically that it was more tractable to drug treatment rather than to social or psychological interventions.

But it seems safe to say most people would tend to assume so. In a 2012 talk, psychologist Russell Barkley told listeners "ADHD is due to neurogenetic deficits, and that means that medication is absolutely justifiable."[480]

This type of thinking goes back a long way. In a 1996 commentary, psychologist Steven Faraone, one of the world's leading experts on ADHD genetics and a member of the Biederman group, advised that telling parents that ADHD is a genetically-based disorder is a good way to get them to give their kids the drugs:

> *Many parents are reluctant for their children to take psychotropic medication and others find it difficult to maintain the prescribed regimen. Many parents hold naïve beliefs about the etiology of their children's problems; they are quick to attribute them to life circumstances, events in the past, or parental inadequacies... For many psychiatric disorders, genetic data provide the quickest and most convincing means of showing patients how biology plays a role in their condition.[481]*

This idea was expanded to book length by Harold S. Koplewicz, a Professor of Psychiatry at New York University and author of *It's Nobody's Fault: New Hope and Help for Difficult Children*.[482] Dr. Koplewicz begins by heaping scorn on those benighted souls who still believe that a child's problems have anything to do with the actions of his parents:

> *The fact is, when a child has a brain disorder, it is not the parents' fault. A brain disorder is the result of what I call 'DNA Roulette.' In the same way a child comes into the world with a tendency to go gray in his twenties, or like Kenny, beautiful hazel eyes and deep dimples, a child is born with a brain that functions in a particular way because of its chemical composition... **It is brain chemistry***

that is responsible for brain disorders, not bad parenting.[483] *(Emphasis in the original.)*

Dr. Koplewicz goes on to explain:

If bad parenting is what is causing a child's disease, it stands to reason that good parenting can make it better. Unfortunately, that's not how it works. Parents don't cause the disorders, and they can't cure them either.[484]

No doubt that kind of statement is a siren song in a society which has sadly undermined parental authority to the point where many parents feel like their children's frazzled servants. It is also a formulation that effectively slams the door on any serious inquiry into the social and psychological roots of children's problems.

So what is the cause of these children's distress? Dr. Koplewicz sets his readers straight on that point, too:

ADHD has nothing to do with diet or bad parenting.[485]

ADHD is a disorder of the brain.[486]

Neuroimaging techniques—especially magnetic resonance imaging (MRI), positron emission tomography (PET) scans, and single photon emission computer tomography (SPECT)—have demonstrated that children with ADHD have brains that are different from the brains of kids that don't have it.[487]

Fortunately, Dr. Koplewicz and his colleagues stand by, ready to help:

There are more than 200 studies showing that a stimulant called Ritalin (generic name: methylphenidate) works wonders for children with ADHD.[488]

At this point the reader may be wondering if we are setting up the child for a lifetime of failure by saddling him with the idea that he was born with a broken brain that requires long-term treatment with powerful stimulant drugs. This fear is not shared by Dr. Koplewicz, who regales his readers with the tale of Ned, who was "having a terrible time in school." His academic performance was poor, his teacher was complaining about his behavior, none of the other kids wanted to play with him, and even his own parents didn't like having him around.[489]

But all that changed, thanks to Dr. Koplewicz. After young Ned began taking his prescribed forty milligrams of Ritalin a day, his grades were now "terrific," he had lots of friends, and his parents found him a joy to be with. To express his gratitude, Ned invited Koplewicz to his elementary school graduation where the boy was awarded the prize for the best science project. Afterwards, he introduced the good doctor to his grandparents thusly: "This is Dr. Koplewicz. He's my ... my friend."[490]

Are these results typical? Dr. Koplewicz never explicitly says so, but he certainly does nothing to disabuse his readers of this notion.

The book is chock-full of heartwarming little tales like this one. Apparently none of Dr. Koplewicz's patients ever suffers from mania, tics, akathisia, or any of the myriad other toxic effects psychiatric drugs have been shown to exert on developing brains.

In fairness to Dr. Koplewicz, the book isn't just about drugs. He does leaven his work with some child-rearing advice, which seems to center mainly on giving children gold stars for good behavior.[491] (Does anyone really want a kid who is such a sap he can be manipulated by giving or withholding gold stars? It's a measure of how beleaguered some parents today feel that the answer is probably Yes.)

Dr. Koplewicz was one of twenty-two notional authors of SmithKline Beecham's notorious Study 329 of Paxil published in the *Journal of the American Academy of Child and Adolescent Psychiatry*, which reported that the drug was safe and effective for treating major depression in adolescents, even though their own data showed no difference between Paxil and placebo for any of the eight original outcome variables, and that one out of eight youths given the drug suffered from suicidality or self-harming behavior. In plain English, the stuff was totally ineffective and drove the kids crazy to boot.[492] So the sincerity of his professed concern for "difficult children" like Ned may be open to question. But never mind that for now.

The question is: is ADHD a really a genetically-based condition? A 1992 paper by Drs. Faraone and Biederman and several of their colleagues claimed to demonstrate that ADHD is caused by a single co-dominant gene with a low rate of penetrance.[493] No one today, including Faraone and Biederman, believe this. A 2019 review article on the genetics of ADHD by Faraone and another colleague did not even mention the 1992 paper.[494]

Today, psychiatrics genetics experts conceptualize of ADHD as a polygenic disorder, affected by numerous genes, each contributing a tiny bit to one's risk of developing this condition. The psychiatric literature is replete with statements to the effect that "ADHD is seventy percent [or eighty percent, or ninety percent] inherited."[495] But what does it even mean to say that?

"Heritability" means the proportion of population variance in a trait due to genetic variability, as opposed to environmental variability. The concept of heritability was invented by the geneticist Sewall Wright to give agricultural scientists a way to predict the results of controlled breeding experiments on plants and animals on factory farms. But it is an open question as to whether the concept even means anything when applied to human beings.

The figure of ADHD having a heritability of seventy percent (or eighty percent, or ninety percent) comes from family studies, twin studies, and adoption studies. But the same kinds of studies have "proven" that pellagra, tuberculosis, and "hysteria" are also hereditary disorders, so a bit of skepticism seems in order here. Elsewhere I have argued that all of these studies are fatally flawed, in ways that cannot be fixed, and none of them adequately control for environmental variability.[496]

Granted, this is a minority view, but new science of molecular genetics seems poised to put an end to this controversy once and for all. In 1998, clinical psychologist Russell Barkley boldly stated "The day is not far off when genetic testing for ADHD may become available and more specialized medications may be designed to counter the specific genetic defects of the children who suffer from it."[497] How have promises like this worked out for us in real life?

There are two categories of molecular genetics studies we are interested in: copy-number variant studies and genome-wide association studies.[498] Let's take a look at each of these in turn.

Copy-Number Variant Studies

In October of 2010, the *Lancet* published the results of a study of rare large copy number variants said to be associated with ADHD.[499] The term copy number variants (CNV's) refers to repeated sequences of DNA in which the number of copies varies between individuals. The researchers scanned the genomes of 366 children diagnosed with ADHD and 1,047 controls, and found the number of large CNV's (i.e., more than 500 kb in length) was significantly greater in the ADHD kids than in the controls.

Some of these CNV's had previously been found to be associated with schizophrenia and autism as well—which seems to contradict the notion that these conditions are properly regarded as discrete disorders.

Nevertheless, the paper was greeted enthusiastically by the media. Headlines proclaimed:

> *"ADHD is a genetic condition, study says"*[500]

> *"Hyperactive children may suffer from a genetic disorder, says study"*[501]

"Study finds genetic link to ADHD"[502]

The stories also repeated the comforting "It's nobody's fault" mantra. *The Guardian* proclaimed "Parents of hyperactive children should not be blamed for failing to bring up their offspring properly,"[503] while Reuters informed readers "The research should help dispel myths that ADHD is caused by bad parenting."[504] Such formulations may make troubled children and their parents feel better momentarily—but they also exculpate the rest of us from doing something about crowded underfunded schools and offering meaningful help to exhausted and overextended parents.

What exactly did the researchers find? They found that fourteen percent of the ADHD kids had one or more large CNV's, as opposed to seven percent of the controls.[505] In other words, the vast majority of ADHD kids had no CNV's, while some of the controls did. They certainly did not find any kind of genetic anomaly that could be used to diagnose ADHD.

What's more, the index and control groups were not comparable. Thirty-three of the ADHD kids also suffered from intellectual disability, defined as an IQ below seventy, and the rate of CNV's was much higher in these children (thirty-six percent) than in the rest of the ADHD kids. When these thirty-three children were dropped from the analysis, along with fourteen more for whom IQ data was unavailable, the relationship between CNV's and a diagnosis of ADHD persisted, although it was greatly attenuated.

The researchers didn't have any IQ data for the controls, but presumably it was the same as that of the general population, which by definition is one hundred. Even after the children with intellectual disability were dropped from the analysis, the average IQ of the remaining ADHD kids was only eighty-nine.[506] Low IQ is a well-known risk factor for a diagnosis of ADHD,[507] but the researchers did not adequately control for this, instead engaging in a rhetorical sleight of hand—substituting a categorical variable (presence or absence of intellectual disability) for an incremental one (IQ).

Since then several more such studies have been carried out,[508] without producing any findings of clinical significance. None of the CNV's they have found associated with ADHD are found in any more than a tiny minority of index cases, and many of these can be found in normal controls as well. None of the studies adequately controls for IQ—they usually exclude index cases with IQs below some arbitrary cutoff, but none of them employs a set of controls matched to the ADHD subjects for IQ.

To give the reader an idea of just how tiny these reported correlations are, a 2017 paper in *Genome Medicine*[509] reported found a certain copy-number variant was associated with a diagnosis of ADHD, but the "association" was absurdly small. One out of 250 ADHD subjects had the variant, as opposed to one out of a thousand normal controls. In other words, 99.7% of ADHD subjects did not have the variant.

It seems likely that if these researchers have discovered anything here, it was a correlation between CNV's and low IQ, with the ADHD label coming along for the ride.

Anyone who knows anything about life as it is lived knows that kids vary in the speed at which they learn, and that a child forced to sit through classes run at a pace too rapid for him is likely to stop paying attention and/or start acting out—thereby earning himself a diagnosis of "ADHD." Wouldn't hiring more teachers (to enable more individualized learning opportunities for kids) be preferable to continuing to pour money into this kind of research?

Genome-Wide Association Studies

In genome-wide association studies, entire genomes of large number of individuals are scanned for the presence of single-nucleotide polymorphisms, or SNP's. A typical study might look at hundreds, thousands, or even tens of thousands of index and control subjects, and as many as a million or more SNP's, to find ones that are correlated with the condition of interest. In order to eliminate false positives, levels of significance typically are set at $p = 5 \times 10^{-8}$, corresponding to the customary level of $p = 0.05$, divided by one million. These techniques have enabled researchers to go over the human genome with a fine-toothed comb. And what have the researchers found?

The first GWA studies of ADHD found no DNA variants of genome-wide significance. Even a 2010 meta-analysis of studies failed to find any significant results.[510] But in November of 2018, the journal *Nature Genetics* reported the discovery of the first genome-wide significant risk loci for ADHD.[511] The paper listed seventy-one individual authors along with the ADHD Working Group of the Psychiatric Genetics Consortium, the Early Lifecourse and Genetic Epidemiology Consortium, and the 23andMe Research Team. The researchers sequenced the DNA of 20,183 index subjects and 35,191 controls and found twelve genetic loci correlated with a significantly increased risk of a diagnosis of ADHD.

Once again these findings were greeted with enthusiasm. *The Daily Mail* repeated a familiar trope: "Don't blame the parents. ADHD is in our genes."[512] *The Guardian* declared "The findings could help shed light on the biological mechanisms behind ADHD, potentially aiding the development of new drugs,"[513] while the *Economist* informed readers:

> *These findings will not, therefore, lead directly to genetic tests. What they do do, though, is dispel the idea that ADHD is merely bad behavior, or even a mythical condition. And that, of itself, may help to change attitudes toward children who have it, and towards their parents.[514]*

Again, what exactly did the researchers find? The odds ratios for these "significant risk loci" were on the order of 1.198 or even less, meaning a 19.8 percent increase in risk (or even less). Now, the published estimates for the incidence of ADHD vary wildly, but a meta-analysis by Stephen

Faraone and Joseph Biederman and several of their colleagues came up with a figure of 5.3 percent,[515] so let's go with that. Multiply 5.3 percent by 19.8 percent and you get a figure of 0.0105, or a little over a one in a hundred increase in absolute risk. Can a gene associated with a one in a hundred increase in risk serve as a target for drug development?

The piece in the *Guardian* quoted one of the senior authors of the study, Anders Børglum of Aahus University in Denmark, as follows: "Among all the causes that can lead to ADHD, genetic factors account for between 70% and 80%,"[516] presumably a reference to the figures obtained from family, twin, and adoption studies. Dr. Børglum added that all the loci put together accounted for just one percent of the population-wide increase in risk, and, deploying a theme that has become commonplace in psychiatric genetics, averred that the missing genes must be there, somewhere, still waiting to be found:

> *"Those 12 regions are just representing the tip of the iceberg," he said, noting there were likely thousands more to be discovered.*[517]

The possibility that the figures obtained from family, twin, and adoption studies were wildly inflated was not considered. Nor did the article mention that if "thousands" of genes are somehow involved in the development of ADHD, their individual effect sizes must be orders of magnitude tinier than the already puny figure of one in a hundred, or less. This is stretching the notion of cause and effect into meaninglessness.

These genes are not disease genes, as genes for cystic fibrosis or sickle cell anemia or Huntington's disease are. These are simply part of the normal range of human genetic variation.

What do we mean by "A Gene for…?"

As every high school biology student knows, the laws of genetics were discovered by Gregor Mendel, through his tireless experiments with pea plants. Mendel never defined what he meant by a gene for a given trait—he just used an "I-know-it-when-I-see-it" definition. (Actually, the word "gene" had not even been coined back then—Mendel used the term *anlagen*, but that clearly corresponds to our modern notion of a gene.)

In a 2005 paper,[518] Kenneth Kendler, one of the world's leading experts in psychiatric genetics, proposed the following criteria for identifying a gene for a specific trait:

1) Strength of association: If a pea plant has two copies of the gene for wrinkled seeds, it will produce wrinkled seeds, under any of a wide range of conditions—provided it is able to produce seeds at all. The odds ratio, if you like, is infinity, or at least astronomically large. Dr. Kendler proposed a minimum odds ratio of 100:1 for identifying a gene for a specific trait.

2) Specificity of association: The genes that Mendel worked on had very specific effects: one gene affected seed color but not shape or stem length, while another affected seed shape but not color or stem length.

3) Noncontingency of association: The relationship between the gene and the trait is not dependent on other factors, such as exposure to a particular environment or the presence of other genes.

4) Causal proximity: There must be a direct causal link between the gene and the trait in question.

5) Appropriate level of explanation: The formulation "X is a gene for Y" must address the phenomena in question at the most appropriate level. Dr. Kendler provides a hypothetical example: suppose there were a gene that conferred its owner with perfect pitch. Such a gene might well predispose its owner to enjoying the music of Mozart. Would it be appropriate to call this "a gene for liking Mozart?" Hardly. This

hypothesized gene could just as easily increase the likelihood of one enjoying the music of Hadyn, Beethoven, and Brahms as well. Calling it a gene for perfect pitch is both more parsimonious and has greater explanatory power.

Genes for monogenic disorders such as Huntington's disease, cystic fibrosis, and sickle-cell anemia, pass all five of these tests with flying colors. However, not one of the genes said to be associated with ADHD can pass even one of them. The same is true for the genes associated with any of the other "functional disorders" listed in the *DSM*.

Follow the Money

There is no abnormality of brain structure that can be used to diagnose ADHD.

There is no abnormality of brain function that can be used to diagnose ADHD.

There is no gene for ADHD.

There is no credible evidence that the brains of children labeled "ADHD" are different from those of other children.

So to get back to the original question, "Is ADHD a disease?", it just depends on how you define the word "disease." It certainly is not a disease in terms of having any measurable signs.

And how could there be? There could be any number of reasons why a child is having problems with inattention or hyperactivity—lack of discipline, lack of outdoor free play time, a curriculum that is too challenging, or not challenging enough, hunger, fatigue, a chaotic home life, or any of a large number of untreated medical conditions. How could there be a common gene, or a common neural substrate, underlying all these disparate problems?

One may wonder about the clinical utility of phenomena whose mere existence can be demonstrated only after spending enormous sums of money and generating untold petabytes of data—and sometimes not even then. At what point do we start asking whether we really want to continue pouring more billions into this kind of research? If not now, when?

Jay Joseph is a clinical psychologist who has been writing on the subject of psychiatric genetics for over twenty years. He reviewed the myriad problems with ADHD genetics research in a 2000 paper, and in his reply to a critique of that paper by Drs. Faraone and Biederman he wrote "A gene (or genes) for ADHD will not be discovered because it does not exist."[519] Twenty years later that pronouncement has yet to be refuted.

In a 2009 paper he reiterated that position, adding:

> *Psychiatric geneticists and their supporters instead write optimistically about the great strides they have made, and how ADHD genes will soon be identified. They write as if they were searching for the cure for a deadly disease, or the virus causing an epidemic. But ADHD is simply a grouping of socially disapproved behaviors falsely passed off as a disease, and it is questionable whether finding genes would do anything to 'cure' these behaviours.*[520]

When I asked Dr. Joseph why funding agencies continue to pour money into this kind of research, he replied, "Follow the money."

> *The drug companies promote this kind of research because they earn huge profits selling psychiatric medications. They want these conditions to be thought of as brain disorders, as genetic disorders, to justify the use of their products. The drug companies drive a lot of the research, and the U.S. government also promotes genetic and brain disorder explanations of mental disorders.*
>
> *Researchers are promoted and rewarded for doing genetic and brain research, and not so rewarded for doing environmental research. The system promotes genetic and brain disorder explanations, even though there isn't much evidence in favor of these expla-*

> *nations. And even if there were such evidence, environmental factors would still be important.*

Indeed. Instead of asking "Is ADHD a disease?" perhaps we ought to direct our efforts into building institutions that meet actual human needs, rather than drugging children (and, increasingly, adults) to try to make them fit the needs of institutions. But that's not likely to happen until we confront an interlocking network of players who have a vested interest in promoting the disease model of ADHD.

In the next chapter, we will heed Dr. Joseph's admonition to "follow the money" and take a look at some of these players.

CHAPTER TWELVE

THE MONEY TRAIL

The Key Opinion Leader

Probably no man alive has done more to promote the diagnosis and drugging of children for ADHD—and its bastard offspring, pediatric bipolar disorder—than Joseph Biederman.

Dr. Biederman is Chief of the Clinical and Research Programs in Pediatric Psychopharmacology and Adult ADHD at the Massachusetts General Hospital and Professor of Psychiatry at Harvard Medical School. Once, while being deposed in a lawsuit, he gave his rank at Harvard as "Full Professor." Asked if there was anything above that, he replied "God."

In 2002, Dr. Biederman and his colleague Steven Faraone authored the annual report of the Johnson and Johnson Center for Pediatric Psychopathology at Mass General,[521] which discussed plans to study children diagnosed with conduct disorder and comorbid affective disorder: "Further validation of this group will alert physicians to the existence of a large group of children who might benefit from treatment with RISPERDAL." At the time, J&J was the owner of Janssen, which in turn owned the patent rights to Risperdal.

A June 2007 article in the *Boston Globe* noted that Dr. Biederman had taken payments from fifteen different drug companies, and served as a paid speaker or adviser to seven of them, including Eli Lilly, the maker of Zyprexa, along with Janssen.[522] In the same article, Jerrold Rosenbaum, Chief of Psychiatry at Mass General, absolved Biederman of any blame: "For Joe, it is his idea and mission that drive him, not the fees."[523]

In June of 2008, the *New York Times* revealed that Dr. Biederman had earned $1.6 million in consulting fees from J&J and other drugmakers but did not report much of this income to Harvard.[524] Two of Biederman's associates, Thomas Spencer and Timothy Wilens, had also taken over $1 million each in drug company payments.

In addition, the article revealed that in 2000, Dr. Biederman had received a grant from the National Institutes of Health to study the effect of the drug Strattera in children. That same year, he had received over $14,000 in payments from Eli Lilly, the maker of Strattera. At the time, Harvard rules forbade researchers from conducting clinical trials of any drug if they had received more than $10,000 from the drug's manufacturer.[525]

In an email statement, Biederman declared: "My interests are solely in the advancement of medical treatment through rigorous research and study."[526]

Meanwhile Dr. Spencer offered these words in his own exculpation:

> *I am deeply committed to helping children with ADHD and other similar disorders find treatments that can help improve their lives… It was my sincere belief that I was at all times complying with the relevant policies and procedures as to outside income.*[527]

Mass General sent out a missive to its physicians, expressing profound sympathy for Dr. Biederman and his colleagues Spencer and Wilens: "We know this is an incredibly painful time for these doctors and their families, and our hearts go out to them."[528]

The following January, Marcia Angell, author of *The Truth About the Drug Companies*,[529] offered this devastating assessment of Dr. Biederman in an article in the *New York Review of Books*:

> *Thanks largely to him, children as young as two years old are now being diagnosed with bipolar disorder and treated with a cocktail of powerful drugs, many of which were not approved by the Food and Drug Administration (FDA) for that purpose and none of which were approved for children below ten years of age.[530]*

The same article offered this devastating critique of modern medicine:

> *It is simply no longer possible to believe much of the clinical research that is published, or to rely on the judgement of trusted physicians or authoritative medical guidelines. I take no pleasure in this conclusion, which I reached slowly and reluctantly over my two decades as an editor of the New England Journal of Medicine.[531]*

In July of 2011, Mass General announced sanctions against Dr. Biederman, along with Drs. Spencer and Wilens, for violating disclosure rules. All three men were required to undergo unspecified "training," to refrain from all industry-sponsored outside activities for one year, to obtain permission from Harvard and Mass General before engaging in such activities for two years after that, and to face unspecified delays in being considered for promotion and advancement.[532]

In a joint statement, all three men declared "We always believed that we were complying on good faith with the institutional policies and that our mistakes were honest ones."[533]

Two years later, the United States Department of Justice announced that J&J had been ordered to pay $2.2 billion to resolve criminal and civil claims of illegal marketing of its drugs, including Risperdal.[534] In January of 2018, the Philadelphia Court of Common Pleas found the company liable for eight billion dollars in punitive damages after a young man grew breasts after taking the drug.[535]

None of this seems to have slowed Dr. Biederman down. In 2014 the news and information service Thomson Reuters named Biederman as one of the World's Most Influential Scientific Minds. The website for Mass General boasts of his 800 scientific articles, 650 abstracts, and seventy book chapters.[536] He was ranked second-highest producer of high-impact papers in child psychiatry and highest in total citations to his papers on ADHD.

The website also demurely notes that "Dr. Biederman's work is supported by multiple federal and pharmaceutical industry grants."[537]

The Story of Strattera

The evidence base for FDA approval of the new drugs and new drug indications touted by key opinion leaders is for the most part manufactured and controlled by the drug companies who have a fiduciary duty to their stockholders to sell as many drugs as possible. The results are predictable and well-documented: exaggeration of benefits and downplaying or outright concealment of harms.[538]

Consider the case of Eli Lilly's blockbuster drug Strattera. This drug was initially developed by Lilly as a treatment for incontinence and major depression.[539] However, only one small study, on ten patients diagnosed with major depression, was ever published.[540] All of these patients were given chloral hydrate, a sedative, in addition to Strattera. Three of the ten dropped out of the study, and while the remaining ones did exhibit some improvement in depressive symptoms, further research into using the drug as a treatment for depression was shelved.

Strattera was approved by the FDA for treatment of ADHD in children and adults in November of 2002, and released on to the market the following January.[541] Strattera was the first new chemical entity okayed for the treatment of ADHD since the approval in 1975 of Pemoline[542] (that drug was taken off the market in 2005 after being linked to cases of liver damage).[543] Amphetamine and Ritalin had already been on the market for decades, and we have already seen that grave concerns had been raised about the potential of these drugs for addiction and abuse. By contrast, Strattera was touted as a "non-stimulant" remedy for ADHD.

The month before Strattera was released on to the market, no less a luminary than Dr. Biederman himself, along with several of colleagues, published a paper proclaiming the need for this new drug:

> *There are significant limitations to treatment with psychostimu-lants, which are not effective or well tolerated in approximately 30% of school-age children with ADHD. Adverse effects such as insomnia, decreased appetite, and irritability may lead to discon-tinuation or dosage limitations. The lack of adequate full-day treatment often results in recurrence of impairing symptoms at home and in the community. In addition, psychostimulants bear the additional burden of being controlled substances, resulting in concerns about abuse and diversion. For these reasons, there remains a need for safe, effective, and nonstimulant alternatives for the treatment of ADHD in children and adults.[544]*

The research was funded by Eli Lilly and Company. Seventeen of the authors of the paper had served as paid consultants or investigators for Lilly, and five more were employees and shareholders. Not surprisingly, the study concluded that Strattera was indeed a safe and effective nonstimu-lant remedy for ADHD.

A 2009 book chapter by David Cohen and two of his colleagues noted that at the time Strattera was released, there were a total of eleven published Phase II and Phase III studies on the drug, all of them funded by Lilly, and many of the authors of these studies were Lilly employees.[545] In other words, prescribers consulting the scientific literature would be able to find what Lilly wanted them to know about Strattera, and no more than that.

However, shortly after the drug was released, the FDA published on its website many of the documents submitted by Lilly for its New Drug Application for Strattera. These documents contained some interesting revelations. Dr. Cohen and his co-authors note that while the eleven published ADHD studies reported the rate of serious adverse events as 0.7 percent, the FDA documents show a 2.1 percent rate of serious adverse events for ADHD studies and a whopping 7.1 percent for the discontinued incontinence and major depression studies.[546]

In September of 2004, a letter to the editor of *Pediatrics* reported that of 153 consecutive patients treated for ADHD with Strattera, fifty-one, or one out of three, exhibited extreme irritability, aggression, mania, or hypomania.[547] The authors seemed at a loss as to why so many of these children reacted badly, although as a possible explanation they suggested "incompletely treated ADHD with its attendant impulsivity."

Almost exactly a year later, the FDA issued a black-box warning (the strongest sanction short of removing a drug from the market) for increased risk of suicidal thinking in children and adolescents taking Strattera.[548]

Martin Whitely is a former state legislator in Western Australia and a research fellow at the John Curtin Institute of Public Policy. In his 2021 book *Overprescribing Madness*, he recounted some of the adverse event reports for Strattera submitted to the Adverse Drug Reactions Committee:[549]

- A seven-year-old girl who experienced abdominal pain, nausea, migraine headaches, shooting pains, white spots in her visual field, and academic regression along with fecal and urinary incontinence

- A seven-year-old boy who experienced suicidal ideation, mood changes, extreme aggression, and self-harm

- An eight-year-old boy who banged his head against the wall and said he wanted to kill himself

- A nine-year-old boy who became emotionally withdrawn and exhibited abnormal behavior, drooping eyelids, and strange facial expressions

- A nine-year-old boy who exhibited extreme mood swings, anger, violent outbursts, banged his head against the wall, and said he wanted to kill himself

- A nine-year-old boy who experienced suicidal ideation, aggression, and self-harm, and drew pictures of himself hanging from a tree

- A ten-year-old boy who experienced violent outbursts and suicidal thoughts and threatened suicide

- A ten-year-old boy who experienced nausea, depression, aggressive behavior, and suicidal thoughts

- A ten-year-old boy who experienced psychotic symptoms and began talking about killing himself

- A ten-year-old boy who experienced auditory and visual hallucinations, including voices in his head commanding him to murder his sister

- An eleven-year-old boy who experienced a psychotic episode

- An eleven-year-old boy who experienced headaches, stomach cramps, muscle rigidity, and poor concentration, and attempted suicide

- An eleven-year-old boy who became extremely agitated and talked about wanting to die

- An eleven-year-old boy who became depressed and suicidal

- A twelve-year-old girl who experienced anorexia, weight loss, fidgeting, anger outbursts, and ripped out her own fingernails and toenails

- A twelve-year-old boy who experienced strong suicidal ideation and expressed a desire to hang himself

- A thirteen-year-old boy who experienced hostility, aggression, and chest pains

- A thirteen-year-old boy who became angry, withdrawn, socially isolated, impulsive, moody, exhibited physical and verbal aggression to his family, and experienced suicidal ideation

- A thirteen-year-old boy who experienced agitation, suicidal ideation, and threatened to harm his classmates

- A fourteen-year-old girl who experienced suicidal ideation and cut herself with scissors, knives, and razors

- A fifteen-year-old girl who experienced suicidal ideation and began cutting herself to an extent that was described as "life-threatening"

In 2012, the Therapeutic Goods Administration (the Australian equivalent of the FDA) responded to these distressing reports with alacrity, by ceasing to make individual adverse events reports available to the public.[550]

While Strattera may not have benefitted every child who took it, it certainly has been a boon to Eli Lilly's bottom line. Within six months of its release, over one million prescriptions were written for the drug, and market share rose from zero to 12.3 percent.[551] For the year 2016, the drug's last year on-patent, total sales were $535 million in the United States and $854 million worldwide.[552]

The Ghost Writer

The pharmaceutical industry relies on the services of medical writers in order to spin the results of their studies to make their products look as good as possible. These professionals are known colloquially as "ghost writers."

In August of 2011, an essay appeared in *PLoS Medicine* by one self-described "ghost writer," Linda Logdberg.[553] Having earned a PhD in neuroanatomy, Dr. Logdberg found herself unable to secure a tenure-track faculty position, and she decided to seek employment as a medical writer instead.

Initially, Dr. Logdberg enjoyed the job. As a mother of young children she appreciated the flexibility of working at home, the work was interesting, she genuinely believed she was helping people, and the money was good—"really good," she remembers:

Traveling, eating in high-end restaurants, wearing fashionable clothes, and rushing to meet important deadlines—what's not to like?

As it turned out, there was a great deal not to like. Initially, the companies she worked for were small stand-alone firms, owned and run by actual scientists. But these companies went out of business and she found herself working for giant corporations owned by large advertising agencies, having to answer to superiors who had no background in science. While working for one such firm, she was ordered to write a paper extolling the virtues of a new extended-release formula of an ADHD drug.

There already were several competing products on the market, and the drugmaker needed some way of distinguishing its product from the others. This nostrum had a duration of action intermediate between those of short-acting and long-acting ADHD drugs.

Living in an ADHD household, Dr. Logdberg did not think this was a great idea. She could not see the value of a drug whose effects would wear off right around suppertime, a time when tempers flared and arguments were often at their worst.

Dr. Logdberg asked for permission to speak to the notional author of the paper. Her boss sneered "Just write it."

Dr. Logdberg got out of the business, and went to work as a teacher for the Fernbank Science Center, giving presentations to kids ranging in age from Kindergarten through Grade Twelve. Almost all the staff members there had PhD's or at least Master's degrees in science. Fernbank is a program of the Dekalb County School District, which serves a student population that is eighty-nine percent minority.

When I asked her how she found the students, she replied without hesitation: "I loved them. They were great. They were fun to teach. They liked learning, and I liked teaching them."

"It's a wonderful model," she says of the Fernbank project. "On a typical day, I could go out and present 'Everybody smells' to kindergartners, and teach them about the sense of smell, and then I could go do three STD classes in the Middle School."

Dr. Logdberg indicated that she is not anti-med. "I believe in medication if it is given intelligently—like any drug." But when I asked her if her time as a public schoolteacher gave her any insight into the problem of ADHD, she did not hesitate before replying:

> *Schoolteachers should be prohibited from having any input whatsoever into ADHD diagnoses. They have no training or background or interest in psychology. Their solution for the hyperactive kids was to turn the desk to face the wall and have the child miss recess.*
>
> *They would ask these teachers to fill out these checklists. So they would fill out the check sheet, and the parent would take the kid to the pediatrician—a person completely unskilled in diagnosing any kind of emotional ailment. That's like going to a gynecologist for a heart disease.*
>
> *I do get that it's hard to be with forty kids in one classroom— and there was not much space. And there was a lot of belief then that if you take too much time out of the day to deal with things like sports, or recess, it will take time away from learning, and then the kids won't score well on the standardized tests.*

Direct-to-Consumer Advertising

The media profits handsomely from direct-to-consumer advertising of prescription drugs. Between 1998 and 2006, annual spending on direct-to-consumer ads rose from $1.3 billion to $5.4 billion.[554] This is potentially a lucrative area for the drugmakers as well—every dollar spent on direct-to-consumer advertising is believed to generate six dollars in sales.[555]

Let's consider the case of Adderall XR, the extended-release version of Adderall, which was released in 2002, the same year that the patent expired on original-formula Adderall. A 2013 article in the *New York Times* by reporter Alan Schwarz[556] and an accompanying video examined a number of print advertisements for ADHD drugs, including Adderall XR.

One of these ads depicted a young boy toting a soccer ball under one arm and an armful of books under the other, while the caption exhorted parents to "reveal his potential." The message is obvious: Adderall XR isn't changing your child, just "revealing" his better self—scholarly, athletic, well-rounded. The photograph of the child is superimposed upon an image of nerve cells, implying that something awfully important and science-y is going on.

Another featured a lad being enthusiastically embraced by his mother. The boy holds a worksheet bearing the notation "B+" in bright red ink, while the caption exclaims "Finally! Schoolwork that matches his intelligence!"

A third showed a youngster frolicking with his mother, both of them sporting smiles as wide as the Grand Canyon, while the accompanying captions read:

> *David's mother is learning a whole new language*
> *I'm proud of you*
> *Do you want to have your friends over on Saturday?*
> *Let's play a game*
> *Thanks for taking out the garbage*

A pill to make your kid take out the garbage? Seriously? Is that what parents want? Again, it's a measure of how beleaguered some parents feel these days that the answer is probably Yes.

The overall message of these ads is clear: these drugs will improve every aspect of your child's life, including grades, extracurricular activities, peer relations, and family life. In fact, as we have seen, there is no credible evidence that any of these drugs leads to any meaningful long-term benefits to kids.

Schwarz's *NYT* article also noted that nearly every major ADHD drug—Adderall, Concerta, Focalin, Vyvanse, Intuniv, and Strattera—had been touted in ads which resulted in its manufacturer being cited by the FDA for false or misleading advertising, some of them multiple times.[557] But the FDA's efforts in this area may be akin to trying to hold back the wind with a fishnet. For the fiscal year 2009, the FDA had only fifty-nine employees charged with reviewing over 70,000 advertisements submitted to the agency by the drug companies.[558]

Whether these ads have helped parents become better-informed consumers of Shire's patent medicines is an open question, but they certainly don't seem to have diminished that company's revenues. Between 2002 and 2008 (the last full year Adderall XR remained on-patent), sales receipts for Shire's blockbuster drug skyrocketed from less than \$2 billion to over \$8 billion.[559] By the time the patent expired on Adderall XR, Shire's new blockbuster-to-be, Vyvanse, had already been released.

In the previous chapter we saw how time and again the news media have spurned their role as watchdogs to serve as cheerleaders for the latest discovery "proving" the biological basis of ADHD—even though none of these claims has ever held up. Could this lack of serious scrutiny be due to their dependence on drug company largesse to stay in business in a time of falling ad revenues?[560]

A Perverse Set of Incentives

It's not just doctors, drug companies, and the news media who have profited from skyrocketing rates of diagnosis and drugging for ADHD. The law has created a perverse set of incentives for parents and children which favor the ADHD label.

The key piece of legislation which brought this about was the Individuals with Disabilities Education Act (IDEA) of 1990, which mandates special services for children with disabilities.[561] Under the provisions of that act, a child thought to be disabled is entitled to an evaluation and, if deemed necessary, access to special educational services according to an Individualized Education Plan (IEP) tailored to meet the needs of that child.

Originally ADHD was not a covered disability under IDEA, although children so labeled might have been deemed eligible for special services according to any of several other categories covered in the act, such as "other health impairment," "serious emotional disturbance," or "specific learning disability." But in September of 1991, the United States Department of Education issued a "Policy Clarification Memorandum" which specifically included ADHD in the list of covered disabilities.[562]

Now children "disabled" by ADHD could be eligible for any of a variety of special privileges, including reduced class size, one-on-one tutorials, classroom aides and note-takers, tape recorders, and the use of "high-interest" materials.[563] (Why does a student need a psychiatric diagnosis in order to be provided with "high-interest" materials? Shouldn't they all be getting that?) No wonder that enrollment in special education programs skyrocketed in the years following the Policy Clarification Memorandum.[564]

A similar pattern was seen in the United Kingdom, where the number of children diagnosed with special needs rose more than fifty percent from 1995 to 2010, from 12.5% to 20% of schoolchildren.[565] (That twenty percent figure refers to all special needs kids, not just the ones labeled "ADHD.")

During the same period, the proportion of children being drugged for ADHD rose a staggering thirty-three-fold, from 1.5 per 10,000 to 49.9 per 10,000.[566]

Any child—with or without the ADHD label—could probably benefit from any or all of the perks that come with that label. As psychiatrist Lawrence Diller (who is by no means anti-med) points out in his book *Running on Ritalin*,[567] this process has cascading effects. The more money schools spend on special education, the less they have to spend on all of the other students, resulting in overcrowded classrooms, stressed-out teachers, etc. These are precisely the sorts of problems which are guaranteed to push marginal students over the edge into failure—resulting in more students being diagnosed as "ADHD" or "learning disabled," more resources devoted to special education, and so on.

So just how much are we spending to provide extra services to children with the ADHD label? Here's the astonishing answer: nobody knows. A 2015 report prepared by the Education Commission of the States stated:

> *As hard as it may be to believe, there is little information about how much funding school districts in the U.S. are expending on the education of students with disabilities. Most states don't require districts to report their special education expenditures, and those states that do require reporting from districts tend not to require that they provide detailed financial information.*[568]

The report goes on to note that the most recent attempt to tally up the total dates all the way back to the school year 1999-2000, and found that per-pupil spending for general education students was $6,556, while for special education that figure was $12,474—almost twice as much.[569] (Again, the $12,474 figure is for all special education students, not just the ones labeled "ADHD.")

On the other side of the pond, a 2017 report in *Schools Week* noted that the number of special needs pupils sent to private schools in the UK had tripled in just the past six years, at an average annual cost of £52,000 per student (and as high as £129,000 in one county), as opposed to the average annual cost of £20,000 to educate the same special-needs student at state school.[570]

There's more. Here in the USA, families of children labeled ADHD may also be eligible for Supplemental Security Income (SSI) payments. Just two years after the SSI law was changed in 1990 by adding ADHD to the list of eligible diagnoses, the number of new enrollees with the ADHD label increased more than five-fold.[571] (At this point, the reader may recall Carolyn and Michael Riley's efforts to obtain disability payments for their daughter Rebecca, after already procuring them for their other children.)

In addition, students labeled disabled may also be shielded from the consequences of their own misbehavior. Under IDEA, a school could not suspend a "disabled" student for more than ten days, for any reason. Moreover, the courts had ruled that repeated suspensions could be interpreted as evidence of a pattern of discrimination directed at the child.[572] The burden of proof was placed on the school to demonstrate that a student's anti-social behavior was not the result of his "handicap."

In 1997, Congress amended this obviously unworkable rule to allow an emergency forty-five-day suspension of any student for possessing a gun, or bringing drugs to school.[573] The irony of this latter proviso apparently was lost on these Solons.

How has this worked out for us? An August 1997 article in the *New Republic* titled "Defining Disability Down"[574] told the tale of Michael F., a ninth-grader who was earning A's in his honors courses. He also found time to play in his high school band, had written a book, and had successfully completed his bar mitzvah training—all the while battling the scourges of "attention-deficit disorder, language-based specific learning disabilities, neuro-motor dysfunction, and tactile sensitivity." Fortunately, Michael enjoyed the saving graces of an IEP which afforded him special tutoring; extra time on homework, assignments, and tests; permission to stand up, stretch, and/or walk around in class; permission to chew gum or hard candy "to help him concentrate and focus"; access to transcripts of lectures, outlines, and notes; as well as a tape recorder and a laptop computer (this was before such devices became ubiquitous).

But Michael's parents became dissatisfied with the miserly provisions of their son's IEP and demanded more. After their boy received a grade of 65 on his Honors Geometry midterm exam, they excoriated school officials for numerous procedural failings, including neglecting to pursue a math reevaluation of their son, and demanded extended summer tutoring for him in that subject.[575]

One can only wonder what Sabrina Green might have thought had she learned about Michael's plight.[576]

More recently, in September of 2009 a federal judge ordered Williamson County Schools in Tennessee to pay for legal fees incurred by the family of Chase Kildgore in their three-year legal battle with the school district. Young Chase was diagnosed with ADHD in May of 2003, prior to entering the seventh grade. School officials decided the boy was not eligible for special education services but devised an education plan for him, allowing him extra time on homework and tests, organizational help, and "incentives" for completing assignments.

Things got complicated when Chase got into a fight at school. After meeting with the boy's doctor, father, teachers, and counselors, school officials determined the fight was not caused by his ADHD (how such a thing is determined was not explained) and suspended him for twenty days. The punishment was later dropped to ten days of in-school suspension.

Chase's father demanded that the fight be expunged from the boy's disciplinary record, and also that the school district provide his son with three hours a week of tutoring. After an administrative law judge ruled in his favor, the district appealed the ruling to District Court but lost and was ordered to pay the family's lawyers $135,859. An article in the *Tennessean*[577] reported that two more lawsuits were pending against Williamson County Schools, and also that 3,776 children, or thirteen percent of the total student population, were enrolled in special education programs in the school district, at an annual cost of $36.5 million. By then Chase had moved on, and was enrolled as a student at the University of Tennessee.

While IDEA mandates that children labeled "special needs" are entitled to a free "appropriate" public education in the "least restrictive setting," there is no such mandate for children who are not so labeled, and whose parents are faced with the choice of accepting whatever is on offer at the local public school system or nothing at all. And acquiring such a label for one's child is a process that can require time, energy, knowledge and money—requirements guaranteed to stack the deck against the poor and uneducated. It's no wonder the probability of a diagnosis of ADHD correlates positively with income and negatively with racial minority status.[578]

Moreover, many wealthy educated parents no longer see special education as a stigma or a trap, and are willing to spend five- and six-figure sums on legal fees to obtain the special treatment for their children that goes with the disability label.[579] A December 2007 article in the *New York Times* noted that the previous year, the city of New York spent $57 million to provide private education for children so labeled.[580] The city was deluged with so many lawsuits it assembled a unit of ten lawyers to fight these cases, presumably including the one filed by former Viacom CEO Tom Freston, who demanded the city pay for private education for his "learning-disabled" son.

The year before this, Freston had been fired by Viacom, with a $100.8 million golden parachute to cushion his fall from grace.[581]

In her book *We've Got Issues*, author Judith Warner details the struggle of one mother, a former government employee who quit her job in order to have more time to lobby to have her child labeled with ADHD and "sensory integration issues." She finally succeeded and was able to enroll him in private school, at the taxpayers' expense, where the boy thrived. The mother asked rhetorically, "How do parents who aren't educated and obnoxious get anything done for their kids?"[582]

How indeed?

Students with the ADHD label may also be eligible for extra time taking the Scholastic Aptitude Test (SAT) as well. A 2019 article in the *Vanderbilt Law Review* subtitled "Affirmative Action for the Elites?" noted some astonishing findings:

> *In prosperous regions such as Beverly Hills and La Jolla, nearly 10 percent of students taking the SATs received extra time; by contrast, of the 1,439 students taking the SATs in inner-city regions including Roosevelt, Garfield, and Inglewood, not a single one received any accommodations.*
>
> *142 high schools in America—43 private schools and 99 public—are responsible for 24 percent of all accommodated test takers, though they comprise considerably less than 1 percent of the nation's high schools.*
>
> *In one school, an incredible 46 percent of all students taking the SATs received accommodations.[583]*

(In fairness, it should be noted these figures refer to students labeled with any kind of "learning disability"—not just ADHD.)

The perks don't stop after graduating from secondary school. Students with the ADHD label may be eligible for extra time to take the Law School Admission Test (LSAT) and even the Medical College Admission Test (MCAT).[584] Unfortunately, no one has yet figured out a way to give all these ADHD-afflicted aspiring docs extra time after they begin the practice of medicine and then find themselves facing a patient who presents to the emergency room with, say, a traumatic brain injury or a cardiac arrest.

Patient Advocacy

As the number of children diagnosed with ADHD soared, so did the membership rolls of Children and Adults with Attention-Deficit Hyperactivity Disorder (CHADD). Founded in 1987, CHADD is far and away the largest "patient advocacy organization" for children and adults with ADHD. According to their 2018 annual report:

> *CHADD improves the lives of people affected by ADHD by providing support, training, education, and advocacy for millions of children and adults in the United States living with ADHD, their families, educators, and healthcare professionals.*[585]

Early in its history, CHADD became embroiled in a controversy when the organization petitioned congress to have Ritalin declassified as a Schedule II drug with a high potential for abuse and addiction. The petition stated that Ritalin is "a beneficial and relatively benign medication which assists millions of children daily" and is not "dangerous and addictive." What the petition did not mention was that CHADD had received nearly $900,000 in contributions from Ciba-Geigy, the manufacturer of Ritalin.

This inconvenient truth was brought to light by the PBS news magazine *The Merrow Report*. In a 1995 op-ed piece in the *New York Times*,[586] reporter John Merrow quoted Ciba-Geigy's director of public information as saying that CHADD is "essentially a conduit for us," adding "We're getting big information out there." The same article quoted Dr. Harvey Parker, one of the co-founders of CHADD, who described the organization as "absolutely independent," adding that they recommend Ritalin "because it works, plain and simple," and that the group did not use any Ciba-Geigy money to lobby for the loosening of restrictions on Ritalin.

Since that episode CHADD has grown into an organization with an annual budget of $2.5 million a year. How much of that comes from the drug companies is not easy to find out—the group's website coquettishly notes that "We rely on many sources of funding to support the activities of the organization," but a comprehensive list of those sources is not provided.

Nevertheless, a dash through that website is instructive. A fact sheet titled "About ADHD" informs readers that "Without identification and proper treatment, ADHD may have serious consequences, including school failure, family stress and disruption, depression, problems with relationships, substance abuse, delinquency, accidental injuries, and job failure."[587] Which of these bad outcomes is reduced by "identification and proper treatment" is never mentioned.

Also, note the author's choice of words: family stress and disruption are consequences of ADHD—not the causes of the complaints that fall under that diagnostic label. The familiar refrain of "It's nobody's fault" rears its head again.

Another fact sheet tells us that "Medication is recognized by the scientific community as the primary treatment to reduce the symptoms of ADHD."[588] As evidence for this pronouncement, the paper cites the MTA Study fourteen-month follow-up—ignoring the eight-year follow-up which found no benefit from medication for any of twenty-four outcome variables. This paper cites other sources from as recently as 2013, so it seems unlikely that the author could have missed the MTA eight-year follow-up, which was published in 2009.

The organization's "Public Policy Agenda for Children and Adolescents" states that "CHADD supports the fact that researchers have an obligation to disclose their sources of funding of their research..."[589] This is an admirable sentiment, but the reader may be forgiven for wondering why the group apparently does not apply this principle to themselves.

Finally, the website boasts of an "ADHD Centers Directory," which provides "contact information for clinics which have specific experience and expertise in diagnosing and treating ADHD..." One of these fonts of expertise is Tufts Medical Center, where little Rebecca Riley was diagnosed and drugged for ADHD.

CHAPTER THIRTEEN

EXPANDING THE MARKET: ADULT ADHD

A Chronic Condition

Originally, the various ill-defined syndromes that later came to be subsumed under the diagnostic umbrella of "ADHD" were assumed to be conditions that children could be expected to grow out of. This theme recurs frequently in the psychiatric literature of the mid-twentieth century:

> *"In later years this syndrome tends to wane spontaneously and disappear."*[590]

> *"Medication may be required only for a brief period, long enough to get a new set of behavior patterns started."*[591]

> *"The 'hyperkinetic behavior syndrome' tends to disappear by adulthood."*[592]

> *"Children with hyperactivity generally manifest their symptoms throughout their elementary school years. From ages 13–15, their hyperactivity begins to lessen."*[593]

> *"In fact, it is usual for the problems to diminish or disappear around the time of puberty."*[594]

But starting in the 1970's, this syndrome began to be seen as a chronic condition requiring lifelong medication. Paul Wender, "The Dean of ADHD," was instrumental in this paradigm shift.

In a 1979 book chapter titled "The Concept of Adult Minimal Brain Dysfunction,"[595] Dr. Wender discussed the difficulties inherent even in defining this syndrome, beginning with this caveat: "There is currently no adequate term for the disorder, and there will be none in the near future,"[596] adding "With regard to signs and symptoms, *I believe* the following constitute the major attributes of the disorder..."[597] (Italics in the original.)

Dr. Wender follows with this list: 1) Attentional deficits, 2) Motor abnormalities, 3) Deficits in impulse control, 4) Altered interpersonal relations, 5) Altered emotional reactivity, and 6) Cognitive abnormalities. The aforementioned may manifest themselves as any or all of the following complaints: hyperactivity, clumsiness, impaired sphincter control, low frustration tolerance, social impulsivity, being too independent, not being independent enough, obstinacy, negativism, stubbornness, imperviousness, hyperreactivity, overexcitability, irritability, hot-temperedness, dysphoria, sadness, low self-esteem, and social transgressions including stealing, lying, fire-setting, sexual acting out, and lawbreaking.[598]

Dr. Wender's description of the category of "cognitive abnormalities" is especially interesting:

> *These include* **hard-to-characterize** *abnormalities in cognition (variously called dyslogia, sometimes identified as concreteness or lack of ability to abstract) and* **a nebulous cluster** *of cognitive—not perceptual—impairments referred to under the phrase 'learning disabilities.'*[599] *(Emphasis added.)*

Dr. Wender goes on to acknowledge that there are no known biological signs underlying the grab-bag of complaints falling under the rubric of minimal brain dysfunction, and then offers this statement in exculpation: "MBD is in no more parlous shape than any other psychiatric syndrome."[600] No argument there.

In a series of papers, Dr. Wender and his colleagues reported success in short-term trials in treating adults said to be suffering from this ill-defined syndrome with a variety of drugs: pemoline, methylphenidate, tricyclic antidepressants, and monoamine oxidase inhibitors. They found that at least sixty percent of patients exhibited moderate-to-marked improvement on these drugs, as opposed to ten percent of placebo patients.[601]

"Improvement," in this context, meant improvement in the eyes of the treating clinician, not the patient himself, as Dr. Wender and his colleagues made clear:

> *These patients are considerably lacking in 'outsight.' They are unaware of how their symptoms impact on other people and are often non-perceptive to the changes in symptoms that are produced by the medication. Accordingly, they underestimate the effect of medication and frequently discontinue it despite the fact that they may manifest a considerable therapeutic response.*[602]

Out of a Darkness

The first article in the popular media on adult ADHD, titled "Out of a Darkness," ran in the *New York Times* on 11 October 1987.[603] The author, freelance photographer and picture editor Frank Wolkenberg, began the piece by recounting a pivotal moment in his life at the age of thirty as he was lying awake in bed, contemplating suicide.

> *I faced the repetition of an intolerable pattern. Its motif was one of bright hopes that tarnished, quick starts that came to nothing, leaving behind debts, bitterness, and disappointment.*

> *By my late 20's I was no stranger to seemingly inexplicable failures. Some were romantic, others professional, all unnecessary and many inexcusable.*[604]

Some readers might surmise that Wolkenberg suffered from a disease known as "being in your twenties," but that was not how he saw it:

> *The ADD syndrome is generally believed to stem from a dysfunction of genetic origin, most likely from a failure in the system of the brain that fine-tunes attention.*
>
> *Studies such as those being conducted by Dr. Alan Zametkin at the National Institute of Mental Health, using sophisticated new neuro-imaging technology, may soon make it possible to locate where in the brain the dysfunctions occur.*[605]

More than thirty years later, these promises remain entirely unfulfilled. But never mind that for now. Luckily for the author, he was able to obtain a diagnosis of adult ADHD and a prescription for Ritalin and goes on to describe the effects the drug has had on him—most of which seem to be related to the flattening of affect which is a well-known effect of stimulant drugs.[606] Whether this represent a step up is a question only Frank Wolkenberg can answer.

On July 26, 1993, *Newsweek* ran a piece on adult ADHD by Geoffrey Cowley titled "The Not-Young and Restless,"[607] which told the story of thirty-eight-year-old Gary Roy, who spent thirteen years in college without ever taking a degree and who since then has held "over 128" jobs. As a child, Roy had been diagnosed as "hyperactive" and later was diagnosed with manic depression and treated with lithium, which only made his condition worse. But, after being diagnosed with adult ADHD at the University of Massachusetts Medical Center (where psychologist Russell Barkley was serving as clinic director) and taking his prescribed medication, he was able to obtain his ham radio license and become a civil defense radio supervisor.

We have already seen that mania is an extraordinarily well-documented toxic effect of the stimulant drugs commonly prescribed for hyperactivity. When Roy was diagnosed as "hyperactive" as a child, was he prescribed these drugs, and could this have been the cause of his problems? Author Cowley never considers these questions.

But then again, a healthy skepticism towards the drugmakers was never Cowley's strong point. Three years earlier, *Newsweek* had run another article by him titled "The Promise of Prozac,"[608] which read like a love letter to Eli Lilly's blockbuster drug. The cover illustration for that story depicted a group of supplicants gazing skyward at a larger-than-life Prozac capsule (or "pulvule," as Lilly called it) hovering over the landscape.

Two months after Cowley's article on adult ADHD ran, *American Health* ran a piece titled "Pay Attention,"[609] which extolled the benefits that stimulant drugs confer on the "lucky ones" who get diagnosed and drugged for adult ADHD, while painting a poignant picture of their undiagnosed and undrugged peers:

> *The less fortunate, not knowing what afflicts them, drift from job to job and place to place, never really settling down. Their relationships tend to be short and stormy. Their lives often become a sad jumble of dead ends, wrong turns, frustration and failure. They are more likely to abuse alcohol or drugs, get into accidents or trouble with the law, develop psychiatric disorders, or commit suicide.[610]*

So is there any evidence the drugs reduce the likelihood of any of these unfortunate outcomes? There is, if you count the word of the Dean of ADHD as evidence:

> *I've had patients finish school, get promoted rather than get fired and give up self-destructive behavior. Their spouses say the difference is like day and night, as if they were married to a different person.[611]*

The piece also quoted another eminent doctor who had this to say:

We're not sedating or tranquilizing people, we're making them normal. It's like giving insulin to diabetics.[612]

As the Twig is Bent

In the years that followed interest in adult ADHD soared, with the Biederman group leading the way, warning us in a series of papers about the dire consequences of "adult ADHD": divorce, multiple marriages, reduced income, psychological maladjustment, antisocial behavior, drug addiction, nicotine dependence, mood disorders, anxiety disorders, educational underattainment, occupational underattainment, job insecurity, traffic violations, and arrests.[613]

No child receives a diagnosis of ADHD unless his behavior is considered a problem by somebody—and it shouldn't come as a surprise that problem children sometimes grow up to be problem adults. As the twig is bent, so grows the tree. People have known this for ages. That is not the question here.

And anyone can take a stimulant drug and very likely will experience increased focus and powers of concentration and, if he is so inclined, can attribute all of his life's failures to his doctors' failure to diagnose and treat his adult ADHD. No one has ever disputed this. That is not the question here either.

The question is, does drugging adults diagnosed with ADHD reduce the likelihood of any of the above-mentioned dire consequences and lead to meaningful improvements in the quality of life? In a 1996 paper, Dr. Biederman and his colleagues reviewed the trials of stimulant drugs for adults diagnosed with this condition.[614] Only nine trials had been performed, with none of them lasting for longer than six weeks. The question remained unanswered.

A dozen years later, a study by the Biederman group did provide an answer to the question[615]—although perhaps not the answer the experts wanted. The study looked at 410 adults diagnosed with ADHD who were randomized to either Strattera or placebo. At the six-month mark, the difference between the treatment group and the placebo group on the primary outcome, the Endicott Work Productivity Scale, was a paltry six-tenths of a point—on a scale of zero to one hundred.

Subject were also assessed via the Clinical Global Improvement Scale. A difference of one point on this scale is deemed the minimum necessary to be noticeable to a treating clinician. In this case, the difference was a mere one-tenth of a point—with the difference favoring placebo.[616]

The Doyen of Adult ADHD

Psychiatrist Edward Hallowell is the doyen of adult ADHD, a position he has staked out for himself by means of several books along with innumerable articles, lectures, and interviews. Along with his colleague John Ratey, he authored the first book about adult ADHD intended for a general audience, *Driven to Distraction*,[617] published in 1994 (throughout the book they use the term "ADD" rather than the then-recently coined "ADHD").

Drs. Hallowell and Ratey encounter the same difficulties their colleagues who came before them experienced in delimiting the boundaries of this ill-defined syndrome, regardless of what it is called. According to Hallowell and Ratey, ADD can manifest itself in not paying enough attention, or paying too much attention; in being oversexed, or undersexed; in being too active, or being too quiet. Symptoms of ADD can include cocaine abuse, consumption of pornography, "addiction" to crossword puzzles—or all three.[618] On the very first page of the book, the authors themselves state, with perhaps more candor than they intended, "Once you catch on to what this syndrome is all about, you'll see it everywhere."[619]

Throughout the book, the authors speak of ADD as something one has or does not have, like a rock in a basket. This seems a bit odd, given that they acknowledge that there is no test for ADD, that nearly everybody has some of its symptoms, and that this condition intergrades imperceptibly into normality.[620] Early in the book, they state unequivocally that ADD is caused by a chemical imbalance,[621] although towards the end they admit they do not know what the nature of that imbalance is.[622]

Drs. Hallowell and Ratey both identify themselves as "having" ADD, although, given that both of them managed to graduate from medical school, it is not clear in what sense either of them suffers from a deficit of attention. No matter. This is a condition which, according to them, they "have" alongside such luminaries as Benjamin Franklin, Mozart, Edison, Einstein, and Dustin Hoffmann[623]—although, since they have already acknowledged that there is no biological test for ADD, it is not clear what there is in this case to be "had."

We hear testimonials from patients who have tried medication for this condition and found it turned their lives around:

> *"I feel much more relaxed, more positive, and more on an even keel emotionally…I have more energy in the evenings and am able to think more clearly. In general, I am having more fun."[624]*

> *"I get more done now in a morning than I used to in a week."[625]*

> *"What has happened here is amazing. I'm a new man. My wife is overjoyed."[626]*

Employing a didactic style similar to that utilized by psychiatrist Peter Kramer in his best-selling *Listening to Prozac*, the authors never claim that these results are typical, although they do little to disabuse readers of that notion.

In fairness to Drs. Hallowell and Ratey, they are about more than just drugs:

> *The ADD therapist must offer concrete ways of getting organized, staying focused, making plans, keeping to schedules, prioritizing tasks due, and in general dealing with the chaos of everyday life.*[627]

Elsewhere they advise readers "Do what you are good at, rather than spending all your time trying to get good at what you are bad at."[628]

These points are well-taken, but didn't all this used to be called "growing up?"

We Create an Illness

When I asked Dr. Healy about the upsurge in diagnosing and drugging people for "Adult ADHD," his reply was abrupt: "There is no such thing."

Then I asked him why this diagnostic category had become so popular. This was his answer:

> *The main interest comes from the pharmaceutical companies. The use of stimulants among adults has greatly increased. And you're looking at a bunch of drugs which are not new. You've got a bunch of drugs like methylphenidate and the amphetamines which have been re-formulated in ways so that somebody can take out a patent on the fact that this is in an extended-release formula now, and sell this as a completely new drug, and charge vast amounts of money for drugs that in essence were produced during the 1950's or even earlier.*
>
> *From a community point of view it looks good. There's always been a lot of interest in the public to have stimulant drugs. We figure there are going to be times when these things are going make us more effective, when we're trying to study at university or when we're trying to do jobs like keep up with the stock exchange and the calls are going out and things like that and we think we are going to need to operate at speed and with focus. It's the kind of thing that is a very appealing message to all of us, or most of us. So there*

has always been a public push to use these drugs and it could be for concentration purposes, for weight loss purposes. Among the public at large, this is an attractive kind of drug to have.

And to some extent, because of the way stimulants were used in the 1960's, they ended up being controlled, and the way to get them back to the market, which is a kind of conspiracy of good will between the companies and the regulators and us, is to create 'ADHD.' We don't want to give drugs loosely, for stimulant purposes. They should be restricted to the treatment of illness. So we create an illness which the drug becomes the answer to, and of course there is a moral obligation among us to treat our 'illnesses.'

The Central Challenge of Being Human

The new millennium brought a spate of news stories promoting the diagnosis and drugging of grownups for ADHD.[629] These stories tend to follow a familiar pattern. We are given a list of symptoms of adult ADHD—mood swings, difficulty getting along with others, procrastination, disorganization, feelings of stress, money problems—complaints that are so broad and general that it may be hard for the reader to think of anyone he knows who does not display one or more of them.

Often we are served a soupçon of neurobabble or genobabble to convince us that adult ADHD is a genuine honest-to-gosh biologically-based neurodevelopmental brain disorder,[630] along with a list of sequelae of "untreated ADHD"—divorce, never completing college, chronic underemployment, substance abuse, eating disorders, anxiety, depression, suicidality—deftly sidestepping the question of whether "treatment" reduces the likelihood of any of these outcomes.

Finally, we hear the tale of some troubled person, stumbling through life, miserable and unfulfilled, until finally his adult ADHD was diagnosed and treated, enabling him to live happily ever after. Like Peter Kramer and

Edward Hallowell, the authors of these articles never claim these results are typical, although they do nothing to disabuse their readers of that notion.

The market continues to expand. On 25 February 2020, the *Wall Street Journal* reported that senior citizens as old as eighty-five years are being treated for ADHD.[631] This alarming news becomes even more alarming when you realize the drugs commonly administered for ADHD raise the heart rate and blood pressure. Once considered a transient condition afflicting primarily elementary-school-age children, now ADHD apparently is a chronic disorder requiring cradle-to-grave treatment with powerful stimulant drugs.[632]

And for what purpose? Many of us have known one or more persons with advanced degrees, in their thirties or even beyond, lost and unmoored, working odd jobs, and yet feeling in their bones they were meant for something more. Maybe all these people need is to get diagnosed and drugged for their adult ADHD. Or, perhaps they need to realize that they still have lessons to learn right where they are, before they are ready to move on to bigger and better things.

The central challenge of being human is learning to maximize our strengths and manage our weaknesses. Most of us are works in progress. Probably most of us suffer from one or more of the character defects that fall under the diagnostic rubric of "adult ADHD." It is not clear why we cannot work on these defects without attributing them to some mythical disease entity, the existence of which has never been demonstrated.

CHAPTER FOURTEEN

A SHOCKING PROPOSAL

On Friday, 19 April 2019, the FDA approved the marketing of the first medical device to treat ADHD. Called the Monarch eTNS System ("eTNS" stands for "external Trigeminal Nerve Stimulation"), this device delivers low-voltage electric shocks to a child's forebrain, all night long, while the child is sleeping.[633] The FDA approved the device after a four-week trial published that same month in the *Journal of the American Academy of Child and Adolescent Psychiatry*.[634]

The trial included sixty-two youngsters aged eight through twelve who were randomized either to treatment or to a sham procedure that did not deliver any actual electric shocks. The primary outcome was the score on the clinician-administered ADHD Rating Scale. Compared to the placebo group, kids in the active treatment group exhibited a 4.5-point reduction in their ADHD-RS scores[635]—on a scale of zero to fifty-four.

Nowhere is the magnitude of the effect size explicitly stated in the *JAACP* paper, which instead presents this information in graphical form, with the bottom cut off the graph to make this paltry outcome seem larger than it is.[636]

Adverse events that occurred in the treatment group at a greater frequency than in the placebo group include trouble sleeping, nightmares, drowsiness, fatigue, tingling, and headache. None of these was deemed serious enough to cause the child to be withdrawn from the study.[637] The long-term benefits and harms of this device remain unknown.

A video produced by NeuroSigma describes the protocol for using this device,[638] which is worth examining in some detail:

1) Insert a fully charged battery into the device.

2) Clean the child's forehead with soap and water or an alcohol-based wipe, then make sure the skin is thoroughly dry before applying the electrically conductive patch.

3) Apply the patch to the center of the child's forehead, just above the eyebrows.

4) Connect the lead wire to the patch.

5) Insert the lead wire into the port at the top of the electric pulse generator. (At this point the narrator cautions viewers, "Make sure that all connections are secure. If a connection becomes loose, the device will stop delivering therapy [sic]."

6) Turn the device on and enter the password.

7) Select the proper stimulation channel.

8) Increase the current until it is perceptible to the child but not painful.

9) Lock the device and your child can sleep as normal.

10) The next morning, unlock the device, turn off the power, remove the patch, and store the device.

The video shows a young boy, serenely obedient to his mother as she goes through all the steps of this prolonged setup procedure. She then tucks him into bed and he drifts off to Slumberland, cradling his teddy bear to his bosom. At this point the viewer could be forgiven for wondering how any kid that docile and submissive could have ever received a diagnosis of "ADHD."

You might think any actual boy worth his salt in real life could think up better uses for a teddy bear, like blowing it up with an M-80 firecracker, but never mind that for now. What is going to be the long-term psychological effects of telling children that their brains are so defective that they require this elaborate, ersatz medical ritual, night after night? This is a gigantic uncontrolled experiment.

Then there is the matter of price. The manufacturer's website offers no guidance as to how long the device should be used, but the device itself retails for $980 and the single-use patches cost ten dollars apiece,[639] meaning a single year of "therapy" would cost $4630.

When I asked Dr. Breggin what he thought of the Monarch eTNS System, he did not hesitate before replying:

> *This is a criminal attitude toward children in a number of ways. It teaches the child to be a kind of electrical robot. This is a door that opens the way into horrendous atrocities that resemble the psychosurgery that I successfully opposed in the seventies. It teaches a child to be the product of outside influences, to be the product of devices. It teaches the child the opposite of taking moral, ethical, psychological responsibility for oneself.*
>
> *The single most important thing growing up is learning to take charge of oneself, believing and trusting that we can handle our own emotions and growth, that we can overcome our difficulties focusing, and that we can choose to focus on different things and build our lives in a different direction. Self-determination, autonomy, is the key to life. After we have a feeling of autonomy, an understanding of it, then we can learn to be disciplined, we can learn to be loving, we can learn ethics and all the good things.*
>
> *And this approach to a child teaches the child very early on that they don't have autonomy—they have submissiveness to a machine.*

From the viewpoint of the parent, the parent may get a gratification out of not feeling blamed—the problem has nothing to do with them. But then this robs them of their parental influence.

All that's good, all that's wonderful in parenting is actually eradicated, including a parent's instinctual desire to preserve a child and protect a child's brain. We all know the brain is a delicate organ that needs to be protected. That's why kids wear helmets when they play football or ride bikes. We know a child's brain has to be protected. That's why we don't want them to smoke or drink. We know all that. And this goes against everything good in parenting.

Indeed. We live in a society in which children are exploited as consumers—of manufactured entertainment, of mindless video games, of nutritionally barren junk food, of poisonous psychiatric "medicines"—and now of electric shock machines—as ruthlessly as they once were for their labor. Doesn't anyone have a better idea?

CHAPTER FIFTEEN

INSPIRING
KIDS

For years now pundits have been warning us that public education in America is going to the dogs. The solution? Standardized testing, teaching to the test, piling on homework, lengthening the school day, and cutting back or even eliminating recess—as if sticking the kids' noses in the material long enough will ensure learning. Perhaps most absurdly, even in schools that still allow kids recess, boys who act out in class may be punished by withholding recess—denying them the very opportunity they need to blow off steam and keep them from acting out.

But a handful of schools in Texas and Oklahoma are bucking the trend. A new program called LiiNK (Let's inspire innovation 'N' Kids) has taken a radical approach—giving kids the opportunity to be kids.[640]

LiiNK is the brainchild of Deborah Rhea, a former physical education teacher and track coach and now a Professor of Kinesiology at Texas Christian University. Inspired by her observations of public schools in Finland,[641] Dr. Rhea's program incorporates three essential elements.

The first is increased recess time. In an era in which many schools have cut recess time to twenty or fifteen minutes or eliminated it completely, kids in the LiiNK program are provided an entire hour of unstructured outdoor play time daily, broken down into four fifteen-minute intervals scattered throughout the day. Students never spend more than seventy-five minutes in the classroom without a break.[642] Teachers are not allowed to withhold recess time as punishment for misbehavior. This extra recess time is inserted into the curriculum without lengthening the school day. Instead, the emphasis is on quality of instructional time, rather than quantity.[643]

The second is ethics training. Kids are given daily fifteen-minute Positive Action character curriculum lessons focused on school connectedness, respect for adults, honesty, empathy, and engagement with learning.[644]

The third is teacher training. Teachers are provided three full days of training, focused on changing the teachers' mindsets related to being outdoors and taking time to re-energize themselves and their students.[645] The program is instituted in stages: the first year in grades K-One, then Grade Two, then Grade Three, and finally Grade Four.[646]

How has all this worked out for the kids? At the first school where the LiiNK program was instituted, off-task behaviors in the classroom (movement out of the seat or away from the learning area, talking out of turn, fidgeting, and daydreaming) decreased markedly, as did the incidence of disruptive, self-injurious, and anti-social behaviors. Students' body mass index decreased, as did transition time between the classroom and the playground. Listening comprehension increased, as did the incidence of positive behaviors on the playground—smiling, laughing, jumping, clapping, hopping, skipping, and cheering.[647]

Imagine that—kids who are allowed to play outdoors laugh and smile more.

What about test scores? They went up, too.[648] Granted, the increase was small, but so what? More play time, happier, healthier kids, and increased test scores sounds like a win-win-win.

"The first year is always hard," Dr. Rhea told me.

> *At first when we do the teacher training teachers are all on board,*
> *they're all excited, they're ready to go. Especially your pre-K through*
> *Grade Two. But once fall hits, even your excited pre-K through*

Two teachers are starting to become resistant about week four to six. And in that time period they start feeling the crunch—'I'm not getting as much done as I used to.' And I say to them 'How much do you think the children were really taking in of what you were pushing at them?' It's not until the second year that the pre-K through Grade Two teachers are like 'Yup—we got this.'

Then I asked Dr. Rhea how the program has been received by the parents.

The parents love it. The hardest parents we had to deal with were the very first year in the private school, with the parents who said 'I do not want this to stop my kid from being the Harvard graduate or the Princeton graduate or the Yale graduate.' I said 'Well, can we give it a couple of years? They're only kindergartners. Can we just give it a couple of years and see what happens?' We didn't even hear from them again after the first year, seeing the difference it made in their kids—socially, emotionally, and physically.

How about the kids? "It's been great," she told me, smiling broadly. "When we walk in they say 'Who are you?' and I say something like 'I'm the person who gave you four play breaks a day' and they go 'YAYYY!!'"

Finally, I ask Dr. Rhea if the program is a cure for ADHD. With proper scientific caution, she declined to go that far, although she did state the program reduces the frequency of "ADHD-like" behaviors. But what on earth is ADHD but the name we give to a wide variety of off-task, disruptive, self-injurious, and anti-social behaviors?

CHAPTER SIXTEEN

THE SPIN DOCTORS

We have seen that a favorite rhetorical tactic for proponents of ADHD medications—whether they are writing in the scientific literature or the popular media—is to cite a long list of negative consequences said to result from "untreated ADHD," begging the question of whether drugging children or adults diagnosed with that condition reduces the likelihood of any of these bad outcomes. However, on 27 January 2020, a systematic review and meta-analysis by the Biederman group claimed to demonstrate that ADHD medications do indeed reduce frequency of many of these harms.[649]

One of the most interesting parts of this paper is the disclosure statement, which reports that Dr. Biederman has accepted research funding from Genentech, Lundbeck, Neurocentria, Pfizer, Roche, Shire, and Sunovion—although, the reader is assured, Biederman's interests "are managed by Massachusetts General Hospital and Partners HealthCare in accordance with their conflict-of-interest policies."[650]

But never mind that for now. Let's begin by taking a look at the studies reviewed by Dr. Biederman and his colleagues. Not one of them was a randomized controlled trial. All of them were observational studies relying on data extracted from population-wide data bases or large health insurance claim databases, and either compared individuals who were prescribed ADHD medication with those who were not, or else compared data from the same individual when he was adherent to treatment to when he was not.[651] This kind of study is prone to bias, for a couple of reasons.[652]

Firstly, individuals who seek treatment for a given condition are more likely to engage in other health-promoting behaviors than those who are not. This is called the "healthy user effect." For example, women who seek hormone replacement therapy (HRT) are more likely to exercise, eat a healthy diet, avoid alcohol, and maintain a healthy weight than those who do not.[653]

Secondly, individuals who adhere to a given treatment also are more likely to engage in other health-promoting behaviors. This is known as the "healthy adherer effect."[654] One study found that patients who adhered to statin therapy had lower rates of burns, falls, fractures, motor vehicle accidents, open wounds, poisoning, and workplace accidents than those who did not.[655] Another study, of HRT for women, found that even adherence to placebo was correlated with reduced risk of hip fracture, myocardial infarction, cancer deaths, and all-cause mortality.[656] Apparently, just being the sort of person who takes her medication regularly has a salubrious effect, independent of any actual pharmacological effects.

These sources of bias can completely overwhelm the actual drug effects demonstrated in randomized controlled trials. While observational studies found that women who received hormone replacement therapy had one-third the risk of coronary heart disease of those who did not, randomized controlled trials found that hormone replacement actually increases the risk by twenty-nine percent.[657]

Bearing these precautions in mind, let's take a look at the specific findings of the paper. The conclusion as stated in the abstract informs readers:

> *The majority [of articles reviewed] suggest a robust protective effect of ADHD medication treatment on mood disorders, suicid-*

> *ality, criminality, substance use disorders, accidents and injuries,*
> *traumatic brain injuries, motor vehicle crashes, and educational*
> *outcomes.[658]*

That seems like an odd way of spinning the results, given that the purpose of a meta-analysis is to determine what the overall pattern of data is telling you, rather than the sheer number of studies supporting this or that conclusion. In fact, the authors' own meta-analysis found no significant effect of ADHD medications on suicidality, criminality, substance use disorders, traumatic brain injuries, and motor vehicle crashes.[659] That leaves educational outcomes, mood disorders, and accidents and injuries. How convincing is the evidence that ADHD drugs reduce the likelihood of these bad outcomes?

The conclusion that ADHD medication improves educational outcomes was based on all of two studies with categorical outcomes. Can you do a "meta-analysis" on just two studies?

Moreover, the authors' own literature review uncovered three more studies with available continuous data that showed no drug effect.[660]

The conclusion that ADHD medication reduces the likelihood of mood disorders likewise was based on two studies, one which looked at major depression and the other at bipolar disorder.[661] Can you do a meta-analysis on two studies with two different endpoints?

The conclusion that ADHD medication reduces accidents and injuries was based on six studies.[662] This was the only significant outcome that was based on more than two studies, and the authors of the meta-analysis reported significant heterogeneity in the studies, which suggest that these studies may not all have been measuring the same endpoint.

At this point the reader could be forgiven for concluding that all this constitutes a rather puny haul, coming as it does after decades of research, and given the biases inherent in these studies—and especially so in the light of the MTA Study, a randomized controlled trial, far and away the largest and longest of its kind, carried out by eminently credentialed researchers all of whom were decidedly pro-med and who gave the drugs every chance to work, and which found no long-term benefit of drugging kids for something called "ADHD."[663]

CHAPTER SEVENTEEN

ADHD IN THE TIME OF COVID

Meltdown after Meltdown

Since the COVID-19 pandemic began, schools have been shuttered, after-school sports programs have been canceled, and Zoom meetings substituted for actual human contact. By the end of 2020, three million children had dropped off the radar—they weren't attending school, not even virtually, and no one seemed to know what had become of them.[664] Meanwhile, untold thousands of mommies and daddies have perished from "unintentional injuries" which have soared in the wake of pandemic restrictions,[665] and millions more have lost jobs, homes, or businesses they have worked all their lives to build. How are the children faring under this "New Normal?"

On 29 May 2020, a report published by athenahealth noted that since the pandemic began, new and recurring diagnoses for ADHD for teenage boys, along with new and recurring prescriptions for ADHD meds for that same group, have skyrocketed. Between the week of 9 March through the week of 30 March, the rate of new diagnoses for ADHD for teenage boys rose by a staggering sixty-seven percent, and that of new prescriptions increased by a similar amount. These figures have gone up for teenage girls as well, although for them the increase was much more modest. There was no comparable increase in any of these figures for the same period in the year 2019.[666]

A 16 February 2021 story in NBC News corroborated this, quoting Harold Koplewicz,[667] founder of the Child Mind Institute, who stated that the number of appointments to discuss medication has risen by twenty percent compared to the same period in 2019. Dr. Koplewicz affirmed that the "lion's share" of appointments pertained to ADHD medications. Meanwhile, calls to the CHADD helpline rose by sixty-two percent, and traffic to that organization's website has risen by seventy-seven percent.[668]

The NBC News story also gave readers some insight into the human aspect of all this. The article told the tale of Isabela, a twelve-year-old child who had been a straight-A student before the pandemic began. But when her school shut down and switched to Zoom classes, her grades took a "nosedive."

"It was meltdown after meltdown after meltdown" her mother recalled. The last straw came when Isabela "fell to pieces":

> *She was crying and screaming and hyperventilating and started to get some tics, moving her head and flapping her arms. That's when we started to consider that it might be ADHD.[669]*

Isabela's mother, who already was taking medication for ADHD ("I can't function without it"), took her child to a psychiatrist with the objective of obtaining the same diagnosis:

> *She hopes that with an ADHD diagnosis, Isabela will be able to get a prescription for a stimulant medication—such as Ritalin, Adderall, or Vyvanse—to alleviate her symptoms.[670]*

The same article told the tale of an eight-year-old boy who had received a diagnosis of ADHD the year before but had never been drugged for it. But all this changed after the schools were shut down and the boy was switched to online learning:

He would take an hour to complete four words of a writing assign-
ment. Days would go by when he got "absolutely nothing" done.

> *When [the child and his mother] realized that they were*
> *"looking down the barrel of another year like this," they visited a*
> *psychiatrist who prescribed Ritalin and Metadate.*[671]

What is the source of these children's distress? The athenahealth report quotes pediatrician Vik Mali, of Mali Pediatrics in Sterling, Michigan, as follows:

> *It's hard enough to do [schoolwork] in the classroom. Trying to do*
> *that when a parent is on call for work, and you're expected to do*
> *this on your own, I think it's asking a lot of these kids at various*
> *age levels.*[672]

The NBC News story quotes Devang Patel, a family practice physician in Plainfield, Illinois who specializes in ADHD:

> *Now that [the children] are at home [parents are] trying to make*
> *their kids sit still for just half an hour and seeing how difficult that*
> *is.*[673]

The same story offers these words of wisdom from pediatrician Jenny Radesky, an Assistant Professor at the University of Michigan Medical School:

> *I'm watching kids who used to love school become unenthused and*
> *unmotivated. They need the social environment at school to learn*
> *how to regulate themselves. Without that, they are really strug-*
> *gling.*[674]

Have these eminently credential docs just admitted that the complaints that fall under the diagnostic rubric of "ADHD" are not, after all, caused by a genetically-based brain disease, but rather are completely understandable responses to the circumstances a child finds himself in? And wouldn't changing those circumstances be preferable to drugging the child?

Vast Unintended Harm

In January of 2020, the Drug Enforcement Administration announced that in response to the covid pandemic and associated restrictions, it was temporarily waiving provisions of the Ryan Haight Online Pharmacy Consumer Act, which restricted the online prescription of controlled substances.[675] (The act was named after an eighteen-year-old boy who died of an overdose after buying Vicodin online.) This proved to be a boon for online pharmacies, but perhaps none benefitted so much as Cerebral, a startup which had just been founded earlier that very same month.[676]

Cerebral's website[677] promises "help for anxiety, depression, insomnia, and ADHD" and offers "online prescriber visits, care counseling, and prescriptions delivered to your door." The homepage also touts subscriptions beginning for as little as seven dollars a week and features this message from "Chief Impact Officer" and United States Olympic Team member Simone Biles:

> *I believe everyone should have access to mental health resources and Cerebral gives me the ability to personalize my mental health care experience.*

For the price of a subscription (cancelable at any time) Cerebral offers evaluation, diagnosis, and prescription by a "medical prescriber" (a term the company consistently uses to refer to its nurse practitioner employees), "evidence-based behavioral health counseling," regular telephone/video sessions with an assigned "care counselor," and monthly medication delivery (with the coy disclaimer "if prescribed").[678]

An article that ran 11 March 2022 in *Bloomberg Businessweek* noted that the company declined to state the percentage of patients who receive prescriptions. The piece also claimed that the company's chief medical officer was adamant in meetings with his managers that ninety-five percent of people who see a Cerebral prescriber should get a prescription. He was equally adamant that that figure should never rise to one hundred percent—lest anyone get the impression the company was just a giant online pill mill. [679]

Cerebral markets its services aggressively on Instagram and TikTok, beguiling patients with the message "Have you ever thought you might have ADHD?" Deploying a familiar theme, complaints such as poor planning, disorganization and procrastination—the sorts of problems every human being has to deal with at one time or another—are re-cast as symptoms of a brain disease. In one advertisement, a woman was shown shaking her leg, while viewers were warned that "restless leg syndrome" can be a symptom of ADHD.[680]

Cerebral's free and easy dispensation of prescriptions and lavish spending on advertising are matched by the company's tight-fisted attitude towards its employees. The "care counselors" were in fact fictitious characters, with any of numerous operators being asked to play the role of any given counselor on any given day. One operator claimed she had a roster of one thousand patients and was expected to respond to all queries within twenty-four hours. On a typical day she might handle one hundred queries, and she heard from patients in crisis several times a week. Last August, the company stripped two hundred therapists of their salaries and benefits. The ones who didn't quit were relegated to the ever-growing gig economy, receiving forty to forty-five dollars per session.[681]

All this has proven to be a profitable business model. Between June and December of 2021, the company's valuation quadrupled. Not surprisingly, Cerebral, along with more than three hundred other telehealth providers, is calling for the telehealth waiver to be extended for another two years.[682] An article in *STAT* that ran last December warned readers of "vast unintended harm" if this call goes unheeded.[683]

Marching in Lockstep

I asked Dr. Healy if he saw any parallels between society's response to the complaints that fall under the diagnostic rubric of "ADHD," and society's response to the covid pandemic. This is what he had to say:

The interesting thing about ADHD is the kind of marketing of the condition, which is a bit like the marketing of covid—you know, it's marketing based on fear, if you don't get this treated your child will go on to suicide and a life of crime and all these kind of things.

And that kind of speaks to the fact the people are atomized, our communities are broken.

When we were kids, we used to race out in the fields or climb trees or do this that and the other. Kids were interacting with each other and not just hooked into social media. And we do seem to have become atomized in ways that we weren't before and as such being much more open to being led. It's easier to lead individuals than to lead an entire community. Unless the entire community has been atomized.

What is quite striking across the board is the tendency to shut people like Gretchen LeFever out, the inability to let people research and have careers if it's not fitting in with the pharmaceutical company line. We're all looking very North Korean these days since covid.

That's quite a statement. Do you care to explain what you mean by that?

We do seem to be marching in lockstep. Having been in Europe and behind the Iron Curtain back in the old days, there was a certain freedom of thought over there that you didn't find in the West. You know, people behind the Iron Curtain could see who the enemy was and knew when they had to keep quiet and things like that.

But at the same time you had the sense that they thought their own thoughts, and didn't necessarily believe what they were told by the leadership. And looking at western Europe from eastern Europe you could see all the people in the West that think they're free aren't half as free as they think. They're moving in lockstep but the propaganda is more subtle.

People aren't able to speak out and say things that are not in line with the prevailing wisdom. We used to be much freer to talk about the hazards of things. We used to talk about the harms of treatment and things like that. And now it's almost impossible to, and Kim Jong-Whatever would probably envy our degree of control over the way the population thinks.

These are sobering words indeed. And as we the enter the third year of the covid pandemic, there is every reason to believe the number of children and adults plied with brain-altering drugs will continue to skyrocket—not just in the United States, but all over the world.

CHAPTER EIGHTEEN

ADHD GOES GLOBAL

An American Export

A 2007 review[684] found that the United States, with less than five percent of the world's population, accounted for a staggering eighty percent of the world's total consumption of ADHD meds. The figure was even higher in terms of dollars, with the US accounting for ninety-two to ninety-five percent of total global spending on these drugs.[685] On a per capita basis, the US had more than twice as many prescriptions of ADHD drugs for kids than its nearest rival, Canada.[686] More recently, the 2014 report of the International Narcotics Control Board found that the US still accounted for eighty percent of the total world consumption of methylphenidate.[687]

In addition, we have seen that there is no objective test for ADHD, and that the criteria for diagnosing this condition are hopelessly subjective and context-dependent. Reported incidence rates of ADHD are known to vary by a factor of fifty.[688] In a 1992 study, mental health professionals from four different countries—the United States, Japan, China, and Indonesia—watched videos of four boys, playing both by themselves and with other children, and rated the boys' conduct on an eighteen-item checklist for disruptive behaviors. Clinicians from China and Indonesia found significantly more disruptive behaviors than did their professional colleagues in the United States or Japan, indicating that notions of what is considered "disruptive" behavior vary a great deal between different cultures.[689]

So is ADHD just another American cultural export, like rock and roll or the Super Mario Brothers? A 2007 meta-analysis by the Biederman group[690] purported to debunk this notion. They looked at incidence rates reported in 102 studies comprising 171,756 subjects from North America, Europe, Asia, South America, Oceania, the Middle East, and Africa. The studies employed a variety of criteria to diagnose this condition, including the *DSM-III*, the *DSM-IIIR*, the *DSM-IV*, and the World Health Organization's *International Classification of Diseases* (*ICD-10*).

The *ICD-10* category corresponding to ADHD is called Hyperkinetic Disorder (HKD), and is defined by much stricter criteria. A 2006 study found that one hundred percent of boys diagnosed with HKD also met the criteria for ADHD, while only twenty-six percent of boys diagnosed with ADHD met the criteria for HKD.[691]

The researchers' estimate of the world-wide pooled prevalence of ADD/ADHD/HKD was 5.29%. Moreover, they concluded that most of the variation in incidence rates was due to different diagnostic criteria being employed, and that once they controlled for this, incidence rates were essentially the same throughout much of the world. Significant differences remained between the United States and Africa, between the United States and the Middle East, between Europe and Africa, and between Europe and the Middle East.[692]

The authors then re-analyzed their data by means of an "additional model" which was said to "increase statistical power" and this time they found there were no remaining significant differences in incidence rates, concluding "This finding argues against the view that ADHD/HKD is a culturally-based construct peculiar to the North American culture."[693] These results were replicated by associates of Dr. Biederman in two subsequent meta-analyses.[694]

It is beyond the scope of the present work to comment on the statistical wizardry needed to make a fifty-fold difference in incidence rates disappear. It was all a tempest in a teapot anyway.

There is no convincing evidence of any long-term benefit to drugging children for ADHD. Nor is there any convincing evidence for the existence of a subset of children so labeled who benefit. So the question of whether the incidence of ADHD or HKD (as defined by *DSM-IV* criteria or by any other) is the same throughout the world is a moot point. It is not clear what this would prove if it were true, given there is no non-psychiatric illness that follows this pattern.

The Global Migration of ADHD

While the United States continues to lead the world in prescription for simulant drugs for kids, the rest of the world is catching up with us. In 1993, thirty-one countries had adopted the use of ADHD medications, but by 2003 that number had swollen to fifty-five. Low-use countries exhibited annual growth rates as high as forty-six percent, while moderate-use countries had growth rates of twenty percent.[695]

In a 2014 review,[696] sociologists Peter Conrad and Meredith R. Bergey attributed the global migration of ADHD to five factors: 1) The transnational pharmaceutical industry, 2) The increasing influence of American psychiatry, 3) The adoption of the *DSM* criteria for diagnosing ADHD, 4) The internet, and 5) ADHD advocacy groups. Each of these tends to reinforce the others.

While the United States may be nearing saturation point in terms of ADHD diagnosis and treatment, the rest of world still represents, in the eyes of the drugmakers, a largely untapped market. A review by Global Data gushed:

> *Between 2010 and 2018, the global ADHD market is expected to grow at a CAGR of 8%.*

> *During this forecast period, patents for various drugs such as Adderall XR, Daytrana, Concerta (methylphenidate) Strattera (atomoxetine) and Kapvay are set to expire. However the losses due to the expiry of these patents would be compensated by new drugs entering the market such as Vyvanse and Intuniv. Thus, the global ADHD market will show a steady growth from 2010 to 2018.*[697]

Not to be outdone, the firm Global Industry Analysts noted that "the global market for ADHD drugs is severely constrained by the lack of awareness of the disorder, even in developed countries such as the UK, Germany and Japan." To remedy this dire situation, they called for more marketing and education directed at physicians and, where possible, potential consumers.[698] This call has not gone unheeded.

The ADHD Institute, "an educational platform developed and funded by Takeda," offers "ADHD resources" for "patients, parents, educators, and professionals" with country-specific information for Canada, Germany, Spain, Sweden, and the UK.[699] All these "ADHD resources" were developed by Takeda, which in 2019 acquired Shire PLC, manufacturer of Vyvanse and Adderall XR.

Janssen Global, which markets the ADHD drug Concerta, provides country-specific information on its products for no fewer than fifty different sovereign nations. The website for Xian-Janssen, the company's branch in China, provides these helpful details about Attention Deficit Hyperactivity Disorder:

> *Attention deficit hyperactivity disorder (ADHD) is a chronic disease that affects through one's whole life. ADHD is common in school-age children, will continue to adolescence and adulthood, and has a wide negative influence on one's academic, career and social life.*

> *The etiology and pathogenesis of ADHD is unclear, but there is ample evidence that ADHD is a neurodevelopmental disorder, which is a syndrome caused singly or synergistically by a variety of biological factors (including genetic factors, environmental factors, brain development abnormalities, etc.), psychological factors, and social factors.*
>
> *ADHD is mainly characterized by distraction which does not match with age, reduced attention span, excessive activity and emotional impulses regardless of occasion, accompanied by cognitive impairment and learning difficulties, and intelligence is normal or near normal. The core symptoms of ADHD include attention deficit, hyperactivity and impulsivity.*
>
> *There are two main methods of ADHD management: (1) pharmacological treatment; (2) non- pharmacological treatment: including behavioral therapy, parent training, etc.*
>
> *For more information see your Doctor or Healthcare Professional.*[700]

What is being sold here is not so much a specific drug, nor even a specific diagnosis, as a specific worldview: one in which human distress is the manifestation of a drug-treatable brain disease, and one in which the drugmakers are cast as benevolent, objective sources of information.

Christine Phillips, Senior Lecturer in Social Foundations of Medicine at the Australian National University Medical School, commented:

> *It could be argued that in providing information to teachers, pharmaceutical companies are simply acting as good corporate citizens. Such an argument would carry more weight if these companies also provided education programs addressing autism and dyslexia, two other conditions which impact on educational performance, but which do not have accepted pharmaceutical therapies.*[701]

In addition to autism and dyslexia, she could have added hunger, homelessness, domestic violence, and a whole host of other evils.

ADHD advocacy groups are active online, as well. ADHD Europe offers a position statement "ADHD Myths and Facts,"[702] conveniently translated into French, Spanish, Greek, Italian, and Hungarian." A "Fact Sheet"[703] produced by ADHD Australia warns readers that "ADHD is currently under-diagnosed, particularly in girls and the adult population." The Center for ADHD Awareness Canada informs us that "Overwhelming scientific evidence has led all major medical associations and government health agencies to recognize ADHD as a major medical disorder."[704] The website for ADHD New Zealand instructs teachers on how to spot the signs of this condition and how to communicate their concerns to the parents.[705]

And the website for ADHD UK offers users its "Adult ADHD Self-Screening Tool."[706] Sample questions include "How often do you have trouble wrapping up the final details of a project, once the challenging parts have been done?" "How often do you make careless mistakes when you have to work on a boring or difficult project?" and "How often do you have difficulty keeping your attention when doing boring or repetitive work?" all rated on a five-point Likert scale from "Never" to "Very often." Users who score sufficiently high on this quiz are advised, not to find work that doesn't bore them, but rather to discuss the test results with a clinician.

And that highlights the problem with checklists such as this one: they decontextualize human experience, draining it of any larger meaning and reducing every variety of human distress to a drug-treatable medical disorder.

Global acceptance of this medical model of ADHD likely is facilitated by the large number of international medical graduates who currently fill one-third of residency positions in psychiatry.[707] While many of these residents choose to remain in the United States, those who return to their homelands will have been schooled in the diagnostic categories contained in the *DSM*—and we have already seen that every iteration of that volume has broadened the number of children eligible for that diagnosis.

The latest version of the *ICD, ICD-11*, which came into effect 1 January 2022, has replaced the old category of "Hyperkinetic Disorder" with Attention Deficit Hyperactivity Disorder, bringing the rest of the world into line with American psychiatry. Just as in the *DSM*, this condition is divided into three subtypes: Predominantly Inattentive, Predominantly Hyperactive, and Combined. Whereas hyperactivity was the defining feature of HKD, the new category of ADHD gives equal emphasis to hyperactivity or inattention. The maximum age of onset, previously (and somewhat vaguely) defined as "early onset (usually in the first five years of life)" has been changed to twelve years, again bringing the rest of the world into line with American psychiatry.

No doubt these changes will increase the number of children worldwide considered eligible for stimulant drugs.

The market continues to expand. The following insights come from an April 2020 report from Persistence Market Research, a company which entices customers with its promised "Expertise in Life Sciences and Transformational Health":

> *Rising prevalence of ADHD across the globe, owing to the low threshold of diagnostic criteria, is expected to fuel growth of the global attention-deficit hyperactivity disorder (ADHD) therapeutics market over the forecast period.*
>
> *The COVID-19 pandemic is certainly a difficult time for individuals with attention-deficit hyperactivity disorder, owing to their vulnerability to the distress caused by the pandemic and physical distancing measures. As a result of these measures, individuals with ADHD might exhibit increased behavioral problems. On the back of this, ADHD therapeutics will witness significant growth in sales.*

Increasing introduction of innovative ADHD therapeutic products such as fruit-flavored chewable pills for children will favor the growth of the global attention-deficit hyperactivity disorder therapeutics market.

The attention deficit hyperactivity disorder therapeutics market is expected to grow twofold between 2021 and 2031.[708]

Three Nations

It is beyond the scope of this work to provide an exhaustive account of the history of the ADHD diagnosis in every country in the world where this label is used. Instead, we will take a look at three nations with very different approaches to this label: one of which has embraced the medical model of ADHD almost as enthusiastically as the United States; one in which the medical model has barely begun to penetrate; and one in which that model has encountered stiff resistance but still has penetrated to an extent.

ADHD in Canada

We have already seen that the diagnostic category known as ADHD, and the practice of prescribing stimulant drugs for this condition, is almost exclusively an American invention. However, the switch in emphasis from hyperactivity to inattention (which guaranteed that many more children, including girls, would receive this label) was an initiative that came not from American doctors but from their professional counterparts in Canada, led by clinical psychologist Virginia Douglas and her colleagues at McGill University and Montreal Children's Hospital. Dr. Douglas summarized this work in her 1972 Presidential Address to the Canadian Psychological Association.[709]

All this raises a question: how does one measure attention in a laboratory setting? The way Dr. Douglas and her colleagues went about it was to assess the performance of children labeled "hyperactive" at a variety of tasks, and compared the results with those of their peers not so labeled. The results they obtained were interesting. In one "automated concept learning" task, the performance of children labeled "hyperactive" equaled that of the controls under a continuous reward scheme, but plummeted under an intermittent reward scheme.[710]

In plain English, these boys (almost all of her subjects were boys) were perfectly capable of paying attention to the assigned task when there was something in it for them. So what is being measured here is not attention but rather obeisance to adult authority.

Dr. Douglas herself acknowledged as much, discussing the work of one of her students who observed children's behavior in a classroom setting:

> *She obtained the most consistent differences between hyperactives and normal on a coding category that included "purposive (or goal-directed) behaviour not related to the classroom activity." It is important to note that we are not talking here about random or aimless behaviour. The problem seems to be, rather, that the child's goals and the teacher's goals differ.[711]*

No one is denying this sort of thing can be a problem, especially in an overcrowded classroom supervised by a stressed-out teacher, but it is not clear what is to be gained by regarding such behavior as a manifestation of a brain pathology.

In fairness to Dr. Douglas, she offered a much more balanced view of the value of stimulant drugs than many of her peers, opining that they should be used only when a child's symptoms are "extremely debilitating," adding:

> *Though no cases of addiction have been reported by clinicians working with hyperactive children or adolescents, the possibility cannot yet be dismissed. We have also found greatly increased heart rates in some of the children in our short-term studies; we have*

> *no data as yet on long-term effects. We find, too, that a few of our children become extremely depressed and show strangely flattened affect while on the drugs. Thus, we believe that the drugs should be used only after a very careful evaluation of the child's problems and if they are used, the physician should stay in close contact in order to titrate dosage and to monitor the youngster's response.*

Unfortunately, these words of caution were all but forgotten in the decades to follow.

Of course, while Canadian researchers have played a key role in shaping the modern diagnostic concept of ADHD, the flow of ideas between Canada and its much larger neighbor to the south has by no means been in one direction. In a book chapter aptly titled "In the Elephant's Shadow,"[712] Canadian sociologists Claudia Malacrida and Tiffani Semach discuss the many ways in which American influences have shaped the debate on ADHD in Canada, both in the popular media and in professional forums.

Most of the parenting magazines sold in Canada are of American origin, as are the majority of books about parenting, psychology, and self-help. The lion's share of Canadian television programming is produced in America. Most of the experts quoted in stories about ADHD are American as well.[713]

The ADHD skeptics also get a hearing, but here too the debate is dominated by American voices, notably Dr. Breggin, whose books have sold well in Canada.[714]

In regard to patient advocacy, the picture is mixed. In the 1990's, the American-founded advocacy group CHADD could boast of forty chapters in Canada,[715] but since then the national organization has dissolved. CHADD Vancouver, the last remaining chapter of that organization in Canada, has re-named itself the ADD Vancouver Support Group. As of 19 September 2021, the organization's home page informs readers "Out of concern for our participants and speakers, we have decided to postpone the ADD Vancouver Support Group meetings until further notice." The website's content is rather sparse, and many of the links are broken.[716]

By contrast, the Center for ADHD Awareness Canada (CADDAC) appears to be thriving. Incorporated in 2006 as a national not-for-profit organization, CADDAC lobbies in support of ADHD-related legislation; provides networking between ADHD groups across Canada; sponsors workshops, conferences, and webinars as well as live shows for kids, teens, and adults with ADHD and their families and friends; produces educational materials for individuals and families affected by ADD as well as for medical professionals and educators; promotes the "Canadian ADHD Awareness Week"; and operates an extensive, content-rich website in addition to the organization's Facebook and Twitter pages.

Under "Funding Policy," the organization offers this meaningless disclaimer: "CADDAC only accepts funding for projects that we propose, or that we deem to be of benefit to our patient population such as families or individuals with ADHD,"[717] and then goes to list some of their corporate sponsors, including Takeda Canada and Janssen, not to mention Purdue Pharma, whose subsidiary Adlon Therapeutics is the manufacturer of Adhansia XR.

On 1 September 2021, Purdue Pharma was dissolved by a federal bankruptcy court judge following accusations the company had drastically downplayed the addictive nature of its blockbuster drug oxycontin and actively solicited high-volume prescribers for that product.[718] This is an extreme sanction, one usually reserved for the most egregious corporate offenders.

CADDAC's annual report, "2019 Accomplishments," repeats a familiar bait-and-switch argument: "Left untreated, ADHD can have devastating effects over the course of one's lifetime," going on to mention mood and anxiety disorders, substance use disorders, transportation accidents, suicides, injuries, teenage pregnancies, unemployment, underemployment, and incarceration—neatly sidestepping the question as to whether any of these outcomes is averted by drug treatment.

In regard to the educational and health services industries, here too the influence of the United States is obvious. US professional organizations for doctors, psychiatrists, psychologists, and teachers are much larger than their Canadian counterparts and actively recruit Canadian members, and US drugmakers actively target Canadian doctors for their marketing campaigns.[719]

However, once again Canadians have attempted to put their own unique stamp on things. The Canadian ADHD Resource Alliance (CADDRA) was incorporated as a not-for-profit national organization in 2006. The organization publishes the Canadian ADHD Practice Guidelines; hosts the annual CADDRA ADHD Conference; facilitates an annual ADHD Research Day; lobbies for increased resources for health care professionals and patients; and operates an "eLearning Portal" as a depository for webcasts, audio podcasts, ePosters, and article reviews. Membership is available only to practicing physicians, psychologists, and other health care professionals. The board of directors consists of eight medical doctors and one psychologist.

CADDRA's webpage[720] lists among its sponsors Janssen, Shire Canada, and Purdue Pharma, and offers this curiously defensive statement of self-exoneration:

> *As many medical organizations do, we also receive some funding from pharmaceutical companies through sponsorship of our annual conference and educational grants for specific projects proposed to the funder by CADDRA.*
>
> *Funding is not conditional on incorporating messaging that benefits the company or promotes their products—in fact this is strictly prohibited according to the Rx& D Stakeholder Relations Collaborative Partnership Guiding Principles available on the*

> *Rx& D website. Conference sponsors have no input into the accredited conference program or schedule. CADDRA stipulates in all agreements with corporate, or any other type of funders, that the organization has full control of content and messaging in proposed projects. No outside funding is sought or accepted for development, review and publication of the Canadian ADHD Practice Guidelines. CADDRA continues to work towards diversification of its funding base to obtain financial support for education, training and advocacy projects from a variety of private and public funded sources.*

The first iteration of the Canadian ADHD Practice Guidelines was issued in 2011. The guidelines reviewed similar documents issued by both the United States (the *DSM*, the American Academy of Pediatrics) and United Kingdom (the National Institute for health and Clinical Excellence, the British Association for Psychopharmacology) and noted that the two countries have radically different approaches to this condition. In the UK, medication is used only for extreme cases, as a last resort, while in the US medication typically is the first resort. The CADDRA guidelines called for a "holistic-based care, individualized to the patients," including education for patients and families, behavioral strategies, psychological treatment, and educational accommodations, with medication used as a way to facilitate the other interventions. The clear implication was that the Canadians intended to steer a middle course between those charted by the US and the UK.[721] How has that worked out?

Canadians are proud of their generous federally-funded health care system,[722] which provides access to the services of doctors and other health care professionals. ADHD patients with complex needs can be referred to "centers of excellence." Telehealth and air transport of patients facilitate the delivery of care across that nation's wide-open spaces.[723]

However, public health funding does not cover the services of psychologists, educators, or social workers, which means that low-income patients do not have the same access to non-medical treatment that high-income patients and their families enjoy. ADHD diagnosis and treatment in Canada are managed almost exclusively by medical personal without significant input from teachers, leading Dr. Malacrida and Ms. Semach to conclude "In practice it is unlikely that such interventions will be implemented as part of a sustained, collaborative treatment approach."[724]

This exclusivity of the medical approach is borne out by the fact that the current ADHD Practice Guidelines are available on the CADDRA website—but only to paying members. Despite promises of holistic, patient-based care, the rate of diagnosis and drugging for ADHD in Canada is second only to that of the United States.[725]

ADHD in Ghana

A team of three Dutch researchers—sociologist Christian Bröer, anthropologist Rachel Spronk, and psychotherapist Viktor Kraak—conducted the first study on the clinical use of the ADHD diagnosis in Ghana, or indeed in any sub-Saharan African country besides South Africa.[726] They contacted all the major mental health clinics, private clinics, and university departments and asked them to identify all clinicians who use the ADHD diagnosis. The search yielded ten clinicians (four psychiatrists, four clinical psychologists, and two pediatricians), and the researchers were able to speak to eight of these. Only one of these (a psychiatrist) operated outside the capital city of Accra, and that one was based in Kumasi, the former capital of the Ashanti Empire and Ghana's second largest city. All but one of these clinicians had been educated in Western countries.

The number of children treated for ADHD each year by each of these clinicians ranged from two to several hundred. All but one of the clinicians rendered the diagnosis of ADHD by means of unstructured observations and verbal reports.[727]

In Ghana, all citizens are covered by the National Health Insurance Scheme. ADHD is recognized in the Standard Treatment Guidelines for that nation, and the only medication recommended is methylpheni-date. Nevertheless, that drug is rarely prescribed. Instead, children with the ADHD label commonly are prescribed tranquilizing drugs, notably haloperidol and chlorpromazine, as well as the anticonvulsant carbamaz-epine, the tricyclic antidepressant imipramine, and the "non-stimulant" ADHD drug atomoxetine.[728]

Prescriptions for haloperidol, chlorpromazine, carbamazepine, and imipramine all are subsidized under the National Health Insurance Scheme, whereas those for atomoxetine and methylphenidate are not. The cost of a month's supply of methylphenidate in Ghana is approximately eighty dollars, whereas a month's supply of atomoxetine retails for two hundred dollars. In a nation with an annual per capita GDP of $1,770, obviously these prices are out of reach for all but the wealthiest citizens.[729]

Dr. Bröer and his colleagues surveyed the popular media in Ghana and could find no references to that diagnostic category prior to 2008. Since then there have been a few tentative efforts by NGO's to raise awareness of ADHD in that country. The UK-based CarePlus Ghana has used Janssen's promotional video materials, and in 2010 the Ghanaian African Social Development Foundation, in collaboration with the Dutch National Committee for International Cooperation and Sustainable Development, produced a seminar on ADHD in Ghana.[730]

From the foregoing account it should be obvious that the diagnostic concept of ADHD has barely begun to penetrate the national conscious-ness in Ghana, and there only in a tiny minority of affluent, western-leaning citizens living in that nation's two largest cities. In the rest of the country, childish misbehavior is dealt with as it always has been, through corporal punishment, spiritual interventions, and prayer.[731]

In theory, public education in Ghana is free, but in practice many children end up staying home due to their parents' inability to afford school fees or supplies.[732] Child labor is still a huge problem in that country,[733] and the reader could be forgiven for wondering whether efforts to raise "ADHD awareness" should be considered a priority.

ADHD in France

The history of ADHD in France—or *TDAH*, for *Trouble du Déficit de l'Attention avec Hyperactivité*, the name by which that diagnostic category is known there—has been documented in a 2018 book chapter by French sociologists Madeleine Akrich and Vololona Rabeharisoa and a 2019 review article by sociologist Manuel Vallée of the University of Auckland.[734]

Ciba-Geigy made Ritalin available in France in 1975—fourteen years after that drug was placed on the market in the United States. A number of onerous restrictions were placed on the drug, which was classified as a "narcotic" with a high potential for abuse and dependency. The first prescription had to be written in hospital, by a specialist—i.e. a psychiatrist, neurologist, or pediatrician—and had to be renewed by the treating physician every twenty-eight days. Only three hospitals in the entire country had permission to distribute the drug, and parents could obtain only a week's supply at a time.[735]

Not surprisingly, demand for Ritalin remained low—so low, in fact, when Ciba-Geigy's license to distribute the drug in France expired in 1985, the company didn't bother to renew it for ten years.[736]

Slowly, the tide began to turn. The first book on this subject published in France, *L'Hyperactivité chez l'Enfant*, by Michel Dugas, was released in 1987.[737] In 1995, Ciba-Geigy's license to distribute the drug was renewed, at the behest of a cadre of French pediatricians and neurologists who lobbied the have the drug made available again—but only for the most seriously impaired children. Some of the restrictions previously imposed were lifted—the drug was made available at all hospital pharmacies, and parents could now obtain an entire month's supply at a time.

The French advocacy group HyperSupers was founded in 2002 to provide information and support for patients and their families. Since then the number of books, news articles, and scientific papers about ADHD has soared.[738]

The tone of the articles has changed as well. Akrich and Rabeharisoa report that between 1998 and 2004, two-thirds of the papers published expressed doubts about the validity of this diagnostic category, with one researcher sarcastically referring to ADD as "American Democratic Disability." But three-fourths of papers published between 2005 and 2012 treated the condition as a bona fide neurological disorder.[739]

In 2011, psychologist Stephen Faraone, in collaboration with two French researchers, published the first (and still the only) estimate of the incidence of ADHD in that country.[740] Using information gleaned from telephone interviews, the researchers concluded that 3.5% of children had a diagnosis of ADHD, with a preponderance of boys bearing that diagnosis, concluding "Our work suggests that the epidemiology of ADHD in France is similar to the epidemiology of ADHD as reported by other countries." This may have had the effect of reinforcing the position of this diagnostic category in the minds of some as a "real" disease.[741]

As acceptance of the diagnostic category of ADHD has risen in France, so have prescriptions for Ritalin. Sales of that drug have risen from 50,000 boxes in 2000 to 280,000 in 2008 to 500,000 in 2013.[742] By 2017, annual consumption had soared to over 800,000 boxes.[743] Nevertheless, a report issued that year by the ASNM (the Agence Nationale de Sécurité du Médicament et des Produits de Santé, the French equivalent of the FDA) claimed that several times as many children could benefit from Ritalin as the number currently receiving it, and an article in *Le Figaro* lamented the under-prescription of that drug.[744]

In July of 2021, the ANSM reported that the regulations restricting the prescribing of Ritalin have been widely ignored, with thirty percent of treatment recommendations carried out by independent doctors, both specialists and generalists.[745] The rule that the initial prescription had to be obtained in hospital was officially waived in September of that year.[746]

The slow but growing acceptance of the medical model of ADHD by no means has eclipsed alternative approaches to that condition. Indeed, French psychiatry has a long-standing tradition of treating the complaints that fall under the diagnostic rubric of "mental illness" with empathy and compassion. This psychodynamic approach, with its emphasis on individual case histories rather than symptom checklists and symptom suppression, dates at least as far back as the Eighteenth Century, with Phillippe Pinel's efforts to humanize care at the Salpêtrière[747] and continues to this day.

In 1983, the FFP, or the Fédération Française de Psychiatrie, released the first edition of the *CFTMEA*, or the *Classification Française des Troubles Mentaux de l'Enfant et de l'Adolescent*, as an explicit reaction to the APA's newly released *DSM-III*. Revised versions of this document were released in 1988, 2000 and 2012.[748] A number of factors make a less likely that children will be diagnosed and/or drugged for ADHD when the French criteria are used.

Firstly, the French criteria are more restrictive, excluding inattention without hyperactivity and stipulating that the problems be of sustained duration—thereby limiting the number of children who will receive the diagnosis in the first place. Secondly, the lack of a symptom checklist may encourage clinicians to conceptualize a child's problems in a broader psychological and social context. The *CFTMEA* explicitly encourages clinicians to consider psychological factors such as "emotional, educational, social and cultural deficiencies as well as bad treatments and negligence." To the extent that they succeed at addressing these factors, fewer children will be judged as needing medication. Finally, this multidisciplinary approach to etiology may tend to promote a multidisciplinary approach to treatment, one in which stimulant medication is seen as a last resort, rather than a first resort.[749]

Many French psychiatrists continue to view medication warily, as a distraction from the real business of finding out what is going on in a child's world that is so distressing. In 2005, *Le Monde* ran a piece on

ADHD which quoted Bernard Golse, head of the psychiatry unit at a children's hospital in Paris:

> *With Ritalin, the mystery remains unsolved since the meaning of the disorder still has to be worked out in regard to each child's history*[750].

This multiplicity of approaches is reflected in the actions of the advocacy group HyperSupers, which tends to take an agnostic view regarding the nature of that condition and a eclectic approach to treatment.[751] In 2011, that group conducted the first and only survey of how French children and their families deal with ADHD and found that thirty-nine percent of patients were engaged in psychotherapy, twenty-seven percent in speech and language therapy, and nineteen percent in psychomotor therapy. Forty-four percent of these children had received an individualized education plan at their schools, while twenty percent had been excluded from school at least once, thirty percent had repeated at least one grade, and half of the parents reported having a difficult or very difficult relationship with teachers.[752]

In 2014, a working group composed of pediatricians, neurologists, psychologists, speech therapists, teachers, health care administrators, and disability administration officers released a position paper intended to provide guidelines for the Ministère de la Santé for the organization of care for children with learning impairments, including ADHD. The report called for a multi-pronged approach, with children divided into three tiers. The first would include those with difficulties that call for light intervention; the second would include children with ADHD of medium intensity; while the third would include complex or severe cases. The report also acknowledged that the expertise needed to effect such a division was lacking—doctors and teachers were insufficiently trained, while evidence for the efficacy of therapies was generally absent.[753]

The debate of the working group highlighted the uncertainties and divisions that characterize the debate over ADHD in France, with some members calling for the abolition of diagnosis in favor of individual history while others, in a stunning example of flipping the script, cautioned that the emphasis on psychological and social factors could lead to dangerous underdiagnosis of ADHD in children from disadvantaged backgrounds.[754]

Given the diversity of views in France regarding the nature of the complaints which fall under the diagnostic rubric of ADHD, it is little wonder that while prescriptions for Ritalin have skyrocketed in recent years, per capita consumption of the drug remains less than five percent of what it is in the United States.[755]

In October of 2021, the French government held a two-day conference on mental health and psychiatry which an article by the news network France24 described as "an attempt to rejuvenate a failing branch of the French medical establishment."[756]

The article quoted child psychiatrist Marie-José Durieux who lamented the decline of French psychiatry:

> *Just 30 years ago, psychiatry was practiced with a lot of interest and excitement. We associated psychiatry with imaginative sciences like philosophy, psychoanalysis, sociology and literature.*

Dr. Durieux blamed the decline on drugs and that American import, the *DSM*. "Medication alone is not enough to solve existential problems," she averred. Whether these concerns will lead to lasting changes remains to be seen.

Finding the Right Niche for Ourselves

When I asked Dr. Healy why Europe and the rest of the world has yet to embrace the disease model of ADHD to the extent that North America has, he related that reluctance to the Jungian concepts of introversion and extraversion—concepts which, he says, never really caught on here.

In an essay, Dr. Jung characterized the introvert as reflective, with a tendency toward caution, while the extravert is prone to impulsivity and novelty seeking.[757] The psychiatrist Hans Eysenck conceptualized the two types as lying at opposite ends of a continuum, and suggested that the avoidant behavior of the introvert, and the novelty-seeking of the extravert, reflect largely inborn differences in arousability, with the nervous system of extravert being less arousable, while that of the introvert more so.[758]

Modern research has since confirmed that the introversion-extraversion dichotomy is biologically-based. Scores on introversion-extraversion scales predict individual responses to anaesthesia.[759]

Dr. Healy explained:

> *The ones who come along talking about being anxious or depressed, they're the introverts, and the ones coming along figuring they've got ADHD and that they need meds for their ADHD are the extraverts. Half of the people come along to me and complain about having too much focus. And the other half are people who come along and say It seems I don't have focus enough.*

Dr. Healy explained that these different personality styles used to be seen as part of the normal range of human variation, rather than as pathologies in need of medical treatment:

> *There's some of us who focus more than we should, and need to loosen up, and there's others who maybe aren't as quite focused and there are times when the answer may be they need to focus more. And, you know, the world needs people who can focus well, and also those who maybe don't focus quite as much.*

He went on to tell the story of a patient of his, a young man studying at university who was bright, personable, had big ideas, and knew how to get other people excited about his ideas. This young man dreamed of being an entrepreneur, and he got into his head the idea that the way to do that was to study business and get a job at a giant corporation and work his way up the career ladder. But he found his coursework required him to spend long hours working on spreadsheets—a task which bored him and failed to inspire him. So he began taking ADHD meds to improve his concentration, and he did manage to finish his degree and get a job at a giant corporation, only to find himself doing—more spreadsheets!

You will never become an entrepreneur while working at a corporation like this. The idea of getting on with life is to find the right niche for ourselves. And if you're more extraverted and you've got a loose kind of focus, you're going to be more creative and entrepreneurial, and you don't want to go into corporations. On the other hand, if you're more introverted, more of a detail person, spreadsheets may be just the thing for you.

But whether you're introvert or extravert, really both types are up against the same kind of problem, which is: These days the world doesn't want people to be varied. It's wants us to be homogenous, it's got to be pro forma tick boxes, we all have to be meeting the same quality standards. The idea of a team has gone out the window, you know, the idea that we need people who can score goals and people who can make sure the other team don't score goals. That's all gone out the window. We just want everybody to fit into the same mold which isn't a good situation for either introverts or extraverts, okay?

In Europe there's probably a little more understanding of this way of speaking. There's no one over here that talks this way. Over here people are a lot more categorical. You know, this is why DSM-III to some extent worked so well, with a bunch of labels. The people over here want their labels, they don't want to take these things away.

It's a curious kind of situation. People like me who want to tell people that they're not mentally ill but they're actually pretty capable, they've had a bad deal from life but they've done all too well coping with it—I mean they're not mentally ill in the sense of brokenness, and they probably know the drugs are going to disable rather than enable them—that kind of message doesn't go down all that well. And this is not drug company crooks or ADHD experts bringing it, it's the way the world is going, and as with a bunch of these things, the world seems to go that way a lot quicker in the United States than anywhere else.

Late Capitalism and the *DSM*

But why is the rest of the world going that way? If it's not just drug company crooks and ADHD experts bringing it, then what is? In search of more answers, I called James Davies, a former psychotherapist who is currently a Reader in Medical Anthropology at Roehampton University in London and the author of *Sedated: How Modern Capitalism Created Our Mental Health Crisis.*[760] Here is what he had to say:

> *One of the areas that interests me is the extent to which our mental health sector has colluded with the current style of economy under which we all now live, which has been variously termed late capitalism, neoliberalism, new capitalism, etc. Our mental health sector has in some sense become an agent of late capitalism, serving its needs at the expense of those people seeking help. And so one of the reasons why the interventions of psychiatry have become so popular in the last thirty years—and mostly psychopharmaceutical interventions—is because these interventions slot with the aims and directives of late capitalism; serving this paradigm very well.*
>
> *Firstly, these interventions have been hugely profitable, with the global psychiatric drug market now worth over $25 billion each year. This has made a lot of people very wealthy, including shareholders and, to lesser extent, those mental health professionals*

and organizations in receipt of industry money. In this sense, medicalization has transformed suffering into a commodity from which profit can be derived.

Psychiatric interventions also depoliticize suffering—they target the self rather than the circumstances in which people are caught up. The ideology that underpins the prescribing of these drugs depoliticizes distress as well. It tells us we are struggling with internal dysfunctions that need 'treating,' rather than from natural protests against bad circumstances that need to be addressed and changed. So the philosophy supports a kind of political quietism that's good for the status quo.

The underpinning philosophy also decollectivizes suffering. If suffering points to a malfunction within the self, so there's no good in coming together with others to explore the collective nature of one's distress, which could potentially lead to groups coming together and lobbying for change. Our paradigm, to some extent, inoculates from that process, dispersing any communal suffering into self-residing dysfunctions.

I could go on, but there are a number of different ways in which the mental health sector serves current neoliberal arrangements. And I think this can explain why mental health interventions, psychopharmaceutical interventions, have flourished exponentially over the last thirty to forty years, despite these interventions having presided over a period where mental health outcomes have not only flatlined but, according to some measures, have actually got worse. So the reason why psychiatric drugs have proliferated is not due to their outcomes (which are generally poor) but because they serve late capitalist directives and aims.

The rest of the world has followed the lead of the US, with the regulatory agencies co-opted by the industries they were purported to regulate.

This has created an autocatalytic process which has spread from the US and the UK to the rest of the world:

> *So, for example, the financial services regulatory agencies in the UK and the US—who set the rules for banking behavior—were run and funded by the financial sector itself—which led to very lenient regulation, as you'd expect. This in turn was the major driver of the economic crisis of 2007-2008, which was essentially caused by the fraudulent behavior that the agencies did absolutely nothing about.*
>
> *The same dynamic still operates in the pharmaceutical sector, where, since the 1980s, pharmaceutical regulation has been gradually handed over to the pharmaceutical industry itself. In the UK, the drug regulator is now 100% funded by fees by the pharmaceutical industry. It's also been run by ex-industry professionals (e.g. the previous CEO of our regulator—the MHRA - was a director of GlaxoSmithKline for seven years prior to his appointment). So there is a hugely problematic revolving door policy.*
>
> *In addition, all the national regulatory agencies now literally compete with each other for licensing fees from the pharma companies. These fees are needed to pay salaries and keep these organizations afloat. And of course you are more likely to attract licensing fees if your regulatory processes are relatively lenient vis-a-vis your competitor.*
>
> *So, there's been a kind of market in the regulatory sector that has incentivized lenient regulation, as that brings in market fees. This has created a race to the bottom in terms of regulatory standards, one favouring pharma interests over the interests of patients to be prescribed drugs that are safe and effective.*

Along with "deregulation" (which turned out to be a code word for regulatory capture), the paradigm of late capitalism touted slashing of funding and increased surveillance of the public sector—two actions which helped stoke the demand for ADHD drugs:

> *I think we've seen that hugely in the school population. In the UK we have a real problem in the schools right now because we've cut funding a huge amount since in particular 2008 and 2009, with the financial crisis which was, in my view, caused by deregulation. We've cut school funding so teachers are under duress, class sizes are bigger, but at the same time we are cutting funding, we have put more and more pressure on schools to deliver good outcomes.*
>
> *So schools are under pressure. They've got to demonstrate efficacy and good educational outcomes, and they have to hit draconian government targets to avoid various government sanctions. But they're having to this without adequate resources. So they're caught in a terrible situation, which leads them to reach anywhere for some respite. And special needs labels, diagnostic labels, are a really good resource. If you characterize the kids in the class who are disruptive as having a special needs or behavioural problem, then you get resources in, to help those kids, and special dispensations which help you in the league tables. The system therefore incentivizes educators to medicalize child behaviour. And so they become victims just as much as the kids, because they are often using these labels to solve other policy problems about which they feel entirely impotent.*
>
> *Some could counter by asking what's wrong with medicalization? Some kids need more help—and psychiatric labels bring that, right? My response is that, while I agree that many of these children will need additional support, this can be achieved without medicalizing children. These labels have stigmatizing effects that can compound children's problems. Also, medicalization opens the door to medication—which is why about seventy percent of these kids who get these labels end up on psychotropic drugs. And we*

know the problems associated with children taking psychotropic drugs. So the door is opened to forms of intervention that aren't necessarily actually helpful. In the end they may become very detrimental to the kid in question.

What about adult ADHD?

Well, I think it's the same mechanism at play when you look at any behavior that society sees as problematic. So depression is stigmatized in neoliberal societies because depression costs economies money. It slows people down. They become introspective. They often don't work at their optimum. They will ask questions that people who aren't depressed probably won't. It is an economically inconvenient experience from the standpoint of employers or the State.

ADHD is similar along those lines. Further, if you can locate the cause of your predicament in something that's apparently gone awry within you, then you acquit yourself from a lot of responsibility for why things have gone awry, and also you acquit your community, the people around you, from responsibility. That's very consoling.

In some cases it can also be in a strange way consoling to parents if the reason for the child's challenging behavior is because they've got some diagnosable mental disorder. This gives them the reassurance of having an answer, of now knowing what is wrong. Now presumably the doctors can help. Some may also experience the label as a green light to no longer wonder about what may be wrong at home, or whether you're working too hard, or arguing too much, or not giving the kid the right food, or adequate play time. Maybe you no longer have to worry about the effects of living in deprivation and working all hours to pay the rent. I mean there's so many situational factors here that can account for why a child is experienced as difficult, or why an adult isn't fitting in.

Do you think these drugs actually make adults more productive in the workplace?

Oh, they've certainly been marketed in that way. But there is a problem, since in most cases, suffering is the organism's protest against something that has gone wrong and needs to be addressed. So if you ignore the suffering or try to medicalize it or medicate it away, then often you're denying yourself a process of learning and introspection that's necessary in order to get to the next stage of your maturation.

In our society we've lost touch with the notion that suffering is part and parcel of what is means to grow as a human being. It is part of the process of waking up and growing up—even acute suffering. If you cut off that idea, and cease using suffering productively in that respect, then you're denying yourself growth, and growth leads to ways of operating in the world that are more healthy for everyone—for the workplace, for your colleagues, for your friends, your family, as a parent, as a sibling, as a husband, as a wife, and so forth. So sedating the mechanisms by which people grow and learn is really not helpful in the long run.

If they're not helpful, why do people continue to take them?

I think people have been sold the idea that suffering is a useless encumbrance best swiftly removed. That's what capitalism tells us. It tells us that suffering is antithetical to life. And by the way, here's a product that you can take to help you avoid it. Lots of industries thrive on the narrative that suffering is useless but can, fortunately, be consumed away. And people find that idea attractive.

And of course you can have sympathy when people are overworked and underpaid and under duress. The last thing they want is to start to suffer, in addition to all their other problems, you know? And so the idea that there is a drug that you can take that can acquit you from this issue that is debilitating and difficult and painful, is a very attractive one, but ultimately one that regularly backfires.

If suffering leads to growth, why would anybody not want that, for himself or others?

Well, most organizations don't want people 'to grow' and 'to evolve'—they just want them to turn up every day on time and do their job, which I understand. But, a lot of the jobs out there in modern society, as the data show, are uninspiring and deadening—experienced as meaningless. The last thing employers want are people sitting down and thinking about the meaning of their work, because they'd have an existential crisis and rebel or possibly leave the corporation. They want functional people who accept the reality with which they are presented and do the job set them.

And so we have a terrible crisis right now in our workplace economy, where two-thirds of the adults now identify as dissatisfied with, and/or emotionally disengaged from, the work they do. About forty percent believe that their jobs are completely meaningless, that the world wouldn't miss these jobs if they disappeared overnight. They don't give anything of value to the world but people do them because, you know, it pays the rent and what else can they do?—well, I suppose they can always take a drug, which is what they are told.

Sankofa

After I finished speaking to Dr. Davies, I could not help but reflect on how similar his views on psychiatric drugs in general, and stimulant drugs for children in particular, were to those of Dr. Breggin—despite these two men coming from two very different points along the political spectrum.

May I be allowed a personal observation here? If my experience with the Critical Psychiatry movement has taught me anything, it is this: the fact that someone is skeptical of the value of psychiatric interventions and the disease model of "mental illness" tells you nothing about where that person stands on other issues. Such a person may be far right, or far left, or anywhere in between. What unites these folks is a conviction that we could do a better job than we are doing in creating institutions that meet actual human needs.

Perhaps this movement has the potential to evolve into something bigger. And perhaps all these disparate viewpoints from all along the political spectrum have something to contribute toward that task.

The people of Ghana have a saying, *San ko fa*, which literally means "Return, go, take." It is an admonition to remember the past and extract the lessons to be learned to help us move forward towards a brighter future. Perhaps that is something we all need to do.

CHAPTER NINETEEN

SEARCH IN YOUR HEART

Memories

Springfield Elementary School, where I began my formal education more than fifty years ago, stands alongside Route 212 in Pleasant Valley PA, right next to the Trinity United Church of Christ. I can hear the carillon bells playing, a melody from a time that seems at once fantastically remote and eerily familiar, as long-slumbering memories begin to stir. On an early Sunday morning in October, not another soul is in sight, but in my mind's eye I can see scores of children, running, laughing, shouting, playing, fulfilling their childhoods.

It seems as if we were in constant motion back then—climbing up to the top of the sliding board, whizzing down, and scurrying back around for another go, swinging on the swings, going up and down on the see-saw, clambering around on the monkey bars, taking turns pushing each other on the merry-go-round. After school we played tag or hide-and-go-seek, or rode our bikes, or climbed trees, or explored the nearby woods. In the summertime I kept an aquarium stocked entirely with creatures I had collected from the local streams and ponds—tadpoles, minnows, whirligig beetles, water striders, snails, flatworms, and my pride and joy—two crayfish, each of which I had daringly plucked from the water with my own fingers before sprinting home with my prize. In the wintertime, we would tote our sleds to a nearby farm, drag them up to the top of the hill and go zooming down, only to drag them back up again, and again, and again.

I have returned here, to the playground of my childhood, to gain some insight into the question: What is behind the explosive increase in diagnosis and drugging of children for something called "ADHD?" Are there really millions of children out there who were born with an "organic brain disorder" that requires daily drug treatment—or can the answer be found in the ways society has changed over the years?

When I was a boy, children were expected to sit quietly in class—and they did so, most of the time—but they also were allowed to run free during gym class, during recess, and then again after school for the rest of the day, every day, until dark. None of us had perfect parents, but you didn't need to be a perfect parent back then, because if you were a parent society had your back. Grownups were in charge, and everybody knew it. Even the juvenile delinquents knew it. They would break the rules when grownups weren't looking, but even they would not have dreamed of directly challenging grownup authority.

Every evening we ate dinner together as a family, all seated around the eight-foot dining table, patterned after an old Shaker design, which my grandfather had built with his own two hands. After dinner, we had television—a little black-and-white job—but with only three channels, which had to be all things to all people, most of the time there wasn't even anything on that a little kid would want to watch. Laptops and smartphones didn't exist then—not even in the realm of science fiction. Instead, we occupied ourselves with books or board games, or—believe it or not—talking to each other.

Back then it was taken for granted that any man willing and able to work hard would be able to find steady employment, and would be paid enough to afford the house and the car and wife and the kids. Public and private organizations valued loyal employees, and worked hard to earn and keep that loyalty. The guaranteed student loan program did not exist, and any competent person could work his or her way through college and graduate owing nothing.

There wasn't anything like the relentless pressure to consume there is now. I wore hand-me-down clothes from my older brothers, and my mother cut my hair until I was sixteen years old. Tattoos were for drunken sailors, or assorted lowlifes. The phrase "designer jeans" did not exist in the English language. The family sedan or station wagon was a device for getting from one place to another, period—gigantic gas-guzzling SUV's with cupholders and padded armrests and touch-screen video monitors were undreamt-of.

On those rare occasions that we needed medical attention, we availed ourselves of the services of the respected town doc, whose daughter attended the local public high school right alongside the rest of us. There was no such thing as direct-to-consumer advertising for drugs, for ADHD or any other condition.

I never even heard of ADHD—or "hyperactivity," as it was then known—until I was a senior in high school. I was appalled to learn that grownups were giving speed to little kids. I've changed my mind about a lot of things since, but that isn't one of them.

A National Disaster

Instead of teaching children wisdom, temperance, fortitude, and justice, we school them in "mental health awareness," encouraging them to think of themselves as fragile creatures whose brains can go haywire at any time, for no apparent reason—and to look for succor in a bottle of pills. Nearly fifty years ago, psychologist L. Alan Sroufe raised concerns that these drugs are a "chemical cop-out" and a distraction from looking for real solutions to real problems. Since then we have devolved into a drug-obsessed dystopia

Philip K. Dick could not have imagined in his worst nightmares. Total annual spending on ADHD treatments now exceeds twenty billion dollars.

And it isn't just stimulant drugs whose consumption has skyrocketed—prescriptions for antidepressant and antipsychotic drugs for youths have skyrocketed as well.[761] And what are we getting for all this relentless drugging?

The kids are not all right. The proportion of youths afflicted with often crippling depression and bipolar disorder has soared, along with the youth suicide rate and overdose death rate.[762]

This is not what happens when treatments work.

Even some of the biggest names in the field now seem appalled by the monster they have helped create. The late C.K. Conners, author of the Conners Comprehensive Behavior Rating Scale and one of the principal investigators of the MTA study, called skyrocketing rates of ADHD diagnosis "a national disaster of dangerous proportions."[763] Roger Griggs, the pharmaceutical company executive who introduced Adderall in 1994, has referred to stimulant drugs as "nuclear bombs" whose use is warranted only under extreme circumstances.[764] And Edward Hallowell, the doyen of adult ADHD, has warned "We are pathologizing boyhood… Schools want these little goody-goodies who sit still and do what they're told— these robots—and that's not who boys are."[765]

As if all this were not enough, a 7 January 2020 article in *Business Insider* discussed parents who are treating their children's "ADHD" with "medical marijuana."[766] The piece did not mention what the people who thought this was a good idea had been smoking.

The following year, a review paper in the March/April issue of the *Harvard Review of Psychiatry*[767] noted that the risk of Parkinson's disease was elevated a staggering six-to-eight times in individuals who had been prescribed stimulant medication for ADHD. Studies in animal models have shown that amphetamine and methamphetamine produce the same changes in the brain—including protein misfolding—that are associated with Parkinson's. (Interestingly, Ritalin does not produce these effects.)

The reader will note that most of the Hill criteria for establishing cause and effect have been satisfied here. In plain English, these drugs are causing Parkinson's disease. Children ingesting these substances today may be suffering these ill effects decades from now.

On 2 April 2021, the pharmaceutical firm Supernus announced the FDA had approved the so-called "orphan drug" Qelbree (viloxazine) for the treatment of ADHD. In a press statement, the CEO of Supernus proclaimed "Qelbree provides prescribing physicians and patients living with ADHD a therapy that is not a controlled substance with proven efficacy and a tolerable safety profile."[768] The full prescribing information for Qelbree warns of somnolence, headache (including migraine headache with aura), decreased appetite, fatigue, pyrexia, nausea, vomiting, insomnia, irritability, and suicidal thoughts and behaviors.[769]

The dystopian nightmare Peter Schrag and Diane Divoky warned us about almost half a century ago—with its sinister hybrid of mind control and round-the-clock surveillance—has become today's humdrum reality. But even they probably never could have imagined today's Covid Republic with children muzzled and taught to fear the very air they breathe, in addition to being plied with brain-altering drugs.

What started out as a perhaps well-intentioned effort to aid seriously disturbed kids—many of them in institutional settings, many of them with a demonstrated history of brain damage—has metastasized into the wholesale drugging of millions of children and adults. Concomitant with this has arisen a vast industry of neuroimaging and genome-wide association studies that has generated mountains of data without producing a single finding that has benefitted a single patient—but which does serve to lend the whole enterprise a veneer of scientific respectability.

A recent NIMH grant application proposed "to investigate the role of frontostriatal glutamatergic metabolism in medication-naive children with ADHD using proton magnetic resonance spectroscopy at 7.0 Tesla." What is this supposed to tell us about how to teach a child to read? Or how to raise children to grow up to be strong, self-reliant adults? This is an industry that has lost all sight of what it means to be human.

And yet, a residential program for boys with behavior problems (later opened to girls as well) reported great success in treating problem children, without any drugs at all.

The children enrolled in this program were a far cry from the kid-who-fidgets-too-much or the kid-who-daydreams-too-much. All of the children had suffered from encephalitis due to infection or brain trauma, and while their intelligence had been unaffected, these kids had serious problems in their relations with others. They defied authority, set fires, tormented other children, stole, vandalized property, spat on people, suffered from insomnia, wandered the streets at night, and acted out sexually. They were hyperkinetic, easily distracted, and showed marked emotional lability. These behaviors were found to be completely refractory even to severe punishment.[770]

The program emphasized order, structure, discipline, and kindness. In addition to their schoolwork, the children were provided with psycho-therapy, occupational therapy (basket weaving, carpentry, gardening, etc.), regular chores, and an hour of exercise a day in either the pool or the gym, along with hours of unstructured indoor and outdoor play time every day.[771]

Of the first eighty-five children to pass through this program, eighty of them displayed moderate or marked improvement in their behavior. The children gained insight into their problems, their sleep disorders went away, and they learned how to get along with their brothers and sisters and other children.[772]

Although, sadly, most of these children regressed when released to their home environments[773]—indicating that the brain lesions they had suffered from were not the only source of their problems.

The outcomes for this program were published in 1935—two years before Charles Bradley came forward with his study on the effects of dosing problem children with amphetamine at the Emma Pemberton Bradley Home.

Unconditional Love

When we look at the young, not just of our own species but those of our closest relatives, the monkeys and apes—and probably all species of mammals—hyperactivity is the norm. The young ones are constantly running, playing, exploring their environment, learning to take control of their environment. That is normal. What is decidedly abnormal is the flattening of affect and hyperfocus on boring tasks induced by stimulant drugs.

I asked Dr. Breggin what it was about the process by which people become psychiatrists that seems to select for those who regard the normal as abnormal, and the abnormal as normal. This was his reply:

> *There's been a very big shift in who goes into psychiatry. It used to be that many of us who went into psychiatry knew we had personal problems, we benefitted from therapy, and so in medical school we learned we can find help with ourselves, we love to help other people, and so you go into practice.*
>
> *People like that were kind and caring, and while they had their own array of human difficulties, they were smart enough to get into medical school. Now, if you become a psychiatrist, you have been engaged in nothing like therapy. It's not taught in medical school, it's not taught in most psychiatric residencies. You have to believe in primarily drugs, or only drugs.*
>
> *So then they end up with the idea that anything you have, like ADHD, is a chronic disorder, and we have to jump in to treat it, the earlier the better, even though none of the drugs have been*

proven to have any positive long-term effects—and they're all proven to be disastrous long-term.

There are no primitive societies which try to educate their children by roping them all off in segregation from the rest of the adults, in an area where they couldn't relate to nature, being lectured to by the most boring person in the tribe all day long. That has never been done before. And so it is entirely abnormal to ask children to spend a lot of their day doing very boring things under very confined circumstances, often without proper nutrition, always without nearly enough exercise.

Children have always learned by doing things with adults. In all cultures, including our own, children are just full of energy, hard to pin down, they want to run around and do things, and it takes a skill to engage them—a loving skill. Not force, but an exciting adult to lovingly engage them and keep their attention.

Now people like [child psychiatrist Harold] Koplewicz can't make a living doing this. They don't know how to do this. They don't understand it. They understand power.

Then I asked Dr. Breggin why Dr. Koplewicz's message of "It's nobody's fault" seems to resonate with so many people. This was his reply:

Often, when we ourselves are in trouble, we just don't want it to be our fault—but perhaps even more so when we've harmed other people. Then we really don't want it to be our fault. So the big market for books like Koplewicz's is that parents in particular want to say that they're not to blame for their kids' problems. Now what they miss in doing that is taking credit for healing, helping, and promoting the growth of their children.

The way I approach these issues in my practice is I start out and I say 'I'm not even in the beginning going to deal with how these problems originated in the family, because those are complex, and we may not have to examine them. What I'm going to help you do as parents is to use your enormous influence with your child in order to help your child grow, and heal, and overcome.'

And what happens in that process, where they learn to maintain unconditional love, where they learn to guide a child more by positives than by negatives in discipline, where they learn the power of encouragement, they learn to build a relationship with the child, because without a relationship you can't influence a child in a positive, loving, caring direction. The child has to want to please you—not to feel at war with you.

So I start out with my helping of the family by establishing a principle of respect. That means all communications will become respectful. That can be learned very quickly. Once respectful relating is established—everybody usually gets it in the first session—then I talk with them about unconditional love, which means you really search in your heart and find the love you have for one other.

ADD Vancouver Support Group. Accessed September 19, 2021. addvancouver-support.ca

ADHD Australia. "What is ADHD." Accessed September 10, 2021.https://www.adhdaustralis.org/about-adhd/what-is-attention-deficit-hyperactivity-disorder-adhd/

ADHD Europe. "ADHD Myths and Facts." Accessed September 10, 2021. https://adhdeurope.eu/awareness/myths-and-facts

ADHD Institute. Accessed September 10, 2021. https://adhd-institute.com

ADHD New Zealand. "Managing ADHD in Schools." Accessed September 10, 2021. https://www.adhd.org/nz/adhd-in-schools.html

ADHD UK. "Adult ADHD Self-Screening Tool." Accessed September 10, 2021. https://adhduk.co.uk/adult-adhd-screening-survey/

ADHD-200 Consortium. "The ADHD-200 Consortium: A Model to Advance the Translational Potential of Neuroimaging in Clinical Neuroscience." *Frontiers in Systems Neuroscience* 6, Article 62 (September 2012): 1-5. https://doi.org/10.3389/fnsys/2002.00062

Adhopia, Vic. "Children with ADHD Have Some Smaller Brain Regions, Study Shows." Canadian Broadcasting Corporation, February 16, 2017. cbc.ca/news/health/adhd-brain-structures-1.3983919

Adler, Leonard A., Thomas J. Spencer, Janet L. Ramsey, Roy Tamura, Douglas Kelsey, Susan G. Ball, Albert J. Allen, and Joseph Biederman.

"Functional Outcomes in the Treatment of Adults with ADHD." *Journal of Affective Disorders* 11, no. 6 (May 2008): 720-727. https://doi.org/10.1177/1087054707308490

Agence Nationale de Sécurité du Médicament et des Produits de Santé. "Méthylphénidate: Données d'Utilisation et de Sécurité d'Emploi en France." July 4, 2021. https://ansm.sante.fr/actualities/methylphenidate-donees-dutilisation-et-de-securite-demploi-en-france

Akrich, Madeleine, and Vololona Rabeharisoa. "The French ADHD Landscape." In *Global Perspectives on ADHD: Social Dimensions of Diagnosis and Treatment in Sixteen Countries*, edited by Meredith R. Bergey et al., 233-260. Baltimore: Johns Hopkins University Press, 2018.

Allen, Scott. "Backlash on Bipolar Diagnosis in Children." *Boston Globe*, June 17, 2007, A1, RA8.

Amhad, Farida B., and Robert N. Anderson. "The Leading Causes of Death in the US for 2020." *JAMA*, published online March 31, 2021. https://doi.org/10.1001.jama.2021.5649

Angell, Marcia. *The Truth About the Drug Companies*. New York: Random House, August 24, 2004.

Angell, Marcia. "Drug Companies and Doctors: A Story of Corruption." *New York Review of Books*, January 15, 2009. nybooks.com/articles/2009/01/15/drug-companies-doctorsa-story-of-corruption

Arcos-Burgos, Mauricio, and Maximillian Muenke. "Toward a Better Understanding of ADHD: *LPHN3* Gene Variants and the Susceptibility to Develop ADHD." *ADHD Attention Deficit Hyperactivity Disorders* 2, no. 3 (November 2010): 139-147. https://doi.org/10.1007/s12402-0030-2

Arria, Amelia M., Kevin E. O'Grady, Kimberly M. Caldeira, Kathryn B. Vincent, and Eric D. Wish. "Nonmedical Use of Prescription Stimulants and Analgesics: Associations with Social and Academic Behaviors among College Students." *Journal of Drug Issues* 38, no. 4 (Fall 2008): 1045-1060.

Aubusson, Kate. "'I Thought I Was a Loser, Now I Have the Answer': Rise in Adult ADHD." *Sydney Morning Herald*, November 3, 2019. https://www.smh.com.au/national/i-thought-i-was-a-loser-now-i-have-the-answer-rise-in-adult-adhd-20191101-p536kn.html

Bacon, John. "Ritalin Drug Abuse on the Rise." *USA Today*, August 3, 1988.

Bachmann, Christian J., Lise Aagard, Mehmet Burcu, Gerd Glaeske, Luuk
J. Kalverdik, Irene Peterson, Catharina C.M. Schuiling-Venninga, et al.
"Trends and Patterns of Antidepressant Use in Children and Adolescents
from Five Western Countries, 2005-2012." *European Neuropsychopharmacology* 26, (2016): 411-419. https://doi.org/10.1016/j.euroneuro.2016.02.001

Baney, Libby, Jillian Brady, and Sarah Lloyd Stevenson. "The Future of
Telehealth and the Ryan Haight Act Post-Pandemic." National Association
of Boards of Pharmacy, April 22, 2021. https://nabp.pharmacy/news/blog/
the-future-of-telehealth-and-the-ryan-haight-act-postppandemic/

Barclay, Dorothy. "A Turn for the Wiser." *Pediatrics* 23, no. 4 (April 1959):
759-760.

Barkley, Russell A. *Hyperactive Children: A Handbook for Diagnosis and Treatment.*
New York: Guilford Press, October 27, 1981.

Barkley, Russell A. "Attention-Deficit Hyperactivity Disorder." *Scientific
American* 279, no. 3 (September 1998): 66-71.

Barkley, Russell A. "This is How You Treat ADHD Based off Science."
September 23, 2014. https://www.youtube.com/watch?v=_tpB-B8BX-
k0&t=189s

Barkley, Russell A., and 20 Co-Endorsers. "Critique or Misrepresentation? A
Reply to Timimi et al." *Clinical Child and Family Psychology Review* 7, no. 1
(March 2004): 64-69. https://doi.org/10.1023/b:ccfp.0000020193.48817.30

Barkley, Russell A., Edwin H. Cook, Adele Diamond, Alan Zametkin, Anita
Thapar, Ann Teeter, Arthur D. Anastopoulos, et al. "International Consensus
Statement on ADHD." *Clinical Child and Family Psychology Review* 5, no. 2
(June 2002): 89-111. https://doi.org/10.1023/a:1017494719205

Barkley, Russell A., and Charles E. Cunningham. "Do Stimulant Drugs Improve
the Academic Performance of Hyperkinetic Children?" *Clinical Pediatrics* 17,
no. 1 (January 1978): 85-92. https://doi.org/10.1177/000992287801700112

Basu, Nisha, and Jonathan Bush. "Archaic In-Person Exam for Digital
Prescribing is Holding Back Health Care Innovation." *STAT*, December

8, 2021. https://www.statnews.com/2021/12/08/archaic-in-person-exam-law-barrier-digital-prescribing-health-care-innovation/

Baumeister, Alan A. "Is Attention Deficit/Hyperactivity Disorder a Risk Syndrome for Parkinson's Disease?" *Harvard Review of Psychiatry* 29, no. 2 (March/April 2021): 142-158. https://doi.org/10.1097. HRP/0000000000000283

Baumeister, Alan, and Mike F. Hawkins. "Incoherence of Neuroimaging Studies of Attention Deficit/Hyperactivity Disorder." *Clinical Neuropharmacology* 24, no. 1 (2001): 2-10. https://doi.org/10.1097/00002826-200101000-00002

Baumgartner, Anna, Mark L. Wolraich, and Mary Dietrich. "Comparison of Diagnostic Criteria for Attention Deficit Disorders in a German Elementary School Sample." *Journal of the American Academy of Child and Adolescent Psychiatry* 35, no. 5 (May 1995): 629-638. https://doi.org/10.1097/00004583-199505000-00015

Beall, Marsh F. "Disenchanted Students." *Science* 175, no. 4018 (January 1, 1972): 123. https://doi.org/10.1126/science.175.4918.123-b

Bell, Joseph N. "The Family that Fought Back." *McCall's*, May 1977, 26, 30, 32, 34, 36, 40.

Bercovici, Jeff. "Fired Yahoo Exec's $109M Golden Parachute Was One of the Biggest Ever." *Forbes*, January 16, 2014. https://www.forbes.com/sites/jeffbercovici/2014/01/16/fired-yahoo-execs-109m-golden-parachute-was-one-of-the-biggest-ever/#73e36b094a4f

Berenson, Alex. *Tell Your Children: The Truth About Marijuana, Mental Illness, and Violence.* New York: Free Press, 2019.

Bergstrom, K., and B. Bille. "Computed Tomography of the Brain in Children with Minimal Brain Damage: A Preliminary Study of 46 Children." *Neuropädiatrie* 9, no. 4 (November 1978): 378-384. https://doi.org/10.1055/s-0028-1091497

Beau-Lejdstrom, Raphaelle, Ian Douglas, Stephen J.W. Evans, and Liam Smeeth. "Latest Trends in ADHD Drug Prescribing Patterns in Children in the UK: Prevalence, Incidence, and Persistence." *BMJ Open* 6, June 13, 2016. https://doi.org/10.1136/bmjopen-2015-010508

Bhatara, Vinod, Michael Feil, Kimberly Hoagwood, Benedetto Vitiello, and Bonnie Zima. "Trends in Combined Pharmacotherapy with Stimulants for Children." *Psychiatric Services* 53, no. 3 (March 2002): 244. https://doi.org/10.1176/appi.ps.53.3.244

Biederman, Joseph, and Steven V. Faraone. "The Johnson and Johnson Center for Pediatric Psychopathology at the Massachusetts General Hospital." 2002.

Biederman, Joseph, Stephen V. Faraone, Eric Mick, Janet Wozniak, Lisa Chen, Cheryl Oullette, Abbe Marrs, et al. "Attention-Deficit Hyperactivity Disorder and Juvenile Mania: An Overlooked Comorbidity?" *Journal of the American Academy of Child and Adolescent Psychiatry* 35, no. 8 (August 1996): 997-1008. https://doi.org/10.1097/00004583-199608000-00010

Biederman, Joseph, Stephen V. Faraone, Thomas J. Spencer, Eric Mick, Michael C. Monuteaux, and Megan Aleardi. "Functional Impairments in Adults with Self-Reports of Undiagnosed ADHD: A Controlled Study of 1001 Adults in the Community." *Journal of Clinical Psychiatry* 67, no. 4 (April 2006): 524-540. https://doi.org/10.4088/jcp.v67n0403

Biederman, Joseph, Stephen V. Faraone, Thomas J. Spencer, Timothy E. Wilens, Dennis Norman, Kathleen A. Lapey, Eric Mick, Belinda Krifcher Lehman, and Alysa Doyle. "Patterns of Psychiatric Comorbidity, Cognition, and Psychosocial Functioning in Adults with Attention Deficit Hyperactivity Disorder." *American Journal of Psychiatry* 150, no. 12 (December 1993): 1792-1798. https://doi.org/10.1176/ajp.150.12.1792

Biederman, Joseph, John H. Heilenstein, Douglas E. Faries, Nora Galil, Ralf Dittman, Graham J. Emslie, Christopher J. Kratochvil, et al. "Efficacy of Atomoxetine versus Placebo in School-Age Girls with Attention-Deficit/Hyperactivity Disorder." *Pediatrics* 110, no. 6 (December 2002): 1-7. https://doi.org/10.1542/peds.110.6.e75

Biederman, Joseph, Michael C. Monuteaux, Eric Mick, Thomas J. Spencer, Timothy E. Wilens, Julie M. Silva, Lindsey E. Snyder, and Stephen V. Faraone. "Young Adult Outcome of Attention Deficit Hyperactivity Disorder: A Controlled 10-Year Follow-Up Study." *Psychological Medicine* 36, no. 2 (February 2006): 167-179. http://doi.org/10.1017/S0033291705006410

Biederman, Joseph, Michael C. Monuteaux, Thomas J. Spencer, Timothy E. Wilens, Heather A. MacPherson, and Steven V. Faraone. "Stimulant Therapy and Risk for Subsequent Substance Use Disorders in Male Adults with ADHD: A Naturalistic Controlled 10-Year Follow-Up Study." *American Journal of Psychiatry* 165, no. 5 (May 2008): 597-603. https://doi.org/10.1176/appi.ajp.2007.07091486

Biederman, Joseph, Carter R. Perry, Ronna Fried, Roselinde Kaiser, Chrystina R. Dolan, Steven Schoenfeld, Alysa E. Doyle, Larry J. Seidman, and Stephen V. Faraone. "Educational and Occupational Underattainment in Adults with Attention-Deficit/Hyperactivity Disorder: A Controlled Study." *Journal of Clinical Psychiatry* 69, no. 8 (August 2008): 1217-1222. https://doi.org/10.4088/jcp.v69n0803

Biederman, Joseph, Timothy E. Wilens, Thomas J. Spencer, and Steven V. Faraone. "Pharmacotherapy of Attention-Deficit/Hyperactivity Disorder Reduces Risk for Substance Use Disorder." *Pediatrics* 104, no. 2 (August 1999): 1-5. https://doi.org/10.1542/peds.104.2.e20

Birmaher, Boris. "Longitudinal Course of Pediatric Bipolar Disorder." *American Journal of Psychiatry* 164, no. 4 (April 2007): 537-539. https://doi.org/10.1176/ajp.2007.164.4.537

Blum, Andrew. "Legal Attack on Ritalin Expands." *National Law Journal*, November 23, 1987.

Bodkin, Henry. "ADHD is a Brain Disorder, Not a Label for Poor Parenting." *Daily Telegraph*, February 16, 2017. https://www.telegraph.co.uk/science/2017/02/15/adhd-brain-disorder-not-label-poor-parenting-say-scientists/

Boland, Heidi, Maura DiSalvo, Ronna Fried, K. Yvonne Woodworth, Timothy Wilens, Stephen V. Faraone, and Joseph Biederman. "A Literature Review and Meta-Analysis on the Effects of ADHD Medications on Functional Outcomes." *Journal of Psychiatric Research* 123, (April 2020): 21-30. https://doi.org/10.1016/j.jpsychires.2020.01.006

Bond, Earl A., and G.E. Partridge. "Post-Encephalitic Behavior Disorders in Boys and Their Management in a Hospital." *American Journal of Psychiatry* 83, no. 1 (July 1926): 25-103. https://doi.org/10.1176/ajp.83.1.25

Bond, Earl A., and Lauren H. Smith. "Post-Encephalitic Behavior Disorder: A Ten-Year Review of the Franklin School." *American Journal of Psychiatry* 92, no. 1 (July 1935): 17-33. https://doi.org/10.1176/ajp.92.1.17

Boseley, Matilda. "Tik Tok Accidently Detected My ADHD. For 25 Years Everyone Missed the Warning Signs." *Guardian*, June 3, 2021. https://www.theguardian.com/commentisfree/2021/jun/04/tiktok-accidently-detected-my-adhd-for-23-years-everyone-missed-the-warning-signs

Boseley, Sarah. "Hyperactive Children May Suffer from Genetic Disorder, Says Study." *Guardian*, September 29, 2010. https://www.theguardian.com/society/2010/sep/30/hyperactive-children-genetic-disorder-studya

Bradley, Charles. "The Behavior of Children Receiving Benzedrine." *American Journal of Psychiatry* 93, no. 4 (November 1937): 578-585.

Bradley, Charles. "Benzedrine and Dexedrine in the Treatment of Children's Behavior Disorders." *Pediatrics* 5, no. 1 (January 1950): 24-37.

Breggin, Peter R. *Toxic Psychiatry: Why Therapy, Empathy, and Love Must Replace the Drugs, Electroshock, and Biochemical Theories of the "New Psychiatry."* New York: Saint Martin's Griffin, 1991.

Breggin, Peter R. "Risks and Mechanisms of Action of Stimulants." In *NIH Consensus Development Conference on Diagnosis and Treatment of Attention Deficit Hyperactivity Disorder*, 105-119. Bethesda, MD: National Institutes of Health, 1998.

Breggin, Peter R. *Talking Back to Ritalin*. Cambridge, MA: Perseus Publishing, 2001.

Breggin, Peter R., and Ginger R. Breggin. *Talking Back to Prozac: What Doctors Aren't Telling You About Prozac and the New Antidepressants*. New York: Saint Martin's Press, 1994.

Bröer, Christian. "Exploring the ADHD Diagnosis in Ghana." In *Global Perspectives on ADHD: Social Dimensions of Diagnosis and Treatment in Sixteen Countries*, edited by Meredith R. Bergey et al., 354-375. Baltimore: Johns Hopkins University Press, 2018.

Brooks, Karen. "No Small Burden." *Fort Worth Star-Telegram*, July 17, 2000.

Brooks, Megan. FDA Clears Chewable Methylphenidate (QuilliChew) for ADHD." MedScape, December 7, 2015. https://www.medscape.com/viewarticle/855572

Brown, Matthew R.G., Gagan S. Sidhu, Russell Greiner, Nasimeh Asgarian, Meysam Bastani, Peter H. Silverstone, Andrew J. Greenshaw, and Serdar M. Dursun. "ADHD-200 Global Competition: Diagnosing ADHD Using Personal Characteristic Data Can Outperform Resting State fMRI Measurements." *Frontiers in Systems Neuroscience* 6, (September 28, 2012): 1-22. https://doi.org/10.3389/fnsys.2012.00069

Brown, Walter A. "Charles Bradley, M.D." *American Journal of Psychiatry* 155, no. 7 (July 1998): 968. https://doi.org/10.1176/ajp.155.7.968

Brygo, Julien. "La Pilule de l'Obéissance." *Le Monde Diplomatique*, December 2019. https://www.monde-diplomatique.fr/2019/12/BRYGO/61087

Butcher, James. "Cognitive Enhancement Raises Ethical Concerns." *Lancet* 362, no. 9378 (July 12, 2003): 132-133. https://doi.org/10.1016/s0140-6736(03)13897-4

CDC. "Mental Health Surveillance Among Children—United States, 2005-2011." May 17, 2013. https://www.cdc.gov/mmwrhtml/su6202a1.htm

CDC. "Fatal Injury Reports: National, Regional, and State 1981-2016." Page last updated February 19, 2017. https://webappa.cdc.gov/sasweb/ncipc/mortrate.html

CHADD. "Annual Report FY18." Accessed April 27, 2020. chadd.org/wpcontent/uploads/2019/01/AnnReport-FY18.pdf

CHADD. "About ADHD." Accessed April 27, 2020. chadd.org/about-adhd/overview

CHADD. "Position Paper on Controlled Substance Measures." Accessed April 27, 2020. chadd.org/about-adhd/overview/

CHADD. "Public Policy Agenda for Children and Adolescents." Accessed April 27, 2020. chadd.org/wp-content/uploads2018/06/Public-Policy-Agenda-for-Children-Adolescents.pdf

CNN. "ADHD Is a Genetic Condition, Study Says." September 29, 2010. thechart.blogs.cnn.com/2010/09/29/adhd-is-a-genetic-condition-study-says/

Canadian ADHD Resource Alliance. Accessed September 19, 2021. https://www.caddra.ca

Canadian Press. "Poll: Canadians are Most Proud of Universal Medicare." Sunday, November 25, 2012. https://www.ctvnews.ca/canada/poll-canadians-are-most-proud-of-universal-medicare-1.1052929

Castellanos, Francis Xavier, Patti P. Lee, Wendy Sharp, Neal O. Jeffries, Deanna K. Greenstein, Liv S. Clasen, Jonathan D. Blumenthal, et al. "Developmental Trajectories of Brain Volume Abnormalities in Children and Adolescents with Attention-Deficit/Hyperactivity Disorder." *JAMA* 288, no. 14 (October 9, 2002): 1740-1748. https://doi.org/10.1001/jama.288.14.1740

Castellanos, Francis Xavier, and Erica Proal. "Large-Scale Brain Systems in ADHD: Beyond the Prefrontal-Striatal Model." *Trends in Cognitive Science* 16, no. 1 (January 2012): 17-26. https://doi.org/10.1016/j.tics.2011.11.007

Center for ADHD Awareness Canada. "ADHD Facts—Dispelling the Myths." Accessed September 10, 2021. https://caddac.ca/understanding-adhd/in-general/facts-stats-myths/

Cerebral: Expert Help for Your Emotional Health. 2022. https://cerebral.com

Chess, Stella. "Diagnosis and Treatment of the Hyperactive Child." *New York State Journal of Medicine* 60, 2379-2385.

Chiles, Adrian. "My Treatment for ADD Changed My Life, so Why Can't I Stop Worrying About It?" *Guardian*, September 30, 2020. https://www.theguardian.com/society/2020/sep/30/my-treatment-for-add-changed-my-life-so-why-cant-i-stop-worrying-about-it

Chouinard, G., L. Annable, J. Bradwejn, A. Labonte, B. Jones, P. Mercier, and M.-C. Belanger. "An Early Phase II Clinical Trial with Followup of Tomoxetine (LY139603) in the Treatment of Newly Admitted Depressed Patients." *Psychopharmacology Bulletin* 21, no. 1 (1985): 73-76. https://doi.org/10.1007/BF00427436

Claridge, Gordon, and David Healy. "The Psychopharmacology of Individual Differences." *Human Psychopharmacology: Clinical and Experimental* 9, no. 4 (July/August 1994): 285-298. https://doi.org/10.1002/hup.470090408

Clark, Laura J., and Deborah J. Rhea. "The LiiNK Project: Comparisons of Recess, Physical Activity, and Positive Emotional States in Grades K-2 Children." *International Journal of Child Health and Nutrition* 6, no. 6 (2017): 54-61. https://doi.org/10.3389/feduc.2018.00009

Clements, Sam D., and John E. Peters. "Minimal Brain Dysfunction in the School-Age Child." *Archives of General Psychiatry* 6, (1962): 17-29.

Clymer, Adam. "Senate Passes Bill on Teaching the Disabled." *New York Times*, May 15, 1997.

Cohen, David, Shannon Hughes, and David J. Jacobs. "The Deficiencies of Drug Treatment Research: The Case of Strattera™." In *Rethinking ADHD: From Brain to Culture*, edited by Sami Timimi and Jonathan Leo, 313-333. New York: Palgrave MacMillan, 2009.

Colpaert, Francis C., Carlos J.E. Niemegeers, and Paul A. Janssen. "Discriminative Properties of Cocaine: Neuropharmacological Characteristics as Derived from Stimulus Generalization Experiments." *Pharmacology, Biochemistry, and Behavior* 10, no. 4 (April 1979): 535-546. https://doi.org/10.1016/0091-3057(79)90229-6

Conant, James Bryant. *Slums and Suburbs*. New York: McGraw Hill, 1961.

Conners, C. Keith. "A Teacher Rating Scale for Use in Drug Studies with Children." *American Journal of Psychiatry* 126, no. 6 (December 1969): 884-888. https://doi.org/10.1176.ajp.126.6.884

Conners, C. Keith. "Attention-Deficit/Hyperactivity Disorder—Historical Development and Overview." *Journal of Attention Deficit Disorders* 3, no. 4 (January 2000): 173-191.

Conners, C. Keith, and Leon Eisenberg. "The Effects of Methylphenidate on Symptomatology and Learning in Disabled Children." *American Journal of Psychiatry* 120, (November 1963): 458-464.

Connors, Amanda L. "Big Bad Pharma: An Ethical Analysis of Physician-Directed and Consumer-Directed Marketing Tactics." *Albany*

Law Review 73, no. 1 (September 2009): 243-282. https://doi.
org/10.1162/156265160360706615

Conrad, Peter, and Meredith R. Bergey. "The Impending Globalization of
ADHD: Notes on the Expansion and Growth of a Medicalized Disorder."
Social Science and Medicine 122, (December 2014): 31-43. https://doi.
org/10.1016/j.socscimed.2014.10.019

Conrad, Peter, and Deborah Potter. "From Hyperactive Children to ADHD
Adults: Observations on the Expansion of Medical Categories." *Social
Problems* 47, no. 4 (November 2000), 567-568.

Convey, Eric. "Mass. General Disciplines Three Psychiatrists." *Boston Business
Journal*, July 1, 2001. bizjournals.com//boston/news/2011/07/01/mass-gen-
eral-punishes-three-html

Corrigan, Michael W. *Debunking ADHD: 10 Reasons to Stop Drugging Kids for
Acting Like Kids*. Lanham: Rowman and Littlefield, 2015.

Cortese, Samuele, Nicoletta Adamo, Cinzia Del Giovane, Christina
Mohr-Jensen, Adrian J. Hayes, Sara Carucci, Lauren Z. Atkinson, et
al. "Comparative Efficacy and Tolerability of Medications for Attention-Deficit Hyperactivity Disorder in Children, Adolescents, and
Adults: A Systematic Review and Network Analysis." *Lancet Psychiatry*
5, no. 9 (September 2018): 727-737. https://doi.org/10.1016/S2215-
0366(18)30269-4

Cosgrove, Lisa, and Sheldon Krimsky. "A Comparison of DSM-IV and DSM-5
Panel Members' Financial Associations with Industry: A Pernicious
Problem Exists." *PLoS Medicine* 9, no. 3 (March 2012): 1-4. https://doi.
org/10.1371//journal/pmed.1001190

Counts, George S. "The Real Challenge of Soviet Education." *Educational Forum*
12, no. 3 (March 1959): 261-268.

Cowan, Alison Leigh. "Amid Affluence, a Struggle over Special Education." *New
York Times*, April 24, 2005.

Cowart, Virginia S. "The Ritalin Controversy: What's Made This Drug's
Opponents Hyperactive?" *JAMA* 259, no. 17 (May 6, 1988): 2521-2523.

Cowley, Geoffrey. "The Promise of Prozac." *Newsweek*, March 26, 1990, 38-41.

Cowley, Geoffrey. "The Not-Young and the Restless." *Newsweek*, July 26, 1993, 48.

Cramer, Maria. "DSS Dropped Inquiry Before Girl, 4, Was Found Dead." *Boston Globe*, February 8, 2007, A1, B4.

Cressman, Alex M., Erin M. MacDonald, Anjie Huang, Tara Gomes, Michael J. Paterson, Paul A. Kurdyak, Muhammad M. Mamdani, and David N. Juurlink. "Prescription Stimulant Use and Hospitalization for Psychosis and Mania." *Journal of Clinical Psychopharmacology* 35, no. 6 (December 2015): 667-671. https://doi.org/10.1097/JCP.0000000000000406

Crunchbase. "Cerebral." Accessed March 14, 2022. https://www.crunchbase.com/organization/cerebral

Curtis, Jeffrey, Joseph C. Larson, Elizabeth Delzell, M. Alan Brookhart, Suzanne M. Cadarette, Rowan Chlebowski, Suzanne Judd, Monika Safford, Daniel H. Solomon, and Andrea Z. LaCroix. "Placebo Adherence, Clinical Outcomes and Mortality in the Women's Health Initiative Randomized Hormone Therapy Trials." *Medical Care* 49, no. 5 (May 2011): 427-435. https://doi.org/10.1097/MLR.0b013e18207ed9c

D'Agostino, Ryan. "The Drugging of the American Boy." *Esquire*, May 27, 2014. https://www.esquire.com/news-politics/a32858/drugging-of-the-american-boy-0414/

Daily Mail. "Don't Blame the Parents. ADHD is in Our Genes." November 27, 2018, 5.

Davids, Anthony, and Jack Sidman. "A Pilot Study—Impulsivity and Delayed Gratification in Future Scientists and in Underachieving High School Students." *Exceptional Children*, December 1962, 170-174.

Davies, James. *Sedated: How Modern Capitalism Created Our Mental Health Crisis*. London: Atlantic Books, 2021.

Davis, Nicola. "Scientists Find Genetic Variants That Increase the Risk of ADHD." *Guardian*, November 26, 2018. https://amp.theguardian.com/society/2018/nov/26/scientists-find-genetic-variants-that-increase-risk-of-adhd

Demeter, Christine A., Lisa D. Townsend, Michael Wilson, and Robert A. Findling. "Current Research in Child and Adolescent Bipolar Disorder." *Dialogues in Clinical Neuroscience* 10, no. 2 (June 2008): 215-228.

Demontis, Ditte, Raymond K. Walters, Joanna Martin, Manuel Matthiesen, Thomas D. Als, Esben Agerbo, Rich Belliveau, et al. "Discovery of the First Genome-Wide Significant Risk Loci for ADHD." *Nature Genetics*, 51, no. 1 (January 2019): 63-75. https://doi.org.10/1038/s41588-018-0269-7

DeSantis, Alan D., and Audrey Curtis Hane. "'Adderall is Definitely Not a Drug': Justifications for the Illegal Use of ADHD Stimulants." *Substance Use and Misuse* 45, 31-46. 10.3109/10826080902858333

DeSantis, Alan D., Seth M. Noar, and Elizabeth M. Webb. "Speeding Through the Frat House: A Qualitative Exploration of Nonmedical ADHD Stimulant Use in Fraternities." *Journal of Drug Education* 40, no. 2 (2010): 157-170. https://doi.org/10.2190/DE.40.2.d

DeSantis, Alan D., Elizabeth M. Webb, and Seth M. Noar. "Illicit Use of Prescription ADHD Medications on a College Campus: A Multimethodological Approach." *Journal of American College Health* 57, no. 3 (November-December 2008): 315-324. https://doi.org/10.3200/JACH.57.3.315-324

Department for Education. "Statistical First Release: Special Educational Needs in England, January 2010." June 23, 2010. https://www.gov.uk/government/statistics/special-educational-needs-in-england-january-2010

Department for Education. "Support and Aspiration: A New Approach to Special Educational Needs and Disability." March 9, 2011. https://www.gov.uk/government/publications/support-and-aspiration-a-new-approach-to-special-educational-needs-and-disability-consultation

Detroit News. "Ritalin Is Safe—and It Works." December 12, 2002.

Diagnosis and Treatment of Attention Deficit Hyperactivity Disorder (ADHD). *NIH Consensus Statement* 16, no. 2 (November 16-18, 1998): 1-37.

Diller, Lawrence H. *Running on Ritalin: A Physician Reflects on Children, Society, and Performance in a Pill*. New York: Bantam Books, 1998.

Diller, Lawrence H. "Bitter Pill." *Psychotherapy Networker*, January/February, 2005, 55-61.

Dillon, Sam. "Special Education Absorbs Resources." *New York Times*, April 7, 1994, A1.

Dillon, Sam. "Comptroller Report Faults Special Education Policy." *New York Times*, June 27, 1994, B3.

Divoky, Diane. "Ritalin: Education's Fix-It Drug?" *Phi Delta Kappan* 70, no. 8 (April 1989): 599-605.

Dormuth, Colin R., Amanda R. Patrick, William H. Shrank, James M. Wright, Robert J. Glynn, Jenny Sutherland, and M. Alan Brookhart. "Statin Adherence and Risk of Accidents: A Cautionary Tale." *Circulation* 119: no. 15 (April 21, 2009): 2051-2057. https://doi.org/10.1161.CIRCULATIO-NAHA.108.824151

Douglas, Virginia I. "Stop, Look, and Listen: The Problem of Sustained Attention and Impulse Control in Hyperactive and Normal Children." *Canadian Journal of Behavioural Science* 4, no. 4 (1972): 259-282.

Eckelberry, R.H.E. "Editorial Comment." *Educational Research Bulletin* 37, no. 8 (November 12, 1958): 221-222.

Economist. "Attention Please: Psychiatric Genetics." 429, no. 9120 (December 1, 2018).

Edwards, Claire, Etaoine Howlett, Madeleine Akrich and Vololona Rabeharisoa. "Attention Deficit Hyperactivity Disorder in France and Ireland: Parents' Groups' Scientific and Political Framing of an Unsettled Condition." *Biosocieties* 9, no. 2 (2014): 153-172.

Elder, Todd E. "The Importance of Relative Standards in ADHD Diagnosis: Evidence Based on Exact Birth Dates." *Journal of Health Economics* 29, (2010): 641-656. https://doi.org/10.1016/j.jhealeco.2010.06.003

Eli Lilly and Company. "Strattera Posts Fastest Launch Ever for a New ADHD Medicine with 1 Million Prescriptions in First Six Months." July 22, 2003. businesswire.com/news/home/20030722005458/Eli-Lilly-Company-Strattera-Posts-Fastest-Launch

Elia, J., X. Gai, H.M. Xie, J.C. Perin, E. Geiger, J.T. Gleissner, M. D'Arcy, et al. "Genome-Wide Copy Number Variation Study Associates Metabotropic Glutamate Receptor Gene Networks with Attention Deficit Hyperactivity Disorder." *Nature Genetics* 44, no. 1 (December 4, 2011): 78-84. http://doi.org/10.1038/ng.1013

Ellington, Careth. "The Children with No Alternative." *Saturday Review*, November 21, 1970, 67.

Erikson, Erik H. "Youth and the Life Cycle." *Children* 7, no. 2 (March/April 1960): 43-49.

Evans, William N., Melinda S. Morrill, and Stephen T. Parente. "Measuring Inappropriate Medical Diagnosis and Treatment in Survey Data: The Case of ADHD among School-Age Children." *Journal of Health Economics* 29, (2010): 657-673. https://doi.org/10.1016/j.jhealeco.2010.07.005

EXPERT REPORTS. "Family Mental Health: Unlocking the Brain's Secrets." *Family Circle*, November 20, 2001.

FDA. "FDA Permits Marketing of First Medical Device for Treatment of ADHD." April 19, 2019. https://www.fda.gov/news-events/press-announcements/fda-permits-marketing-first-medical-device-treatment-adhd

Facher, Lev. "One Night, One Pill, One Tragedy—and a Mother's Mission." *Michigan Daily*, September 8, 2015. michigandaily.com/section/statement/one-night-one-pill-one-tragedy-and-mother's-mission

Faedda, Giovanni L., Ross J. Baldessarini, Trisha Suppes, Leonardo Tondo, Ina Becker, and Deborah S. Lipschitz. "Pediatric-Onset Bipolar Disorder: A Neglected Clinical and Public Health Problem." *Harvard Review of Psychiatry* 3, no. 4 (November-December 1995): 171-195. https://doi.org/10.3109/10673229509017185

Fallon, Richard. "Gallagher Gets 2 Years and $10,000 Fine." *New York Times*, June 16, 1973.

Faraone, Steven V. "Discussion of 'Genetic Influence on Parent-Reported Attention-Related Problems in a Norwegian General Population Twin Sample.'" *Journal of the American Academy of Child and Adolescent Psychiatry* 35, no. 5 (May 1996): 596-598.

Faraone, Stephen V. "Epidemiology of Attention Deficit Hyperactivity Disorder." In *Textbook in Psychiatric Epidemiology Third Edition*, edited by Ming T. Tsuang, 449-462. New York: John Wiley and Sons, 2011.

Faraone, Steven V., Joseph Biederman, W.J. Chen, B. Krifcher, K. Keenan, C. Moore, S. Sprich, and M.T. Tsuang. "Segregation Analysis of Attention Deficit Hyperactivity Disorder." *Psychiatric Genetics* 2, no. 4 (1992): 257-275. https://doi.org/10.1097/00041444-199210000-00004

Faraone, Stephen V., Joseph Biederman, Janet Wozniak, Elizabeth Mundy, Douglas Mennin, and Deborah O'Donnell. "Is Comorbidity with ADHD a Marker for Juvenile-Onset Mania?" *Journal of the American Academy of Child and Adolescent Psychiatry* 36, no. 8 (August 1997): 1046-1055. https://doi.org/10.1097/00004583-199708000-00012

Faraone, Stephen V., and Henrik Larsson. "Genetics of Attention Deficit Hyperactivity Disorder." *Molecular Psychiatry* 24, (2019): 562-575. https://doi.org/10.1038/s41380-018-0070-0

Feinstein, Jessica. "Adderall: The Academic Steroid." *Yale Daily News*, January 24, 2005. https://yaledailynews.com/blog/2005/01/24/adderall-the-academic-steroid/

Fifth Estate. "Chazz Petrella: The Boy Who Should Have Lived." Narrated by Gillian Findlay. CBC. March 27, 2015.

Fleming, Arthur S. "The Philosophy and Objectives of the National Defense Education Act." *Annals of the American Academy of Political and Social Science* 327, (January 1960): 132-138.

Foster, Jill. "Woman Diagnosed with ADHD at 44: 'I Thought It Only Affected Young Boys.'" *Yahoo! Life*, March 15, 2021. https://www.yahoo.com/lifestyle/wioman-diagnosed-adhd-at-44-100037439.html

Franke, B., Stephen V. Faraone, J. Buitelaar, C.H.D. Bau, J.A. Ramos-Quiroga, E. Mick, E.H. Grevet, et al. "The Genetics of Attention-Deficit/Hyperactivity Disorder in Adults, A Review." *Molecular Psychiatry* 17, no. 10 (October 2012): 960-987. https://doi.org.10.1038/mp.2011/138

Frontline. "ADHD Lawsuits." Accessed April 28, 2020. pbs.org/wgbh/pages/frontline/shows/medicating/backlash/lawsuits.html

Frontline. "Federal Laws Pertaining to ADHD Diagnosed Children." Accessed April 28, 2020. pbs.org/wgbh/pages/frontline/shows/medicating/schools/feds.html

Furman, Lydia. "What is Attention-Deficit Hyperactivity Disorder?" *Journal of Child Neurology* 20, no. 12 (December 2005): 994-1002. https://doi.org/10.1 0.1177/088307380502001301

Gadow, Kenneth D. "Effects of Stimulant Drugs on Academic Performance in Hyperactive and Learning Disabled Children." *Journal of Learning Disabilities* 16, no. 5 (May 1983): 290-299. https://doi.org/10.1177/002221948301600509

Gaffey, Conor. "Study Finds Brains of ADHD Sufferers Are Smaller." *Newsweek*, February 16, 2017. https://www.newsweek.com/brains-adhd-sufferers-are-smaller-suggesting-it-physical-disorder-study-557372

Gastaut, Henri. "Combined Photic and Metrazol Activation of the Brain." *Electroencephalography and Clinical Neurophysiology* 2, nos. 1-4 (1950): 249-261. https://doi.org/10.1016/0013-4694(50)90056-3/

Getahun, Darios, and Stephen J. Jacobsen. "Recent Trends in Childhood Attention Deficit Hyperactivity Disorder." *JAMA Pediatrics* 167, no. 3 (March 2013): 282-288. https://doi.org/10.1001/2013.jamapediatrics.401

Giedd, Jay N., Jonathan D. Blumenthal, Elizabeth Molloy, and Francis Xavier Castellanos. "Brain Imaging of Attention Deficit/Hyperactivity Disorder." *Annals of the New York Academy of Sciences* 931, (June 2001): 33-49. https://doi.org/10.1111/j.1749-6632.2001.tb05772.x

Gilbert, Susan. "Study Supports Use of Stimulants for Children with Hyperactivity." *New York Times*, September 16, 1997.

Gizer, Ian R., Courtney Ficks, and Irwin D. Waldman. "Candidate Gene Studies of ADHD: A Meta-Analytic Review." *Human Genetics* 126, (2009): 51-90. https://doi.org/10.1007/s00439-009-0694-x

Glessner, Joseph T., Jin Li, Dai Wang, Michael March, Leandro Lima, Ahshatha Desai, Dexter Hadley, et al. "Copy Number Variation Meta-Analysis as Novel Duplication at 9p24 Associated with Multiple Neurodevelopmental Disorders." *Genome Medicine* 9, no. 1 (September 2017) 1-11. https://doi.org/10.1186/s13073-017-0494-1

Gogenini, R. Rao, April E. Fallon, and Nyapati R. Rao. "International Medical Graduates in Child and Adolescent Psychiatry: Adaptation, Training, and Contributions." *Child and Adolescent Psychiatric Clinics of North America* 19, no. 4 (October 2010): 833-853. https://doi.org/10.1016/j.chc.2010.07.009

Goldberg, Carey. "For the School Nurses, More Than Tending the Sick." *New York Times,* January 28, 1999.

Goldman, Larry, M. Genel, R.J. Bezman, and P.J. Slanetz. "Diagnosis and Treatment of Attention-Deficit/Hyperactivity Disorder in Children and Adolescents." *JAMA* 279, no.14 (April 8, 1998): 1100-1107. https://doi.org/10.1001/jama.279.14.1100

Goldstein, Lisa Fine. "Study: ADHD Drugs Unrelated to Smaller Brain Sizes." *Education Week* 22, no. 7 (October 16, 2002).

Goode, Erica. "Brain Size Tied to Attention Deficit Hyperactivity Disorder." *New York Times*, October 9, 2002.

Gootman, Elissa. "In Special Education Cases, City is Fighting Harder Before Paying for Private School." *New York Times*, December 12, 2007.

Greenhill, Laurence. "Attention-Deficit Hyperactivity Disorder: The Stimulants." *Pediatric Psychopharmacology I* 4, no. 1 (January 1995): 123-168. https://doi.org/10.1016/S1056-4993(18)30455-3

Griffith, Michael. "A Look at Funding for Students with Disabilities." *The Progress of Education Reform* 16, no. 1 (March 2015): 1-6.

Grinspoon, Lester, and Peter Hedblom. *The Speed Culture: Amphetamine Use and Abuse in America.* Cambridge: Harvard University Press, 1974.

Gurciullo, Brianna. "Law Student Died from Lethal Mix of Heroin and Adderall." *GW Hatchet*, March 7, 2013. gwhatchet.com/2013/03/07/law-student-died-from-lethal-mix-of-heroin-adderall

Hahn, Patrick D. *Madness and Genetic Determinism: Is Mental Illness in Our Genes?* New York: Palgrave MacMillan, July 12, 2019.

Hales, D. and R. Hales. "Pay Attention." *American Health*, September 1993, 62-65.

Halikas, James A., Jane Meller, Carolyn Morse, and Marvin D. Lyttle. "Predicting Substance Abuse in Juvenile Offenders: Attention Deficit

Disorder versus Aggressivity." *Child Psychiatry and Human Development* 21, no. 1 (Fall 1990): 49-55. https://doi.org/10.1007/bf00709927

Hallowell, Edward M., and John J. Ratey. *Driven to Distraction*. New York: Pantheon Books, 1994.

Harris, Gardiner, and Benedict Carey. "Researchers Fail to Reveal Full Drug Pay." *New York Times*, June 8, 2008.

Harris, Margaret, Summit Chandran, Nabonita Chakraborty, and David Healy. "The Impact of Mood Stabilizers on Bipolar Disorder: The 1890's and 1990's Compared." *History of Psychiatry* 16, no. 4 (2005): 423-434. https://doi.org/10.1177/0957154X05052088

Harrison, Alysson Granger. "Adults Faking ADHD? You Must Be Kidding!" *ADHD Report* 14, no. 4 (August 2006): 1-7. https://doi.org/10.1521/adhd.2006.14.4.1

Harrison, Alysson Granger, Melanie J. Edwards, and Kevin C.H. Parker. "Identifying Students Faking ADHD: Preliminary Findings and Strategies for Detection." *Archives of Clinical Neuropsychology* 22, (2007): 577-588. https://doi.org/10.1016/j.acn.2007.03.008

Haslip, Gene R. "ADD/ADHD Statement of Drug Enforcement Administration at the Conclusion of the Conference on Stimulant Use in the Treatment of ADHD." Drug Enforcement Administration, December 10-12, 1996.

Hawking, Tom. "Tuning Out the Static: It Took 40 Years before I Found Out That I Have ADHD." *Guardian*, July 9, 2019. https://www.theguardian.com/commentisfree/2019/jul/10/tuning-out-the-static-it-took-40-years-before-I-found-out-that-i-have-adhd

Healy, David. "Shaping the Intimate: Influences on the Experience of Everyday Nerves." *Social Studies of Science* 34, no. 2 (April 2004): 219-245. https://doi.org/10.1177/0306312704042620

Healy, David. *Mania: A Short History of Bipolar Disorder*. Baltimore: Johns Hopkins University Press, 2008.

Healy, David. *Pharmageddon*. Berkeley and Los Angeles: University of California Press, 2012.

Healy, David. *The Decapitation of Care.* Toronto: Samizdat Health Writer's Co-operative, 2021.

Healy, David. *Shipwreck of the Singular: Healthcare's Castaways.* Toronto: Samizdat Health Writer's Co-operative, 2021.

Healy, David, Joanna LeNoury, and Julie Wood. *Children of the Cure: Missing Data, Lost Lives, and Antidepressants.* Toronto: Samizdat Health Writer's Co-operative, 2020.

Hedegaard, Holly, Arialdi M. Miniño, and Margaret Warner. "Drug Overdose Deaths in the United States, 1999-2017." NCHS Data Brief, no. 329 (November 2018). cdc.gov/nchs/data/databriefs/db329-h.pdf

Hellander, Martha E. "Children with Bipolar Disorder." *Journal of the American Academy of Child and Adolescent Psychiatry* 38, no. 5 (May 1999): 495.

Henderson, Theodore, and Keith Hartman. "Aggression, Mania, and Hypomania Induction Associated with Atomoxetine." *Pediatrics* 114, no. 3 (September 2004): 895. https://doi.org/peds.2004-1140

Henkhaus, Luke. "Autopsy Reveals Details in Phi Gamma Delta Student's Death." *Battalion*, December 13, 2018. thebatt.com/news/autopy-reveals-details-in-phi-gamma-delta-student-death/article_0b91df28-ff0d-11e8-bf03-0bddd1d01ea3.html

Hentoff, Nat. "The Drugged Classroom." *Evergreen Review*, December 1970, 31-33.

Hentoff, Nat. "Drug-Pushing in the Schools: The Professionals." *Village Voice*, May 25, 1972, 20.

Hickey, Phil. "In Defense of Antipsychiatry." Behaviorism and Mental Health, April 25, 2019. http://behaviorismandmentalhealth.com/2019/04/25/in-defense-of-anti-psychiatry/

Hill, Austin Bradford. "The Environment and Disease: Association or Causation?" *Proceedings of the Royal Society of Medicine* 58, no. 5 (May 1965): 295-300.

Hinshaw, Stephen P., and Richard M. Scheffler. *The ADHD Explosion: Myths, Medication, Money, and Today's Push for Performance.* Oxford: Oxford University Press, March 3, 2014.

Hinshaw, Stephen P., Richard Scheffler, Brent D. Fulton, Heidi Aase, Tobias Banachewski, Wenhong Cheng, Paulo Mattos, et al. "International Variation in Treatment Procedures for ADHD: Social Context and Recent Trends." *Psychiatric Services* 62, no. 5 (May 2011): 459-464. https://doi.org/10.1176/ps.62.5.pss6205_0459

Hitti, Miranda. "FDA Issues Advisory on ADHD Drug Strattera." WebMD, September 29, 2005. webmd.com/add-adhd/childhood-adhd/news/20050929/fda-issues-advisory-on-adhd-drug-strattera#1

Hodges, Lauren. "A Quiet and 'Unsettling' Pandemic Toll: Students Who've Fallen Off the Grid." National Public Radio, December 29, 2020. https://www.npr.org/2020/12/29/948866982/1-quiet-and-unsettling-panedmic-toll-students-whove-fallen-off-thegrid

Hoffman, Jan. "Purdue Pharma is Dissolved and Sacklers Pay \$4.5 Billion to Settle Opioid Claims." *New York Times*, September 2, 2021.

Holland, Josephine, and Kapil Sayal. "Relative Age and ADHD Symptoms, Diagnosis, and Medication—A Systematic Review." *European Child and Adolescent Psychology* 28, (November 2019): 1417-1429. https://doi.org/10.1007/s00787-1229-6

Hoogman, Martine, Janita Bralten, Derrick P. Hibar, Maarten Mennes, Marcel P. Zwiers, Lizanne S.J. Schweren, Kimm J.E. van Hulzen, et al. "Subcortical Brain Volume Differences in Participants with Attention Deficit Hyperactivity Disorder in Children and Adults: A Cross-Sectional Mega-Analysis." *Lancet Psychiatry*, published online February 15, 2017. https://doi.org/10.1016/S2215-0366(17)30049-4

House of Commons. "Education and Skills: Third Report." July 6, 2006. https://publications.parliament.uk/pa/cm200506/cmselect/cmeduski/478/47802.htm

Hoyt, Palmer. "What is Ahead for Our Schools?" *Grade Teacher* 76, (October 1958): 20-21.

Huxley, Nancy J., and Ross J. Baldessarini. "Disability and Its Treatment in Bipolar Disorder Patients." *Bipolar Disorders* 9, nos. 1-2 (2007): 183-196. https://doi.org/10.1111/j.1399-5618.2007.00430.x

HyperSupers TDAH France. "Fin de la Prescription Initiale Hospitaliére (PIH) pour le Méthylphenidate." September 13, 2021. https://tdah-france.fr

International Narcotics Control Board. "Report 2014." Tuesday, March 3, 2015. https://www.incb.org/incb/en/publications/annual-reports/annual-report-2014.html

Jachimowicz, Gina, and R. Edward Geiselman. "Comparison of Ease of Falsification of Attention Deficit Hyperactivity Disorder Diagnosis Using Standard Behavioral Scales." *Cognitive Sciences Online* 2, (2004): 6-20.

Jacob, Susan, Dawn M. Decker, and Timothy S. Hartshorne. *Ethics and the Law for School Psychologists*. Hoboken: John Wiley and Sons, August 1, 2016.

Jacobvitz, Deborah, L. Alan Sroufe, Mark Stewart, and Nancy Leffer. "Treatment of Attentional and Hyperactivity Problems in Children with Sympathomimetic Drugs: A Comprehensive Review." *Journal of the American Academy of Child and Adolescent Psychiatry* 29, no. 5 (September 1990): 677-688. https://doi.org/10.1097/00004583-199009000-00001

James, Susan Donaldson. "Adderall Abuse Alters Brain, Claims a Young Life." ABC News, November 5, 2010. abcnews.go.com/Health/MindMood-News/Adderall-psychosis-suicide-college-students-abuse-study-drugs/story?id=12066619

Jarick, I., A.-L. Volckmar, S. Pechlivanis, T.T. Nguyen, M.R. Dauverman, S. Beck, Ö. Albayrak, et al. "Genome-Wide Analysis of Rare Copy Number Variations Reveals *PARK2* as a Candidate Gene for Attention-Deficit/Hyperactivity Disorder." *Molecular Psychiatry* 19, no. 1 (January 2014): 115-121. https://doi.org/10.1038/mp/2010.29

Joachim, Heinrich. *The Papyrus Ebers*. Translated by Cyril P. Bryan. Chicago: Ares Publishers, 1930.

Joseph, Jay. "Not in Their Genes: A Critical View of the Genetics of Attention-Deficit Hyperactivity Disorder." *Developmental Review* 20, no. 4 (December 2000): 539-567. https://doi.org/10.1006.drev/.2000.0511

Joseph, Jay. "Problems in Psychiatric Genetic Research: A Reply to Faraone and Biederman." *Developmental Review* 20, no. 4 (December 2000): 582-593. https://doi.org/10.1006/drev.2000.0518

Joseph, Jay. "ADHD and Genetics: A Consensus Reconsidered." In *Rethinking ADHD: From Brain to Culture*, edited by Sami Timimi and Jonathan Leo, 58-91. New York: Palgrave MacMillan, 2009.

Jung, Carl. *Two Essays on Analytical Psychology*. Translated by R.F.C. Hull. Princeton: Princeton University Press.

Juvenile Bipolar Research Foundation. 2015. https://www.jbrf.org/

Kahn, Eugen, and Louis H. Cohen. "Organic Drivenness: A Brain-Stem Syndrome and Experiences." *New England Journal of Medicine* 210, no. 14 (April 5, 1934): 748-756.

Kasanin, Jacob. "The Affective Psychoses in Children." *American Journal of Psychiatry* 10, no. 6 (May 1931): 897-926.

Kebir, Oussama, Karim Tabbane, Sarojini Sengupta, and Ridha Joober. "Candidate Genes and Neuropsychological Phenotypes in Children with ADHD: Review of Association Studies." *Journal of Psychiatry and Neuroscience* 34, no. 2 (2009): 88-101.

Kelland, Kate. "Study Finds Genetic Link to ADHD." Australian Broadcasting Company, September 30, 2010. abc.net.au/news/2010-09-30/study-finds-genetic-link-to-adhd/228092

Keiffer, Elizabeth. "The Miracle That Misfired." *Good Housekeeping*, January 1974, 83, 111, 115.

Kendler, Kenneth S. "'A Gene For…': The Nature of Gene Action in Psychiatric Disorders." *American Journal of Psychiatry* 162, no. 7 (July 2005): 1243-1252. https://doi.org/10.1176/appi.ajp.162.7.1243

Kennedy, Roger L.J. "The Prognosis of Sequelae of Epidemic Encephalitis in Children." *American Journal of Diseases of Children* 28, (1924): 158-172.

Keshavan, Meghana. "Tasty and Easy to Take, a New ADHD Drug Alarms Some Psychiatrists." *STAT*, May 23, 2016. https://www.statnews.com/2016/05/23/adhd-drug-concerns/

Kline, Mitchell. "ADHD Case Grabs Attention." *Tennessean*, September 25, 2009.

Kluger, Jeffrey, Sora Song, Dan Cray, Jeffrey Ressner, Jeanne DeQuine, Melissa Sattley, Cristina Scalett, and Maggie Sieger. "Young and Bipolar." *Newsweek*, August 19, 2002.

Knowles, Asa S. "For the Space Age: Education as an Instrument of National Policy." *Phi Delta Kappan* 39, no. 7 (April 1958): 305-310.

Kooij., J.J.S., D. Bijlenga, R. Jaeschke, I. Bitter, J. Balázs, J. Thome, G. Dom, et al. "Updated European Consensus Statement on Diagnosis and Treatment of Adult ADHD." *European Psychiatry* 56, (2019): 14-34. https://doi.org/10.1016.j.europsy.2018.11.001

Koplewicz, Harold S. *It's Nobody's Fault: New Hope and Help for Difficult Children.* New York: Times Books, 1996.

Kowalczyk, Liz. "Psychiatrist to Suspend Practice, Denies Wrong-Doing." *Boston Globe*, February 8, 2007, B4.

Krabbe, E.E., E.D. Thoutenhoofd, M. Conradi, S.J. Pijl, and L. Batstra. "Birth Month Indicator as a Predictor of ADHD Medication Use in Dutch School Classes." *European Journal of Special Needs Education* 29, no. 4 (2014): 571-578. https://doi.org/10.1080/08856257.2014.943564

Kwasman, Alan, Barbara J. Tinsley, and Heidi S. Lepper. "Pediatricians' Knowledge and Attitudes Concerning Diagnosis and Treatment of Attention Deficit and Hyperactivity Disorders." *Archives of Pediatric and Adolescent Medicine* 149, (November 1995): 1211-1216. https://doi.org/10.1001/archpedi.1995.02170240029004

Ladd, Edward T. "Pills for Classroom Peace." *Saturday Review*, November 21, 1970, 66-68.

Lahey, Benjamin B., William E. Pelham, Andrea Chronis, Greta Massetti, Heidi Kipp, Ashley Ehrhardt, and Steve S. Lee. "Predictive Validity of ICD-10 Hyperkinetic Disorder Relative to DSM-IV Attention Deficit Hyperactivity Disorder Among Younger Children." *Journal of Child Psychology and Psychiatry* 47, no. 5 (2006): 472-479. https://doi.org/10.1111/j.1469-7610.2005.015900.x

Lambert, Lane. "Rebecca Riley's Doctor on the Defense." *Enterprise*, April 10, 2010. https://www.enterprisenews.com/x1661778235/Rebecca-Riley-s-doctor-on-the-defense

Lambert, Lane. "Case Closed: Carolyn Riley's Murder Conviction Also Upheld in Rebecca Riley's Death." *Patriot-Ledger*, May 2, 2014. https://www.patriotledger.com/article/20140502/NEWS/140508819

Lambert, Nadine M., and Carolyn S. Hartsough. "Prospective Study of Tobacco Smoking and Substance Dependencies among Samples of ADHD and Non-ADHD Participants." *Journal of Learning Disabilities* 31, no 6 (November/December 1998): 533-544. https://doi.org/10.1177.002221949803100603

Laufer, Maurice W., and Eric Denhoff. "Hyperkinetic Behavior Syndrome in Children." *Journal of Pediatrics* 50, no. 4 (April 1957): 463-474. https://doi.org/10.1016/S0022-3476(57)80257-1

Laufer, Maurice W., Eric Denhoff, and Gerald Solomons. "Hyperkinetic Impulse Disorder in Children's Behavioral Problems." *Psychosomatic Medicine* 19, no. 1 (1957): 38-49.

Lavelle, Daniel. "'I Assumed It Was All My Fault': The Adults Dealing with Undiagnosed ADHD." *Guardian*, September 5, 2017. https://www.theguardian.com/society/2017/sep/05/i-assumed-it-was-all-my-fault-the-adults-dealing-with-undiagnosed-adhd

Lavelle, Daniel. "'People with ADHD Can Be Incredibly Valuable at Work.'" *Guardian*, March 18, 2018. https://www.theguardian.com/society/2018/mar/18/people-with-adhd-incredibly-valuable-at-work-diagnosis-support

Lecendreux, Michel, Eric Konofal, and Stephen V. Faraone. "Prevalence of Attention Deficit Hyperactivity Disorder and Associated Features among Children in France." *Journal of Attention Deficit Disorders* 15, no. 6 (August 2011): 516-524. https://doi.org/10.1177/1087054710372491

LeFever, Gretchen L., Keila V. Dawson, and Ardythe L. Morrow. "The Extent of Drug Therapy for Attention Deficit-Hyperactivity Disorder among Children in Public Schools." *American Journal of Public Health* 89, no. 9 (September 1999): 1359-1364. https://doi.org/10.2105/ajph.89.9.1359

LeFever, Gretchen B., Margaret S. Villers, and Ardythe L. Morrow. "Parental Perceptions of Adverse Educational Outcomes among Children Diagnosed and Treated for ADHD: A Call for Improved School/Provider Collaboration." *Psychology in the Schools* 39, no. 1 (January 2002): 63-69. https://doi. org/10.1002/pits.10000

Lenz, Connie. "Prescribing a Legislative Response: Educators, Physicians, and Psychotropic Medication for Children." *Journal of Contemporary Health Law and Policy* 22, no. 1 (2006): 72-106.

Lenzer, Jeanne. "Researcher to be Sacked After Reporting High Rates of ADHD." *BMJ* 330, no. 7943 (March 26, 2005): 691. https://doi. org/10.1136/bmj.330.7493.691

Lenzer, Jeanne. "Researcher Cleared of Misconduct Charges." *BMJ* 331, no. 7521 (October 15, 2005): 865.

Leo, Jonathan, and David Cohen. "Broken Brains or Flawed Studies? A Critical Review of ADHD Neuroimaging Research." *Journal of Mind and Behavior* 24, no. 1 (Winter 2003): 29-55.

Lerner, Craig S. "'Accommodations' for the Learning Disabled: A Level Playing Field or Affirmative Action for Elites?" *Vanderbilt Law Review* 57, no. 3 (2019): 1108-1109.

Lesch, Klaus-Peter, S. Selch, T.J. Renner, C. Jacob, T.T. Nguyen, T. Hahn, M. Romanos, et al. "Genome-Wide Copy Number Variation Analysis in Attention Deficit/Hyperactivity Disorder: Association with Neuropeptide Y Gene Dosage in an Extended Pedigree." *Molecular Psychiatry* 16, no. 5 (May 2011): 491-503. https://doi.org/10.1038/mp.2010.29

Levy, Sol. "Post-Encephalitic Behavior Disorder—A Forgotten Entity: A Report of 100 Cases." *American Journal of Psychiatry* 115, no 12 (June 1959): 1062-1067. https://doi.org/10.1176/ajp.115.12.1062

Li, Dawei, Pak C. Sham, Michael J. Owen, and Lin He. "Meta-Analysis Shows Significant Association between Dopamine System Genes and Attention Deficit Hyperactivity Disorder (ADHD)." *Human Molecular Genetics* 15, no. 14 (2006): 2276-2284. https://doi.org/10.1093/hmg/ddl152

Liao, Sharon. "Why Are ADHD Medicines Controlled Substances?" WebMD. Last reviewed May 10, 2017. https://www.webmd.com/add-adhd/features/ adhd-medicines-controlled-substances#1

LiiNK Project. "What Is Liink Project?" 2020. liinkproject.tcu/about-us/what-is-liink-project/

LiiNK Project. "Logic Behind LiiNK." 2020. liinkproject.tcu.edu/about-us/logic-behind-liink

Lish, Jennifer D., Susan Dime-Meenan, Peter C. Whybrow, R. Arlen Price, and Robert M.A. Hirschfeld. "The National Depressive and Manic-Depressive Association (DMDA) Survey of Bipolar Members." *Journal of Affective Disorders* 31, no. 4 (August 1994): 281-294. https://doi.org/10.1016/0165-0327(94)90104-x

Locy, Toni. "Fight over Ritalin is Heading to Court." *USA Today*, September 15, 2000.

Loe, Irene M., and Heidi M. Feldman. "Academic and Educational Outcomes of Children with ADHD." *Journal of Pediatric Psychology* 32, no. 6 (2007): 643-654. https://doi.org/10.1016/j.ambp.2006.05.005

Logdberg, Linda. "Being a Ghost in the Machine: A Medical Ghostwriter's Point of View." *PLoS Medicine* 8, no. 8 (August 2011): 1-2. https://doi.org/10.1371/journal.pmed.1001071

Long, Mark, and Paul Barrett. "Lawsuit Is Filed Against Novartis over Children's Use of Ritalin in Texas." *Wall Street Journal*, May 15, 2000.

Low, K. Graff and A.E. Gendaszek. "Illicit Use of Psychostimulants among College Students: A Preliminary Study." *Psychology, Health, and Medicine* 7, no. 3 (2002): 283-287. https://doi.org/10.1080/13548500220139386

MTA Cooperative Group. "A 14-Month Randomized Clinical Trial of Treatment Strategies for Attention-Deficit/Hyperactivity Disorder." *Archives of General Psychiatry* 56, (December 1999): 1073-1084. https://doi.org/10.1001/archpsyc.56.12.1073

Maclay, Kathleen. "Educator Nadine Lambert Dies in Accident." UC Berkeley, May 4, 2006. Berkeley.edu/news/media/releases/2006/05/04_Lambertobit.shtml

Mahler, Don. "The Hyperactive Child." *Exceptional Children* 38, (October 1971): 161.

Malacrida, Claudia, and Tiffani Semach. "In the Elephant's Shadow: The Canadian ADHD Context." In *Global Perspectives on ADHD: Social Dimensions of Diagnosis and Treatment in Sixteen Countries*, edited by Meredith R. Bergey et al., 34-53. Baltimore: Johns Hopkins University Press, 2018.

Mann, E.M., Y. Ikeda, C.W. Mueller, A. Takahashi, K.T. Tao, E. Humris, B.L. Li, and D. Chin. "Cross-Cultural Differences in Rating Hyperactive-Disruptive Behaviors in Children." *American Journal of Psychiatry* 149, no. 11 (November 1992): 1539-1542. https://doi.org/10.1176/ajp.149.11.1539

Mascret, Damien. "Le Ritaline, entre Sous-Prescription et Abus." *Le Figaro*, May 17, 2017. https://sante/lefigaro.fr/article/ritaline-entre-sous-prescription-et-abus

Massachusetts General Hospital. "About Joseph Biederman, MD." massgeneral.org/psychiatry/doctors/17789/Joseph-Biederman.

Maugh, Thomas H. "Use of Drug to Calm Children Rises Sharply, Study Reports." *Los Angeles Times*, October 21, 1988. https://www.latimes.com/archives/la-xpm-1988-10-21-mn-4509-story.html

Maynard, Robert. "Omaha Pupils Given Behavior Drugs: 5 to 10 Percent of Pupils Given Drugs to Improve Behavior." *Washington Post*, June 29, 1970.

Mazoué, Aude. "French Psychiatry Has Gone Downhill in Part Because of American Influence." France24, October 3, 2021. https://www.france24.com/en/france/20211003-french-psychiatry-has-gone-downhill-in-part-because-of-american-influence

McCabe, Sean Esteban, John R. Knight, Christian J. Teter, and Henry Wechsler. "Non-Medical Use of Prescription Stimulants among US College Students: Prevalence and Correlates from a National Survey." *Addiction* 99, (2005): 96-106. 10.1111/j.1360-0443.2005.00944.x

McDonnell, Mary Ann, and Janet Wozniak. *Is Your Child Bipolar?* New York: Bantam Books, 2008.

McGough, James J., and James T. McCracken. "Assessment of Attention Deficit Hyperactivity Disorder: A Review of Recent Literature." *Current Opinion in Pediatrics* 12, no. 4 (August 2000): 319-324. https://doi.org/10.1097/00008480-200008000-00006

McGough, James J., Alexandra Sturm, Jennifer Cowen, Kelly Tung, Giulia C. Salgari, Andrew F. Leuchter, Ian A. Cook, Catherine A. Sugar, and Sandra K. Loo. "Double-Blind, Sham-Controlled, Pilot Study of Trigeminal Nerve Stimulation for Attention-Deficit/Hyperactivity Disorder." *Journal of the American Academy of Child and Adolescent Psychiatry* 58, no. 4 (April 2019): 403-411. https://doi.org/10.1016/j.jaac.2018.11.013

Meier, Barry. "Suits Charge Conspiracy by Maker and Doctors' Group to Expand Ritalin Use." *New York Times*, September 14, 2000.

Merrow, John. "Reading, Writing, and Ritalin." *New York Times*, October 21, 1995.

Millchap, J. Gordon. "Etiologic Classification of Attention-Deficit Hyperactivity Disorder." *Pediatrics* 121, no. 2 (February 2008): 358-365. https://doi.org/10.1542/peds/2007-1332

Molina, Brooke S.G., Kate Flory, Steven P. Hinshaw, Andrew R. Greiner, L. Eugene Arnold, James M. Swanson, Lily Hechtman, et al. "Delinquent Behavior and Emerging Substance Use in the MTA at 36 Months: Prevalence, Course, and Treatment Effects." *Journal of the American Academy of Child and Adolescent Psychiatry* 46, no. 8 (August 2007): 1028-1040. https://doi.org/10.1097/chi.0b013e318068d96

Molina, Brooke S.G., Stephen P. Hinshaw, L. Eugene Arnold, James M. Swanson, William E. Pelham, Lily Hechtman, Betsy Hoza, et al. "Adolescent Substance Use in the Multimodal Treatment Study of Attention-Deficit/Hyperactivity Disorder (ADHD) (MTA) as a Function of Childhood ADHD, Random Assignment to Childhood Treatments, and Subsequent Medication." *Journal of the American Academy of Child and Adolescent Psychiatry* 52, no. 3 (March 2013): 250-263. https://doi.org/10.1016/jaac.2012.12.014

Molina, Brooke S.G., Stephen P. Hinshaw, James M. Swanson, L. Eugene Arnold, Benedetto Vitiello, Peter S. Jensen, Jeffrey N. Epstein, et al. "The MTA at 8 Years: Prospective Follow-up of Children Treated for Combined-Type ADHD in a Multisite Study." *Journal of the American Academy of Child and Adolescent Psychiatry* 48, no. 5 (May 2009): 484-500. https://doi.org/10.1097/CHI.0b013e31819c23d0

Montero, Douglas. "I Was Told to Dope." *New York Post*, August 7, 2002.

Montero, Douglas. "School Pill-oried: Parents Forced to Drug Kids." *New York Post*, August 9, 2002.

Moreno, Carmen, Gonzalo Laje, Carlos Blanco, Huiping Jiang, Andrew B. Schmidt, and Mark Olfson. "National Trends in the Outpatient Diagnosis and Treatment of Bipolar Disorder in Youth." *Archives of General Psychiatry* 64, no. 9 (September 2007): 1032-1039. https://doi.org/10.1001/archpsyc.64.9.1032

Mosendz, Polly, and Caleb Melby. "ADHD Drugs are Convenient to Get Online. Maybe Too Convenient." *Bloomberg Businessweek*, March 11, 2022. https://apple.news/AOO9s4XqrSb6GSEbpcvALJg

Moss, Deborah Cassens. "Ritalin under Fire." *ABA Journal*, November 1, 1988, 19.

National Defense Education Act of 1958. H.R. 13427. 85th Congress.

Neale, Benjamin M., Sarah E. Medland, Stephan Ripke, Philip Asherson, Barbara E. Franke, Klaus-Peter Lesch, Stephen V. Faraone, et al. "Meta-Analysis of Genome-Wide Association Studies of Attention-Deficit/Hyperactivity Disorder." *Journal of the American Academy of Child and Adolescent Psychiatry* 49, no. 9 (September 2010): 884-897. https://doi.org/10.1016/j.jaacp.2010.06/008

NeuroSigma. "Monarch External Trigeminal Nerve Stimulation System (eTNS) for ADHD." November 26, 2019. https://www.youtube.com/watch?v=qP2l5wU0Zb8

New York Times. "Black Representative Calls Colleague 'Leading Racist.'" February 9, 1972.

Newsweek. "Pep Pills for Pupils." July 13, 1970, 60-62.

Novartis. "Plaintiffs Withdrawal in New Jersey Marks Fifth and Final Dismissal of All Class Actions Filed Against Maker of Ritalin in 2000." March 7, 2002. webarchive.org/web/20030628102148/http://pharma.us.novartis.com/newsroom/pressReleases/releeaseDetail/jsp?PRID=187

Novotny, Lia. "More Pediatricians Talking About ADHD During COVID-19." athenahealth, May 29, 2020. https://athenahealth.com/knowledge-hub/

clinical-trends/more-pediatricians-talking-about-ADHD-during-COVID-19

Olfson, Mark, Carlos Blanco, Linxu Liu, Carmen Moreno, and Gonzalo Laje. "National Trends in the Outpatient Treatment of Children and Adolescents with Antipsychotic Drugs." *Archives of General Psychiatry* 63, (June 2006): 679-685. https://doi.org/10.1001/archpsyc.63.6.679

Olfson, Mark, Marissa King, and Michael Schoenbaum. "Treatment of Young People with Antipsychotic Medications in the United States." *JAMA Psychiatry* 72, no. 9 (September 2015): 867-874. https://doi.org/10.1001/jamapsychiatry.2015.0500

Oulette, Eileen M. "Legal Issues in the Treatment of Children with Attention-Deficit Hyperactivity Disorder." *Journal of Child Neurology* 6, (Supplement 1991): S68-S75.

Papolos, Demetri, and Janice Papolos. *The Bipolar Child*. New York: Broadway Books, 1999.

Parker, Jack, Gill Wales, Nevyne Chalhoub, and Val Harpin. "The Long-Term Outcomes of Interventions for the Management of Attention-Deficit Hyperactivity Disorder in Children and Adolescents: A Systematic Review of Randomized Controlled Trials." *Psychology Research and Behavior Management* 6, (2013): 87-99. https://doi.org/10.2147/PRBM.S49114

Perliss, Roy H., Sachiko Miyahara, Lauren B. Marangell, Stephen L. Wisniewski, Michael Ostacher, Melissa P. DiBello, Charles L. Bowden, Gary S. Sachs, and Andrew A. Nierenberg. "Long-Term Implications of Early Onset in Bipolar Disorder: Data from the First 1000 Participants in the Systematic Treatment Enhancement Program for Bipolar Disorder (STEP-BD)." *Biological Psychiatry* 55, no. 9 (May 1, 2004): 875-881. https://doi.org/10.1016/j.biopsych.2004.01.022

Perman, Einar S. "Speed in Sweden." *NEJM* 283, (October 1, 1970): 760-761. https://doi.org/10.1056/NEJM197010012831410

Perrin, James M. "Changing Patterns of Conditions among Children Receiving Supplemental Security Income Disability Benefits." *Archives of Pediatrics and Adolescent Medicine* 153, no. 1 (January 1999): 80-84. https://doi.org/10.1001/archpedi.153.1.80

Persistence Market Research. "ADHD Therapeutics Market to Expand Twofold by 2030, Deprioritized Status of ADHD in Hospitals Due to Covid-19 Pandemic Surging Market Growth." April 2020. https://www.persistence-marketresearch.com/market-research/attention-deficit-hyperactivity-disorder-therapeutics-market.asp

Peters, John E., et al. *Physician's Handbook: Screening for MBD.*

Pew Research Center. "Despite Subscription Surges for Largest U.S. Newspapers, Circulation and Revenue Fall for Industry Overall." June 1, 2017. pewresearch.org/fact-tank/2017/06/01/circulation-and-revenue-fall-for-newspaper-industry/

Phillips, Christine. "Medicine Goes to School: Teachers as Sickness Brokers for ADHD." *PLoS Medicine* 3, no. 4 (April 2006): 433-435. https://doi.org/10.1371/journal.pmed.0030182

Pierson, Brendan, and Nate Redmond. "Jury Says J&J Must Pay $8 Billion in Case over Male Breast Growth Linked to Risperdal." Reuters, January 17, 2018. reuters.com/article/us-johnson-johnson-risperdal-verdict/jury-says-jj-must-pay-8-billion-in-case-over-male-breast-growth-linked-to-risperdal-idUSKBN1WN2HK

Pichot, P. Circular Insanity, 150 Years on. *Bulletin of the National Academy of Medicine* 188, no. 2 (2004): 275-284.

Pincus, J.H., and G.H. Glaser. "The Syndrome of 'Minimal Brain Damage' in Childhood." *NEJM* 275, no. 1 (July 7, 1966): 27-35. 10.1056/NEJM196607072750106

Pinel, Phillippe. *A Treatise on Mental Alienation.* Translated by Gordon Hickish, David Healy, and Louis C. Charland. Chichester: J. Wiley and Sons, 2008.

Piper, Brian G., Christy L. Ogden, Olapeju M. Simoyan, Daniel Y. Chung, James F. Caggiano, Stephanie D. Nichols, and Kenneth L. McCall. "Trends in Use of Prescription Stimulants in the United States and Territories, 2006 to 2016." *PLoS One*, (November 28, 2016). https://doi.org/10.1371/journal.pone.0206100

Polanczyk, Guilherme, Mauricio Silva de Lima, Bernardo Lessa, Mauricio Silva de Lima, Bernardo Lessa Horta, Joseph Biederman, and Luis Augosto Rhode. "The Worldwide Prevalence of ADHD: A Systematic Review and

Metaregression Analysis." *American Journal of Psychiatry* 164, no. 6 (June 2007): 942-948. https://doi.org/10.1176/ajp.2007.164.6.942

Polanczyk, Guilherme, Erik G. Wilcutt, Giovanni A. Salum, Christian Kieling, and Luis A. Rohde. "ADHD Prevalence Estimates across Three Decades: An Updated Systematic Review and Meta-Regression Analysis." *International Journal of Epidemiology* 43, no. 2 (April 2014): 434-442. https://doi.org/10.1093/ije/dyt262

Pratt, Laura A., Debra J. Brody, and Qiuping Gu. "Antidepressant Use among Persons Aged 12 and over: United States, 2011-2014." NCHS Data Brief, no. 283 (August 2017). cdc.gov/nchs/products/databriefs/db283.htm

Psychology in the Schools. "Erratum." 42, no. 2 (February 2005): 227.

Rapoport, Judith L., Monte S. Buchsbaum, Theodore P. Zahn, Herbert Weingartner, Christine Ludlow, and Edwin J. Mikkelsen. "Dextroamphetamine: Its Cognitive and Behavioral Effects on Normal Prepubertal Boys." *Science* 199, no. 4328 (February 3, 1978): 560-563. https://doi.org/10.1126/science.341313

Rapoport, Judith L., Monte S. Buchsbaum, Herbert Weingartner, Theodore P. Zahn, Christine Ludlow, and Edwin J. Mikkelsen. "Dextroamphetamine: Its Cognitive and Behavioral Effects in Normal and Hyperactive Boys and Normal Men." *Archives of General Psychiatry* 37, no. 8 (August 1980): 933-943. https://doi.org/10.1001/archpsyc.1980.01780210091010

Rapoport, Roger. "Just a Little Pill to Keep the Kid Quiet?" *Los Angeles Times*, April 25, 1971, 38-42.

Reid, Ann H., Sherman McCall, James M. Henry, and Jeffrey K. Taubenberger. "Experimenting on the Past: The Enigma of von Economo's Encephalitis Lethargica." *Journal of Neuropathology and Experimental Neurology* 60, no. 7 (July 2001): 663-670.

Reid, Robert, and Antonis Katsiyannis. "Attention-Deficit/Hyperactivity Disorder and Section 504." *Remedial and Special Education* 16, no. 1 (January 1995): 44-52. https://doi.org/10.1177/074193259501600106

Reinhold, Robert. "Learning Parley Divided on Drugs." *New York Times*, February 6, 1968.

Reynolds, Jennifer Lea. "Are Brains Different for Kids Who Have ADHD?" *US News and World Report*, June 16, 2017. https://usnews677-yahoopartner. tumblr.com/post/161890476983/are-brains-different-for-kids-who-have-adhd

Rhea, Deborah J. "Recess: The Forgotten Classroom." *Instructional Leader* 29, no. 1 (January 2016): 1-4. http://liinkproject.tcu.edu/wp-content/ uploads/2014/11/Rhea-Instructional-Leader-Journal-2016-pub-Recess-LiiNK.pdf

Rhea, Deborah J., and Michelle Baumi. "An Innovative Whole Child Approach to Learning: The LiiNK Project." *Childhood Education* 94, no. 2 (March/ April 2018): 56-63. https://doi.org/10.1080/00094056.2018.1451691

Rhea, Deborah J., and Alexander P. Rivchun. "The LiiNK Project: Effects of Multiple Recesses and Character Curriculum on Classroom Behaviors and Listening Skills in Grades K-2 Children." *Frontiers in Education* 3, (February 15, 2018): 1-10. https://doi.org/10.3389/feduc.2018.00009

Rhea, Deborah J., Alexander P. Rivchun, and Jacqueline Pennings. "The LiiNK Project: Implementation of a Recess and Character Development Pilot Study with Grades K & 1 Children." *TAHPERD Journal*, Summer 2016, 14-17, 35. http://liinkproject.tcu.edu/wp-content/uploads/2016/11/ TAHPERD-Journal-LiiNK-article-2016.pdf

Richters, John E., Eugene Arnold, Peter S. Jensen, Howard Abikoff, C. Keith Conners, Laurence L. Greenhill, Lily Hechtman, et al. "NIMH Collaborative Multisite Multimodal Treatment Study of Children with ADHD: I. Background and Rationale." *Journal of the American Academy of Child and Adolescent Psychiatry* 34, no. 8 (August 1995): 987-1000. https://doi. org/10.1097/00004583-199508000-00008

Rie, Herbert, Ellen D. Rie, Sandra Stewart, and J. Phillip Ambuel. "Effects of Methylphenidate on Underachieving Children." *Journal of Consulting and Clinical Psychology* 44, no. 2 (1976): 250-260. https://doi. org/10.1037//0022-006x.44.2.250

Rosenhan, David L. "On Being Sane in Insane Places." *Science*, 179, no. 4070 (January 19, 1973): 250-258. https://doi.org/10.1126/science.179.4070.250

Rösler, Michael, Thomas Gift, Barrie Merchant, and Frederick Reimherr. "In Memoriam: Paul H. Wender." *ADHD: Attention Deficit and Hyperactivity Disorders* 8, no. 4 (December 2016): 173-174. https://doi.org/1007/s12402-016-0209-2

Rucklidge, Julia J., and Rosemary Tannock. "Psychiatric, Psychosocial, and Cognitive Functioning of Female Adolescents with ADHD." *Journal of the American Academy of Child and Adolescent Psychiatry* 40, no. 5 (May 2001): 530-540. https://doi.org/10.1097/00004583-200105000-00012

Safer, Daniel J. "The Impact of Recent Lawsuits on Methylphenidate Sales." *Clinical Pediatrics* 33, no. 3 (March 1994): 166-168. https://doi.org/1177/000992289403300309

Safer, Daniel J. "Are Stimulants Overprescribed for Youths with ADHD?" *Annals of Clinical Psychiatry* 12, no. 1 (2000): 55-62. https://doi.org/10.1023/a:1009031211900

Safer, Daniel J., and Mark A. Stewart. "Hyperactivity in Children." In *Hyperactive Children: Diagnosis and Management*, edited by Daniel J. Safer and Richard P. Allen, 6-45. Baltimore: University Park Press, 1970.

Safer, Daniel J., Julie M. Zito, and Eric M. Fine. "Increased Methylphenidate Usage for Attention Deficit Disorder in the 1990s." *Pediatrics* 98, no. 6 (December 1996): 1084-1088.

Sagonosky, Eric. "Stampeding Generics Now Expected to Trample Lilly's Now-Off-Patent Strattera." May 31, 2017. fiercepharma.com/lilly-s-adhd-med-strattera-faces-new-generic-competition-from-teva-and-others

Saint Louis Post-Dispatch. "Suit Seeks Damages in School Drug Use." September 10, 1975.

Samea, Fateme, Solmaz Soluki, Vahid Najati, Mojtaba Zarei, Samuele Cortese, Simon B. Eikhoff, Masoud Tahmasian, and Claudia R. Eickhoff. "Brain Alterations in Children/Adolescents with ADHD Revisited: A Neuroimaging Meta-Analysis of 96 Structural and Functional Studies." *Neuroscience and Biobehavioral Reviews* 100, (May 2019): 1-8. https://doi.prg/10.1016/j.neubiorev.2019.02.011

Sandoval, Jonathan, Nadine M. Lambert, and Wilson Yandell. "Current Medical Practice and Hyperactive Children." *American Journal of Orthopsychiatry* 46, no. 2 (April 1976): 323-333. http://dx.doi.org/10.1111/j.1939-0025.1976.tb00932.x

Saul, Richard. "ADHD Does Not Exist." *Time*, March 14, 2014. https://time.com/25370/doctor-adhd-does-not-exist/

Schachar, Russell, and Rosemary Tannock. "Childhood Hyperactivity and Psychostimulants: A Review of Extended Treatment Studies." *Journal of Child and Adolescent Psychopharmacology* 3, no. 2 (1993): 81-97. https://doi.org/10.1089/cap.1993.3.81

Schachter, Howard M., Ba Ham, Jim King, Stephanie Langford, and David Moher. "How Efficacious and Safe is Short-Acting Methylphenidate for the Treatment of Attention-Deficit Disorder in Children and Adolescents? A Meta-Analysis." *CMAJ* 165, no. 11 (November 27, 2001): 1475-1488.

Scheffler, Richard M., Stephen P. Hinshaw, Sepidah Modrek, and Peter Levine. "The Global Market for ADHD Medications." *Health Affairs* 26, no. 2 (March/April 2007): 450-457. https://doi.org/10.1377/hltaff.26.2.450

Schmidt, William E. "Sales of Drug Are Soaring for Treatment of Hyperactivity." *New York Times*, May 5, 1987, C3.

Schrag, Peter and Diane Divoky. *The Myth of the Hyperactive Child and Other Means of Child Control*. New York: Random House, September 1, 1975.

Schreiber, Daniel. "The Dropout and the Delinquent: Promising Practices Gleaned from a Year of Study." *Phi Delta Kappan* 44, no. 5 (February 1963): 215-221.

Schwarz, Alan. "The Selling of Attention Deficit Disorder." *New York Times*, December 15, 2013.

Schürhoff, Franck, Frank Bellivier, Roland Jouvent, Marie-Christine Simeoni, Manuel Bouvard, Jena-Francois Allilaire, and Marion Leboyer. "Early and Late-Onset Bipolar Disorders: Two Different Forms of Manic-Depressive Illness?" *Journal of Affective Disorders* 58, no. 3 (2000): 215-221. https://doi.org/10.1016/s0165-0327(99)00111-1

Scutti, Susan. "Brains of Those with ADHD Show Smaller Structures Related to Emotion." CNN, February 16, 2017. https://www.cnn.com/2017/02/15/health/adhd-brain-scans-study/index.html

Setnik, Jennifer, G. Randall Bond, and Mona Ho. "Adolescent Prescription ADHD Medication Abuse is Rising Along with Prescriptions for These Medications." *Pediatrics* 124, no. 3 (September 2009): 875-880. https://doi.org/10.1542/peds.2008-0931/

Sexton, Joe, and Rachel L. Swarns. "A Slide into Peril, with No One to Catch Her." *New York Times*, November 15, 1997, A1.

Shalit, Ruth. "Defining Disability Down." *New Republic*, August 25, 1997, 16-22.

Shaywitz, Bennett A., Sally E. Shaywitz, Thomas Byrne, Donald J. Cohen, and Steven Rothman. "Attention-Deficit Disorder: Quantitative Analysis of CT." *Neurology* 33, (November 1983): 1500-1503. https://doi.org/10.1212/wnl.33.11.1500

Shillington, Audrey M., Mark B. Reed, James E. Lange, John D. Clapp, and Susan Henry. "College Undergraduate Ritalin Abusers in Southwestern California: Protective and Risk Factors." *Journal of Drug Issues* 36, no. 4 (October 1, 2006): 999-1014. https://doi.org/10.1177/002204260603600411

Shire plc. "Full Year and Fourth Quarter Results Ended 31 December 2002." Accessed May 23, 2020. investors.shire.com/~/media/Files/S/Shire-IR/presentations-webcast/year-2003/q4-presentation-27-02-03.pdf

Shire plc. "Annual Review 2008." Accessed May 23, 2020. investors.shire.com/~/media/Files/S/Shire-IR/annual-interim-reports/archive/shireannualreviewandsummary2008.pdf

Shrank, William H., Amanda R. Patrick, and M. Alan Brookhart. "Healthy User and Related Biases in Observational Studies of Preventive Interventions: A Primer for Physicians." *Journal of General Internal Medicine* 26, no. 5 (May 2011): 546-550. https://doi.org/10.1007/s11606-010-1609-1

Sleator, Esther K., Rina K. Ullmann, and Alice von Neumann. "How Do Hyperactive Children Feel About Taking Stimulants and Will They Tell the Doctor?" *Clinical Pediatrics* 21, no. 8 (August 1982): 474-479. https://doi.org/10.1177/000992288202100805

Smith, Alice K. "'Eggheads of the World Unite!'" *Bulletin of the Atomic Scientists* 14, (1958): 151-152.

Smith, Matthew. *Hyperactive: The Controversial History of ADHD*. London: Reaktion Books, 2014.

Smith, Matthew. "Ritalin at 75: What Does the Future Hold?" *The Conversation*, September 18, 2019. https://theconversation.com/ritalin-at-75-what-does-the-future-hold-121591

Smith, Shannon M., Richard C. Dart, Nathaniel P. Katz, Florence Paillard, Edgar H. Adams, Sandra D. Comer, Aldemar DeGroot, et al. "Classification and Definition of Misuse, Abuse, and Related Events in Clinical Trials: ACTTION Systematic Review and Recommendations." *Pain* 154, no. 11 (November 2013): 2287-2296. https://doi.org/10.1016/j.pain.2013.05/053

Solon, Olivia. "The Great Attention Deficit: More Parents Seek ADHD Diagnosis and Drugs for Kids to Manage Learning." NBC News, February 16, 2021. https;//nbcnews.com/tech/tech-news/great-attention-deficit-more-parents-seek-adhd-diagnosis-drugs-kids-n1257660

Spencer, Thomas J., Joseph Biederman, and Eric Mick. "Attention-Deficit/ Hyperactivity Disorder: Diagnosis, Lifespan, Comorbidities, and Neuro-biology." *Ambulatory Pediatrics* 7, no. 1S (January-February 2007): 73-81. https://doi.org/10.1016/j.ambp.2006.07.006

Spencer, Thomas J., Joseph Biederman, Timothy E. Wilens, Margaret Harding, Deborah O'Donnell, and Susan Griffin. "Pharmacotherapy of Atten-tion-Deficit Hyperactivity Disorder across the Life Cycle." *Journal of the American Academy of Child and Adolescent Psychiatry* 35, no. 4 (April 1996): 409-432. https://doi.org/10.1097/00004583-199604000-00008

Spiegel, Irving. "Jews Call Rarick a Costly Racist." *New York Times*, November 24, 1971.

Sroufe, L. Alan. "Treating Problem Children with Stimulant Drugs." *New England Journal of Medicine* 289, no. 8 (August 23, 1973): 407-413. https://doi.org/10.1056/NEJM197308232890806

Sroufe, L. Alan. "Ritalin Gone Wrong." *New York Times*, January 28, 2012. https://www.nytimes.com/2012/01/29/opinion/sunday/childrens-add-drugs-dont-work-long-term.html

Staufenberg, Jess. "Private Special School Places Cost £480 Million Per Year." *Schools Week*, March 4, 2017. https://schoolsweek.co.uk/private-special-school-places-cost-480-million-per-year/

Stein, Martin T. "FDA Alert: Pemoline Market Withdrawal." NEJM Journal Watch, December 9, 2005. jwatch.org/pa200512090000003/2005/12/09/fda-alert-pemoline-market-withdrawal

Still, George F. "Some Abnormal Psychical Conditions in Children: Lecture I: Delivered on March 4th." *Lancet* 159, no. 4102 (April 12, 1902): 1008-1012.

Still, George F. "Some Abnormal Psychical Conditions in Children: Lecture II: Delivered on March 6th." *Lancet* 159, no. 4103 (April 12, 1902): 1077-1082.

Still, George F. "Some Abnormal Psychical Conditions in Children: Lecture III: Delivered on March 11th." *Lancet* 159, no. 4104 (April 19, 1902): 1163-1168.

Streatfield, Dominic. *Cocaine: An Unauthorized Biography*. London: Virgin, 2003.

Strauss, Valerie J. "Why Some Schools Are Sending Kids Out to Recess Four Times a Day." *Washington Post*, September 13, 2016. https://www.washingtonpost.com/news/answer-sheet/wp/2016/09/13/recess-four-times-a-day-why-some-schools-are-now-letting-kids-play-an-hour-a-day/

Strecker, Edward A. "Behavior Problems in Encephalitis." *Archives of Neurology and Psychiatry* 21, (1929): 137-144.

Substance Abuse and Mental Health Services Administration. "Emergency Department Visits Involving Nonmedical Use of Stimulants among Adults Aged 18 to 34 Increased between 2005 and 2011." *DAWN Report*, August 8, 2013. samhsa.gov/data/sites/default/files/spot103-cns-stimulants-adults/spot103-cns-stimulants-adults.pdf

Sumathi, Reddy. "An Unexpected Diagnosis in Seniors—Doctors Are Identifying ADHD in Older Adults More Often." *Wall Street Journal*, February 25, 2020.

Supernus. "Supernus Announces FDA Approval of Qelbree." April 2, 2021. https://ir.supernus.com/node/12206/pdf

Supernus. "Highlights of Prescribing Information." April 2, 2021. https://www.supernus.com/sites/default/files/Qelbree-Prescribing-info.pdf

Swanson, James M., L. Eugene Arnold, Helena Kraemer, Lily T. Hechtman, Brooke S.G. Molina, Stephen P. Hinshaw, Benedetto Vitiello, et al. "Evidence, Interpretation, and Qualification from Multiple Reports of Long-Term Outcomes in the Multimodal Treatment Study of Children with ADHD (MTA): Part I: Executive Summary." *Journal of Attention Disorders* 12, no. 1 (July 2008): 4-14. https://doi.org/10.1177/1087054708319345

Swanson, James M., L. Eugene Arnold, Brooke S.G. Molina, Margaret H. Sibley, Lily T. Hechtman, Stephen P. Hinshaw, Howard B. Abikoff, et al. "Young Adult Outcomes in the Follow-Up of the Multimodal Treatment Study of Attention-Deficit/Hyperactivity Disorder: Symptom Persistence, Source Discrepancy, and Height Suppression." *Journal of Child Psychology and Psychiatry* 58, no. 6 (June 2017): 663-678. https://doi.org/10.1111/jcpp.12684

Swanson, James M., Glen R. Elliott, Laurence L. Greenhill, Timothy Wigal, L. Eugene Arnold, Benedetto Vitiello, Lily T. Hechtman, et al. "Effects of Stimulant Medication on Rates of Growth across 3 Years in the MTA Follow-Up." *Journal of the American Academy of Child and Adolescent Psychiatry* 46, no. 8 (August 2007): 1015-1025. https://doi.org/10.1097/chi.0b013e3180686d7e

Swanson, James M., Stephen P. Hinshaw, L. Eugene Arnold, Robert D. Gibbons, Sue Marcus, Kwan Hur, Peter S. Jensen, et al. "Secondary Evaluations of MTA 36-Month Outcomes: Propensity Score Analysis and Growth Mixture Model Analysis." *Journal of the American Academy of Child and Adolescent Psychiatry* 46, no. 8 (August 2007): 1003-1014. https://doi.org/10.1097/CHI.0b013e3180686d63

Swanson, James M., Keith McBurnett, Diane L. Christian, and Tim Wigal. "Stimulant Medications and the Treatment of Children with ADHD." *Advances in Clinical Child Psychology* 17, (1995): 265-332.

Szasz, Thomas S. *The Myth of Mental Illness: Foundations of a Theory of Personal Conduct*. New York: Harper & Brothers, 1961.

Szegedy-Maszak, Marianne. "Driven to Distraction." *US News and World Report*, April 26, 2004.

Taylor, Eric. "Syndromes of Attention Deficit and Hyperactivity." In *Child and Adolescent Psychiatry: Modern Approaches*, edited by Michael Rutter, Eric Taylor, and Lionel Hersov, 285-307. Oxford: Blackwell Science, 1994.

Thompson, J.S., Ronald J. Ross, and Samuel J. Horowitz. "The Role of Computed Axial Tomography in the Study of the Child with Minimal Brain Dysfunction." *Journal of Learning Disabilities* 13, no. 6 (June/July 1980): 334-337. https://doi.org/10.1177/00222/1948001300608

Thompson, Stephanie. "Some Parents Are Turning to Medical Marijuana to Treat ADHD Instead of Adderall." *Business Insider* January 7, 2020. https://www.businessinsider.com/adhd-marijuana-adderall-alternative-kids-2020-1?utm_source=feedburner&utm_medium=referral

Time. "Psychiatry on The Couch: To Shake the Blues, Freud's Disciples Seek New Directions." April 2, 1979. http://content.time.com/time/magazine/article/0,9171,916740,00.html

Timimi, Sammi. "ADHD is Best Understood as a Cultural Construct." *British Journal of Psychiatry* 184, no. 1 (January 2004): 8-9. https://doi.org/10.1192/bjp.184.1.8

Timimi, Sammi, Joanna Moncrieff, Jon Jureidini, Jonathan Leo, J. Cohen, D. Whitfield, D. Double, et al. "A Critique of the International Consensus Statement on ADHD." *Clinical Child and Family Psychology Review* 7, no. 1 (March 2004): 59-63. https://doi.org/10.1023/b:ccfp.0000020192.49298.7a

Torrey, E. Fuller. *The End of Psychiatry*. Radnor: Chilton, 1974.

Treadwell, David. "Ritalin Controversy: A 'Miracle Drug' Gets Closer Look." *Los Angeles Times*, December 28, 1987. https://www.latimes.com/archives/la-xpm-1987-12-28-mn-21365-story.html

Twenge, J.M., Thomas E. Joiner, Megan L. Rogers, and Gabrielle N. Martin. "Increases in Depressive Symptoms, Suicide-Related Outcomes, and Suicide Rates among U.S. Adolescents after 2010 and Links to Increased New Media Screen Time." *Clinical Psychological Science* 6, no. 1 (2017): 3-17. https://doi.org/10.1177.216770261117723376

United Nations Information Service. "INCB Sees Continuing Risk in Stimulant Prescribed for Children." March 4, 1997. incb.prg/incb/en/news/press-releases-1996.html

United States Department of Justice. "Johnson and Johnson to Pay More Than $2.2 Billion to Resolve Criminal and Civil Investigations." November 4, 2013. justice.gov/opa/pr/johns-johns-pay-more—22-billion-resolve-criminal-and-civil-investigations

United States Department of Labor. "Child Labor and Forced Labor Reports." 2019. https://dol.gov/agencies/ilab/resources/reports/child-labor/ghana

US News and World Report. "'Pep Pills' for Youngsters." July 13, 1970, 49.

Valenstein, Eliot. *Blaming the Brain: The Truth About Drugs and Mental Health.* New York: Free Press, October 5, 1998.

Vallée, Manuel. "Resisting American Psychiatry." *Advances in Medical Sociology* 12, (2011): 97-98.

Vallée, Manuel. "The Countervailing Forces Behind France's Low Ritalin Consumption." *Social Sciences and Medicine* 238, (August 15, 2019): 1-8. https://doi.org/10.1016/j.socscimed.2019.112492 [Epub ahead of print]

Vastag, Brian. "Pay Attention: Ritalin Acts Much Like Cocaine." *JAMA* 286, no. 8 (August 22/29, 2001): 905-906. https://doi.org/10.1001/jama.286.8.905

Ventola, C. Lee. "Direct-to-Consumer Pharmaceutical Advertising: Therapeutic or Toxic?" *Pharmacy and Therapeutics* 36, no. 10 (October 2011): 669-684.

Vinnedge, Harlan H. "Drugs for Children: The Omaha Program and Resulting Political Involvement." *New Republic*, March 13, 1971, 13-15.

Visser, Susanna N., Melissa L. Danielson, Rebecca H. Bitsko, Joseph R. Holbrook, Michael D. Kogan, Reem M. Ghandour, Ruth Perou, and Stephen J. Blumberg. "Trends in the Parent-Report of Health Care Providers Diagnosed and Medicated ADHD: United States, 2003-2011." *Journal of the American Academy of Child and Adolescent Psychiatry* 53, no. 1 (January 2014): 34-46. https://doi.org/10.1016/j.jaac.2013.09.001

Vitiello, Benedetto. "Psychopharmacology for Young Children: Clinical Needs and Research Opportunities." *Pediatrics* 108, no. 4 (October 2001): 983-989. http://doi.org/10.1542/peds.108.4.983

Volkow, Nora, Yu-Sin Ding, Joanna S. Fowler, Gene-Jack Wang, Jean Logan, John S. Gatley, Stephen Dewey, et al. "Is Methylphenidate Like Cocaine?"

Archives of General Psychiatry 52, (June 1995): 456-463. https://doi. org/10.1001/archpsych.1995.03950180042006

Waldman, Meredith. "Drug Ads Move Online, Creating a Web of Regulatory Challenges." *Nature Medicine* 16, no. 1 (January 2010): 22. https://doi. org/10.1038/nm0110-22

Walker, Sidney. *The Hyperactivity Hoax.* New York: Saint Martin's Press, 1998.

Wallis, Claudia. "Life in Overdrive." *Time*, Monday, July 18, 1994.

Warner, Judith. *We've Got Issues: Children and Parents in the Age of Medication.* New York: Riverhead Books, 2010.

Warren, John B. "Unbalanced Risk-Benefit Analysis of ADHD Drugs." *Lancet Psychiatry* 5, no. 11 (November 2018): 871. https://doi.org/10.1016/S2215- 0366(18)30349-3

Warren, Stafford L. "Implementation of the President's Program on Mental Retardation." *American Journal of Psychiatry* 121, no. 6 (December 1964): 549-554. https://doi.org/10.1176.ajp.121.6.549

Watson, Gretchen LeFever, Andrea Powell Arcona, and David O. Antonuccio. "The ADHD Drug Abuse Crisis on American College Campuses." *Ethical and Human Psychology and Psychiatry* 17, no. 1 (October 2015): 1-16. https:// doi.org/10.1891/1559-4343.17.1.5

Watson, Gretchen LeFever, Andrea Powell Arcona, David O. Antonuccio, and David Healy. "Shooting the Messenger: The Case of ADHD." *Journal of Contemporary Psychotherapy* 44, no. 1 (March 2014): 43-52. https://doi. org/10.1007/s10879-013-9244-x

Weinberg, Warren, and Roger A. Brumback. "Mania in Childhood." *American Journal of Diseases of Childhood* 130, no. 4 (April 1976): 380-385.

Wen, Patricia. "Tufts Settles Suit Against Doctor in Girl's Death for $2.5m." *Boston Globe*, January 25, 2011. http://archive.boston.com/lifestyle/health/ articles/2011/01/25/tufts_settles_suit_against_doctor_in_girls_death_ for_25m/

Wender, Paul H. *The Hyperactive Child.* New York: Crown, 1973.

Wender, Paul H. "The Concept of Adult Minimal Brain Dysfunction." In *Psychiatric Aspects of Minimal Brain Dysfunction*, edited by Leopold Bellak, 1-15. New York: Grune and Stratton, 1979.

Wender, Paul H. *Attention-Deficit Hyperactivity Disorder in Adults*. New York: Oxford University Press, 1998.

Wender, Paul H., David R. Wood, and Fred W. Reimherr. "Pharmacolgical Treatment of Attention Deficit Disorder, Residual Type (ADD-RT) in Adults." *Psychopharmacology Bulletin* 21, no. 2 (1985): 222-231.

Whalen, Carol K., and Barbara Henker. "Stimulant Pharmacotherapy for Attention Deficit/Hyperactivity Disorders: An Analysis of Progress, Problems, and Prospects." In *From Placebo to Panacea: Putting Psychotherapeutic Drugs to Test*, edited by S. Fisher and R.S. Greenburg, 323-356. New York: John Wiley and Sons, 1997.

Whitaker, Robert. *Anatomy of an Epidemic: Magic Bullets, Psychiatric Drugs, and the Astonishing Rise of Mental Illness in America*. New York: Broadway Books, 2010.

Whitaker, Robert, and Michael W. Corrigan. "*Lancet Psychiatry* Needs to Retract ADHD Brain Scan Study." Mad in America, April 15, 2017. https://www.madinamerica.com/2017/04/lancet-psychiatry-needs-to-retract-the-adhd-enigma-study/

White, Y.S., D.S. Bell, and R. Mellick. "Sequelae to Pneumoencephalography." *Journal of Neurology, Neuropsychiatry, and Psychiatry* 36, no. 1 (January 1973): 146-151. https://doi.org/10.1136/pnnp.36.1.146

Whitely, Martin. *Overprescribing Madness: What's Driving Australia's Mental Illness Epidemic?* Melbourne: Wilkinson Publishing, 2021. Kindle.

Whitely, Martin, Melissa Raven, Sami Timmi, Jon Jureidini, John Phillimore, Jonathan Leo, Joanna Moncrieff, and Patrick Landman. "Attention Deficit Hyperactivity Disorder Late Birthdate Effect Common in Both High and Low Prescribing International Jurisdictions: A Systematic Review." *Journal of Child Psychology and Psychiatry* 60, no. 4 (April 2019): 380-391. https://doi.org/10.1111/jcp12991p

Whitney, Jake. "This Researcher Thinks Recess is the Key to Better Test Scores." *D Magazine*, July 10, 2019. https://www.dmagazine.com/front-burner/2019/07/more-recess-better-test-scores-liink-tcu/

Wigal, Tim, James M. Swanson, Roland Regino, Marc A. Lerner, Ihab Soliman, Ken Steinhoff, Suresh Gurbani, and Sharon B. Wigal. "Stimulant Medications for the Treatment of ADHD: Efficacy and Limitations." *Mental Retardation and Developmental Disabilitie*s 5, no. 3 (August 17, 1999): 215-224. https://doi.org/10.1002/(SICI)1098-2779(1999)5:3<215::AID-MRDD8>3.0.CO;2-K

Wilcutt, Eric G. "The Prevalence of *DSM-IV* Attention-Deficit Hyperactivity Disorder: A Meta Analytic Review." *Neurotherapeutics* 9, no. 3 (July 2012): 490-499. https://doi.org/10.1007/s13311-012-0135-8

Wilens, Timothy E., Steven V. Faraone, Joseph Biederman, and Samantha Gunawardene. "Does Stimulant Therapy of Attention-Deficit/Hyperactivity Disorder Beget Later Substance Abuse? A Meta-Analytic Review of the Literature." *Pediatrics* 111, no. 1 (January 2003): 179-185. https://doi.org/10.1542.peds.111.1.179

Williams, Nigel M., Barbara Franke, Eric Mick, Richard J.L. Anney, Christine M. Freitag, Michael Gill, Anita Thapar, et al. "Genome-Wide Analysis of Copy Number Variants in Attention Deficit Hyperactivity Disorder: The Role of Rare Variants and Duplications at 15q13.3." *American Journal of Psychiatry* 169, no. 2 (February 2012): 195-204. https://doi.org/10.I1176/appi.ajp.2011.11060822

Williams, Nigel M., Irina Zaharieva, Andrew Martin, Kate Langley, Kiran Mantripragada, Ragnheidur Fossdal, Hreinn Stefansson, et al. "Rare Chromosomal Deletions and Duplications in Attention-Deficit Hyperactivity Disorder: A Genome-Wide Study." *Lancet* 376, no. 9750 (October 23, 2010): 1401-1408. https://doi.org/10.1016/S0140-6736(10)61109-9

Wilson, Jason. "A New Life: Being Diagnosed with ADHD in My 40s Has Given Me Something Quite Magical." *Guardian*, January 14, 2020. https://www.theguardian.com/society/commentisfree/2020/jan/15/a-new-life-being-diagnosed-wth-adhd-in-my-40s-has-given-me-something-quite-magical

Wolkenberg, Frank. "Out of a Darkness." *New York Times*, October 11, 1987.

Wolraich, Mark L., Jane N. Hannah, Theodora Y. Pinnock, Anna Baumgartner, and Janice Brown. "Comparison of Diagnostic Criteria for Attention-Deficit Hyperactivity Disorder in a County-Wide Sample." *Journal of the American Academy of Child and Adolescent Psychiatry* 35, no. 3 (March 1996): 319-324. https://doi.org/10.1097/00004583-199603000-00013

Work, Henry H. "George Lathrop Bradley and the War over Ritalin." *COSMOS Journal*, September 11, 2001. http://www.cosmosclub.org/web.journals/2001/work.html

Wozniak, Janet, Joseph Biederman, Elizabeth Mundy, Douglas Mennin, and Stephen V. Faraone. "A Pilot Study of Childhood-Onset Mania." *Journal of the American Academy of Child and Adolescent Psychiatry* 34, no. 12 (December 1995): 1577-1583. 10.1097/00004583-199512000-00007

Xian Janssen. "Attention Deficit Hyperactivity Disorder." Accessed September 10, 2021. https://www.xian-janssen.com.cn/en/therapy/adhd

Youngstrom, Eric A., Boris Birmaher, and Robert L. Findling. "Pediatric Bipolar Disorder: Validity, Phenomenology, and Recommendations for Diagnosis." *Bipolar Disorders* 10, no. 1 pt 2 (February 2008): 194-214. https://doi.org/10.1111/j.1399-5618.2007.00563.x

YouTube. "ADHD Consensus Conference—1998." September 3, 2009. https://www.youtube.com/watch?time_continue=7&v=ewTttDY6iB0

Zahn, Theodore P., Judith L. Rapoport, and Christine L. Thompson. "Autonomic and Behavioral Effects of Dextroamphetamine and Placebo in Normal and Hyperactive Prepubertal Boys." *Journal of Abnormal Child Psychology* 8, no. 2 (1980): 145-160. https://doi.org/10.1007/bf00919060

Zepf, Florian D. "Attention-Deficit-Hyperactivity Disorder and Early-Onset Bipolar Disorder: Two Facets of One Entity?" *Dialogues in Clinical Neuroscience* 11, no. 1 (March 2009): 63-72.

Zwi, Morris. "Evidence and Belief in ADHD." *BMJ* 321, no. 7267 (October 21, 2000): 975-976. https://doi.org/10.1136/bmj.321.7267.975

C

D

V

Viloxazine, 246, 289, 361

Vonnegut, Mark, 54, 56

Vyvanse, see Amphetamine, 5, 126, 174, 206, 215

W

Walker, Sidney, 51, 52, 293, 316

Warner, Judith, 98, 99, 179, 270, 293, 328, 346, 360

Watson, Gretchen LeFever, see LeFever, Gretchen, 76, 82, 139, 293, 323, 324, 332

Wender, Paul, 15, 16, 17, 184, 185, 285, 293, 294, 307, 347

Wender's Sign, 17

Whitaker, Robert, 44, 87, 147, 149, 294, 313, 325, 337

Wilens, Timothy J., 76, 164, 165, 255, 256, 288, 295, 333

Wozniak, Janet, 95, 96, 97, 255, 266, 278, 296, 327, 328

ENDNOTES

1 Liz Kowalczyk, "Psychiatrist to Suspend Practice, Denies Wrong-Doing," *Boston Globe*, February 8, 2007, B4.

2 Lane Lambert, "Rebecca Riley's Doctor on the Defense," *Enterprise*, April 10, 2010, https://www.enterprisenews.com/x1661778235/Rebecca-Riley-s-doctor-on-the-defense

3 Heinrich Joachim, *The Papyrus Ebers*, trans. Cyril P. Bryan (Chicago: Ares Publishers, 1930), xiii.

4 Ibid., 162.

5 George F. Still, "Some Abnormal Psychical Conditions in Children: Lecture I: Delivered on March 4th," *Lancet* 159, no. 4102 (April 12, 1902): 1008-1012; George F. Still, "Some Abnormal Psychical Conditions in Children: Lecture II: Delivered on March 6th," *Lancet* 159, no. 4103 (April 19, 1902): 1077-1082; George F. Still, "Some Abnormal Psychical Conditions in Children: Lecture III: Delivered on March 11th," *Lancet* 159, no. 4104 (April 26, 1902): 1163-1168.

6 Still, "Lecture III," 1166.

7 Ibid., 1164.

8 Ibid, 1167.

9 Ann H. Reid et al., "Experimenting on the Past: The Enigma of von Econo-mo's Encephalitis Lethargica," *Journal of Neuropathology and Experimental Neurology* 60, no. 7 (July 2001): 663-670.

10 Edward A. Strecker, "Behavior Problems in Encephalitis," *Archives of Neurology and Psychiatry* 21, (1929): 137-144.

11 Roger L.J. Kennedy, "The Prognosis of Sequelae of Epidemic Encephalitis in Children," *American Journal of Diseases of Children* 28, (1924): 158-172.

12 Eugen Kahn and Louis H. Cohen, "Organic Drivenness: A Brain-Stem Syndrome and Experiences," *New England Journal of Medicine* 210, no. 14 (April 5, 1934): 750.

13 Ibid., 749.

14 Sharon Liao, "Why Are ADHD Medicines Controlled Substances?" WebMD, last reviewed May 10, 2017, https://www.webmd.com/ add-adhd/features/adhd-medicines-controlled-substances#1

15 Henry H. Work, "George Lathrop Bradley and the War over Ritalin," *COSMOS Journal*, September 11, 2001, http://www.cosmosclub.org/web. journals/2001/work.html

16 C. Keith Conners, "Attention-Deficit/Hyperactivity Disorder—Historical Development and Overview," *Journal of Attention Deficit Disorders* 3, no. 4 (January 2000): 173-191.

17 Y.S. White, D.S. Bell, and R. Mellick, "Sequelae to Pneumoencephalography," *Journal of Neurology, Neuropsychiatry, and Psychiatry* 36, no. 1 (January 1973): 146-151, https://doi.org/10.1136/pnnp.36.1.146

18 Conners, "Overview," 179.

19 Charles Bradley, "The Behavior of Children Receiving Benzedrine," *American Journal of Psychiatry* 93, no. 4 (November 1937): 578-585.

20 Charles Bradley, "Benzedrine and Dexedrine in the Treatment of Children's Behavior Disorders," *Pediatrics* 5, no. 1 (January 1950): 24-37.

21 Henri Gastaut, "Combined Photic and Metrazol Activation of the Brain," *Electroencephalography and Clinical Neurophysiology* 2, nos. 1-4 (1950): 249-261, https://doi.org/10.1016/0013-4694(50)90056-3/

22 Ibid., 249.

23 Walter A. Brown, "Charles Bradley, M.D.," *American Journal of Psychiatry* 155, no. 7 (July 1998): 968, https://doi.org/10.1176/ajp.155.7.968

24 Maurice W. Laufer, Eric Denhoff, and Gerald Solomons, "Hyperkinetic Impulse Disorder in Children's Behavioral Problems," *Psychosomatic Medicine* 19, no. 1 (1957): 38-49.

25 Ibid., 38-42.

26 Ibid., 46.

27 Ibid., 40-42.

28 Ibid., 44.

29 Ibid., 46.

30 Ibid., 47-48.

31 Sol Levy, "Post-Encephalitic Behavior Disorder—A Forgotten Entity: A Report of 100 Cases," *American Journal of Psychiatry* 115, no. 12 (June 1959): 1062-1067, https://doi.org/10.1176/ajp.115.12.1062

32 Ibid., 1063.

33 Ibid., 1065-1066.

34 Ibid., 1065-1066.

35 Ibid., 1066.

36 Sam D. Clements and John E. Peters, "Minimal Brain Dysfunction in the School-Age Child," *Archives of General Psychiatry* 6, (1962): 185-197.

37 Ibid., 188.

38 Ibid., 187-188.

39 Ibid., 188.

40 Ibid., 193.

41 Ibid., 194.

42 J.H. Pincus and G.H. Glaser, "The Syndrome of 'Minimal Brain Damage' in Childhood," *NEJM* 275, no. 1 (July 7, 1966): 27-35, 10.1056/NEJM196607072750106

43 Ibid., 28.

44 Ibid., 27.

45 Ibid., 27-32.

46 Ibid., 33-34.

47 C. Keith Conners, "A Teacher Rating Scale for Use in Drug Studies with Children," *American Journal of Psychiatry* 126, no. 6 (December 1969): 884-888, https://doi.org/10.1176.ajp.126.6.884

48 Paul H. Wender, *The Hyperactive Child* (New York: Crown, 1973).

49 Dr. Wender was also one of the main investigators in the Danish Adoption Study, which has been held up as proof of the hereditary nature of schizophrenia, even though the investigators' own data showed no correlation between a diagnosis of schizophrenia and having a schizophrenic birth mother. For more information about the Danish Adoption Study and its numerous methodological problems, see Chapter Five of my book, *Madness and Genetic Determinism: Is Mental Illness in Our Genes?* (New York: Palgrave MacMillan, July 12, 2019).

50 Wender, *Hyperactive Child*, 9.

51 Ibid., 9-26.

52 Ibid., 10, 12.

53 Ibid., 28.

54 Ibid., 57.

55 Ibid., 58.

56 Paul H. Wender, *Attention-Deficit Hyperactivity Disorder in Adults* (New York: Oxford University Press, 1998).

57 Michael Rösler et al., "In Memoriam: Paul H. Wender," *ADHD: Attention Deficit and Hyperactivity Disorders* 8, no. 4 (December 2016): 173-174, https://doi.org/10.1007/s12402-016-0209-2

58 L. Alan Sroufe, "Treating Problem Children with Stimulant Drugs," *New England Journal of Medicine* 289, no. 8 (August 23, 1973): 407-413, https://doi.org/10.1056/NEJM197308232890806

59 Ibid., 407.

60 Ibid., 407. See also Judith L. Rapoport et al., "Dextroamphetamine: Its Cognitive and Behavioral Effects on Normal Prepubertal Boys," *Science* 199, no. 4328 (February 3, 1978): 560-563, https://doi.org/10.1126/

science.341313; Theodore P. Zahn, Judith L. Rapoport, and Christine L. Thompson, "Autonomic and Behavioral Effects of Dextroamphetamine and Placebo in Normal and Hyperactive Prepubertal Boys," *Journal of Abnormal Child Psychology* 8, no. 2 (1980): 145-160, https://doi.org/10.1007/bf00919060; Judith L. Rapoport et al., "Dextroamphetamine: Its Cognitive and Behavioral Effects in Normal and Hyperactive Boys and Normal Men," *Archives of General Psychiatry* 37, no. 8 (August 1980): 933-943, https://doi.org/10.1001/archpsyc.1980.01780210091010

61 Sroufe et al., "Problem Children," 408-409.

62 Ibid., 410.

63 Ibid., 410.

64 Ibid., 410.

65 Ibid., 411.

66 Ibid., 409.

67 Herbert E. Rie et al., "Effects of Methylphenidate on Underachieving Children," *Journal of Consulting and Clinical Psychology* 44, no. 2 (1976): 250-260, https://doi.org/10.1037//0022-006x.44.2.250

68 Rie et al., "Effects," 252.

69 Ibid., 254.

70 Ibid., 256.

71 Ibid., 256.

72 Ibid., 258.

73 Russell Barkley, *Hyperactive Children: A Handbook for Diagnosis and Treatment* (New York: Guilford Press, October 27, 1981).

74 Ibid., 15.

75 Ibid., 210.

76 Matthew Smith, *Hyperactive: The Controversial History of ADHD* (London: Reaktion Books, 2014).

77 Asa S. Knowles, "For the Space Age: Education as an Instrument of National Policy," *Phi Delta Kappan* 39, no. 7 (April 1958): 305-306.

78 Palmer Hoyt, "What is Ahead for Our Schools?" *Grade Teacher* 76, (October 1958): 20.

79 R.H.E. Eckelberry, "Editorial Comment," *Educational Research Bulletin* 37, no. 8 (November 12, 1958): 221.

80 George S. Counts, "The Real Challenge of Soviet Education," *Educational Forum* 12, no. 3 (March 1959): 261.

81 Arthur S. Fleming, "The Philosophy and Objectives of the National Defense Education Act," *Annals of the American Academy of Political and Social Science* 327, (January 1960): 134.

82 Erik H. Erikson, "Youth and the Life Cycle," *Children* 7, no. 2 (March/April 1960): 47.

83 Knowles, "Space Age," 310.

84 Hoyt, "Schools," 21.

85 Eckelberry, "Comment," 222.

86 Counts, "Challenge," 268.

87 Alice K. Smith, "'Eggheads of the World Unite!'" *Bulletin of the Atomic Scientists* 14, (1958): 151-152.

88 Hoyt, "Schools," 21.

89 Eckelberry, "Comment," 222.

90 Hoyt, "Schools," 20.

91 Dorothy Barclay, "A Turn for the Wiser," *Pediatrics* 23, no. 4 (April 1959): 759.

92 National Defense Education Act of 1958, H.R. 13427, 85th Congress.

93 Anthony Davids and Jack Sidman, "A Pilot Study—Impulsivity and Delayed Gratification in Future Scientists and in Underachieving High School Students," *Exceptional Children*, December 1962, 170.

94 Fleming, "Philosophy," 135-136.

95 James Bryant Conant, *Slums and Suburbs* (New York: McGraw Hill, 1961), 51.

96 Daniel Schreiber, "The Dropout and the Delinquent: Promising Practices Gleaned from a Year of Study," *Phi Delta Kappan* 44, no. 5 (February 1963): 217.

97 Stafford L. Warren, "Implementation of the President's Program on Mental Retardation," *American Journal of Psychiatry* 121, no. 6 (December 1964): 550, https://doi.org/10.1176.ajp.121.6.549

98 Marsh F. Beall, "Disenchanted Students," *Science* 175, no. 4018 (January 1, 1972): 123, https://doi.org/10.1126/science.175.4918.123-b

99 Matthew Smith, "Ritalin at 75: What Does the Future Hold?" *The Conversation*, September 18, 2019, https://theconversation.com/ritalin-at-75-what-does-the-future-hold-121591

100 Ibid.

101 C. Keith Connors and Leon Eisenberg, "The Effects of Methylphenidate on Symptomatology and Learning in Disabled Children," *American Journal of Psychiatry* 120, (November 1963): 458-464.

102 Peter Schrag and Diane Divoky, *The Myth of the Hyperactive Child and Other Means of Child Control* (New York: Random House, September 1, 1975), 52, 57.

103 Don Mahler, "The Hyperactive Child," *Exceptional Children* 38, (October 1971): 161.

104 Schrag and Divoky, *Myth*, 58.

105 Ibid., 74

106 John E. Peters et al., *Physician's Handbook: Screening for MBD.*

107 Ibid., 1.

108 Ibid., 5.

109 Ibid., 78.

110 Schrag and Divoky, *Myth*, 89-90.

111 Ibid., 91-92.

112 Ibid., 73.

113 Peter Conrad and Deborah Potter, "From Hyperactive Children to ADHD Adults: Observations on the Expansion of Medical Categories," *Social Problems* 47, no. 4 (November 2000), 567-568.

114 Nat Hentoff, "Drug-Pushing in the Schools: The Professionals," *Village Voice*, May 25, 1972, 20.

115 Schrag and Divoky, *Myth*, 74-75.

116 Ibid., 75-76.

117 Ibid., 49.

118 Ibid., 52.

119 Ibid., 52.

120 Ibid., 52.

121 Robert Reinhold, "Learning Parley Divided on Drugs," *New York Times*, February 6, 1968.

122 Ibid.

123 Ibid.

124 Ibid.

125 Robert Maynard, "Omaha Pupils Given Behavior Drugs: 5 to 10 Percent of Pupils Given Drugs to Improve Behavior," *Washington Post*, June 29, 1970.

126 Ibid.

127 Ibid.

128 Ibid.

129 Ibid.

130 Ibid.

131 Edward T. Ladd, "Pills for Classroom Peace," *Saturday Review*, November 21, 1970, 66.

132 Nat Hentoff, "The Drugged Classroom," *Evergreen Review*, December 1970, 31-33.

133 Hentoff, "Drug-Pushing," 20.

134 *Newsweek*, "Pep Pills for Pupils," July 13, 1970, 60-62.

135 *US News and World Report*, "'Pep Pills' for Youngsters," July 13, 1970, 49.

136 Harlan H. Vinnedge, "Drugs for Children: The Omaha Program and Resulting Political Involvement," *New Republic*, March 13, 1971, 13-15.

137 Keiffer, Elizabeth, "The Miracle That Misfired," *Good Housekeeping*, January 1974, 114.

138 Vinnedge, "Drugs," 14.

139 Ibid., 13.

140 Irving Spiegel, "Jews Call Rarick a Costly Racist," *New York Times*, November 24, 1971; *New York Times*, "Black Representative Calls Colleague 'Leading Racist,'" February 9, 1972.

141 Richard Fallon, "Gallagher Gets 2 Years and $10,000 Fine," *New York Times*, June 16, 1973.

142 Careth Ellington, "The Children with No Alternative," *Saturday Review*, November 21, 1970, 67.

143 Roger Rapoport, "Just a Little Pill to Keep the Kid Quiet?" *Los Angeles Times*, April 25, 1971, 38-42.

144 Ibid., 40-41.

145 Schrag and Divoky, *Myth*, 105-106.

146 Jonathan Sandoval, Nadine M. Lambert, and Wilson Yandell, "Current Medical Practice and Hyperactive Children," *American Journal of Orthopsychiatry* 46, no. 2 (April 1976): 323-333, http://dx.doi.org/10.1111/j.1939-0025.1976.tb00932.x

147 Joseph N. Bell, "The Family that Fought Back," *McCall's*, May 1977, 26, 30, 32, 34, 36, 40.

148 Ibid., 26.

149 Ibid., 32.

150 Ibid., 26.

151 Ibid., 30, 32.

152 Ibid., 30.

153 Ibid., 36.

154 Ibid., 32, 34.

155 Ibid., 34.

156 *Saint Louis Post-Dispatch*, "Suit Seeks Damages in School Drug Use," September 10, 1975.

157 Bell, "Family," 34.

158 Susan Jacob, Dawn M. Decker, and Timothy S. Hartshorne, *Ethics and the Law for School Psychologists* (Hoboken: John Wiley and Sons, August 1, 2016): 241.

159 A search of the *Reader's Guide to Periodical Literature* confirms this. The number of relevant articles about "hyperactivity" peaks in 1975, the year Schrag and Divoky published their book, and falls off sharply after that. A search of the *New York Times* article database reveals the same pattern.

160 Thomas S. Szasz, *The Myth of Mental Illness: Foundations of a Theory of Personal Conduct* (New York: Harper & Brothers, 1961).

161 E. Fuller Torrey, *The End of Psychiatry* (Radnor: Chilton, 1974).

162 D.L. Rosenhan, "On Being Sane in Insane Places," *Science*, 179, no. 4070 (January 19, 1973): 250-258, https://doi.org/10.1126/science.179.4070.250

163 Phil Hickey, "In Defense of Antipsychiatry," Behaviorism and Mental Health, April 25, 2019, http://behaviorismandmentalhealth.com/2019/04/25/in-defense-of-anti-psychiatry/

164 Robert Whitaker, *Anatomy of an Epidemic: Magic Bullets, Psychiatric Drugs, and the Astonishing Rise of Mental Illness in America* (New York: Broadway Books, 2010).

165 *Time*, "Psychiatry on The Couch: To Shake the Blues, Freud's Disciples Seek New Directions," April 2, 1979, http://content.time.com/time/magazine/article/0,9171,916740,00.html

166 Ibid.

167 Whitaker, *Epidemic*, 269-271.

168 Brian J. Piper et al., "Trends in Use of Prescription Stimulants in the United States and Territories, 2006 to 2016," *PLoS One*, November 28, 2018, https://doi.org/10.1371/journal.pone.0206100

169 Esther K. Sleator, Rina K. Ullmann, and Alice von Neumann, "How Do Hyperactive Children Feel About Taking Stimulants and Will They Tell the Doctor?" *Clinical Pediatrics* 21, no. 8 (August 1982): 474-479, https://doi.org/10.1177/000992288202100805

170 Ibid., 477.

171 Ibid., 477.

172 Ibid., 477.

173 Ibid., 477.

174 Ibid., 477.

175 Ibid., 476.

176 Ibid., 478-479.

177 Ibid., 479.

178 Ibid., 479.

179 Mark L. Wolraich et al., "Comparison of Diagnostic Criteria for Attention-Deficit Hyperactivity Disorder in a County-Wide Sample," *Journal of the American Academy of Child and Adolescent Psychiatry* 35, no. 3 (March 1996): 319-324, https://doi.org/10.1097/00004583-199603000-00013

180 Anna Baumgartner, Mark L. Wolraich, and Mary Dietrich, "Comparison of Diagnostic Criteria for Attention Deficit Disorders in a German Elementary School Sample," *Journal of the American Academy of Child and Adolescent Psychiatry* 35, no. 5 (May 1995): 629-638, https://doi.org/10.1097/00004583-199505000-00015

181 Alan Kwasman, Barbara J. Tinsley, and Heidi S. Lepper, "Pediatricians' Knowledge and Attitudes Concerning Diagnosis and Treatment of Attention Deficit and Hyperactivity Disorders," *Archives of Pediatric and Adolescent Medicine* 149, (November 1995): 1211-1216, https://doi.org/10.1001/archpedi.1995.02170240029004

182 Ibid., 1214.

183 Russell A. Barkley and Charles E. Cunningham, "Do Stimulant Drugs Improve the Academic Performance of Hyperkinetic Children?" *Clinical Pediatrics* 17, no. 1 (January 1978): 85-92, https://doi.org/10.1177/000992287801700112

184 Barkley, *Hyperactive Children*, 213.

185 Kenneth D. Gadow, "Effects of Stimulant Drugs on Academic Performance in Hyperactive and Learning Disabled Children," *Journal of Learning Disabilities* 16, no. 5 (May 1983): 290-299, https://doi.org/10.1177/002221948301600509

186 Deborah Jacobvitz et al., "Treatment of Attentional and Hyperactivity Problems in Children with Sympathomimetic Drugs: A Comprehensive Review," *Journal of the American Academy of Child and Adolescent Psychiatry* 29, no. 5 (September 1990): 677-688, https://doi.org/10.1097/00004583-199009000-00001

187 Russell Schachar and Rosemary Tannock, "Childhood Hyperactivity and Psychostimulants: A Review of Extended Treatment Studies," *Journal of Child and Adolescent Psychopharmacology* 3, no. 2 (1993): 81-97, https://doi.org/10.1089/cap.1993.3.81

188 Laurence Greenhill, "Attention-Deficit Hyperactivity Disorder: The Stimulants," *Pediatric Psychopharmacology I* 4, no. 1 (January 1995): 123-168, https://doi.org/10.1016/S1056-4993(18)30455-3

189 James M. Swanson et al., "Stimulant Medications and the Treatment of Children with ADHD," *Advances in Clinical Child Psychology* 17, (1995): 265-332.

190 John E. Richters et al., "NIMH Collaborative Multisite Multimodal Treatment Study of Children with ADHD: I. Background and Rationale," *Journal of the American Academy of Child and Adolescent Psychiatry* 34, no. 8 (August 1995): 987-1000, https://doi.org/10.1097/00004583-199508000-00008

191 Thomas Spencer et al., "Pharmacotherapy of Attention-Deficit Hyperactivity Disorder across the Life Cycle," *Journal of the American Academy of Child and Adolescent Psychiatry* 35, no. 4 (April 1996): 409-432, https://doi.org/10.1097/00004583-199604000-00008

192 Carol K. Whalen and Barbara Henker, "Stimulant Pharmacotherapy for Attention-Deficit/Hyperactivity Disorders: An Analysis of Progress, Problems, and Prospects," in *From Placebo to Panacea: Putting Psychotherapeutic Drugs to Test*, ed. S. Fisher and R.S. Greenburg (New York: John Wiley and Sons, 1997), 323-356.

193 Larry S. Goldman et al., "Diagnosis and Treatment of Attention-Deficit/ Hyperactivity Disorder in Children and Adolescents," *JAMA* 279, no. 14 (April 8, 1998): 1100-1107, https://doi.org/10.1001/jama.279.14.1100

194 Susan Gilbert, "Study Supports Use of Stimulants for Children with Hyperactivity," *New York Times*, September 16, 1997, F10.

195 Sidney Walker, *The Hyperactivity Hoax* (New York: Saint Martin's Press, 1998).

196 Ibid., 6.

197 Peter R. Breggin, *Toxic Psychiatry: Why Therapy, Empathy, and Love Must Replace the Drugs, Electroshock, and Biochemical Theories of the "New Psychiatry"* (New York: Saint Martin's Griffin, 1991).

198 Peter R. Breggin and Ginger R. Breggin, *Talking Back to Prozac: What Doctors Aren't Telling You About the New Antidepressants* (New York: Saint Martin's Press, 1994).

199 Peter R. Breggin, "Risks and Mechanisms of Action of Stimulants," in *NIH Consensus Development Conference on Diagnosis and Treatment of Attention Deficit Hyperactivity Disorder*, National Institutes of Health (Bethesda, MD 1998): 105-119.

200 Ibid., 106.

201 Ibid., 106.

202 Ibid., 106.

203 Ibid., 106.

204 Ibid., 106.

205 Ibid., 106.

206 Ibid., 108.

207 Ibid., 109.

208 Ibid., 110.

209 Ibid., 110.

210 Ibid., 110.

211 Ibid., 110.

212 Ibid., 110.

213 Ibid., 110.

214 Ibid., 111.

215 YouTube, "ADHD Consensus Conference—1998," September 3, 2009,
    https://www.youtube.com/watch?time_continue=7&v=ewTttDY6iB0

216 Diagnosis and Treatment of Attention Deficit Hyperactivity Disorder
    (ADHD), *NIH Consensus Statement* 16, no. 2 (November 16-18, 1998):
    1-37.

217 Ibid., 2.

218 Ibid., 10.

219 Ibid., 10.

220 Ibid., 20.

221 Ibid., 21.

222 Tim Wigal et al., "Stimulant Medications for the Treatment of ADHD:
    Efficacy and Limitations," *Mental Retardation and Developmental Disabil-
    ities* 5, no. 3 (August 17, 1999): 215-224, https://doi.org/10.1002/
    (SICI)1098-2779(1999)5:3<215::AID-MRDD8>3.0.CO;2-K

223 Daniel J. Safer, "Are Stimulants Overprescribed for Youths with ADHD?"
    Annals of Clinical Psychiatry 12, no. 1 (2000): 55-62, https://doi.
    org/10.1023/a:1009031211900

224 Morris Zwi, "Evidence and Belief in ADHD," *BMJ* 321, no. 7267 (October
    21, 2000): 975-976, https://doi.org/10.1136/bmj.321.7267.975

225 Benedetto Vitiello, "Psychopharmacology for Young Children: Clinical
    Needs and Research Opportunities," *Pediatrics* 108, no. 4 (October 2001):
    983-989, http://doi.org/10.1542/peds.108.4.983

226 Howard M. Schachter et al., "How Efficacious and Safe is Short-Acting Methylphenidate for the Treatment of Attention-Deficit Disorder in Children and Adolescents? A Meta-Analysis," *CMAJ* 165, no. 11 (November 27, 2001): 1475-1488.

227 Irene M. Loe and Heidi M. Feldman, "Academic and Educational Outcomes of Children with ADHD," *Journal of Pediatric Psychology* 32, no. 6 (2007): 643-654, https://doi.org/10.1016/j.ambp.2006.05.005

228 Richters et al., "Background," 991.

229 MTA Cooperative Group, "A 14-Month Randomized Clinical Trial of Treatment Strategies for Attention-Deficit/Hyperactivity Disorder," *Archives of General Psychiatry* 56, (December 1999): 1073-1084, https://doi.org/10.1001/archpsyc.56.12.1073

230 Ibid., 1074-1075.

231 Ibid., 1078.

232 Brooke S.G. Molina et al., "The MTA at 8 Years: Prospective Follow-up of Children Treated for Combined-Type ADHD in a Multisite Study," *Journal of the American Academy of Child and Adolescent Psychiatry* 48, no. 5 (May 2009): 484-500, https://doi.org/10.1097/CHI.0b013e31819c23d0

233 Ibid., 489.

234 James M. Swanson et al., "Secondary Evaluations of MTA 36-Month Outcomes: Propensity Score Analysis and Growth Mixture Model Analysis," *Journal of the American Academy of Child and Adolescent Psychiatry* 46, no. 8 (August 2007): 1003-1014, https://doi.org/10.1097/CHI.0b013e3180686d63

235 James M. Swanson et al., "Effects of Stimulant Medication on Rates of Growth across 3 Years in the MTA Follow-Up," *Journal of the American Academy of Child and Adolescent Psychiatry* 46, no. 8 (August 2007): 1015-1025, https://doi.org/10.1097/chi.0b013e3180686d7e

236 James M. Swanson et al., "Evidence, Interpretation, and Qualification from Multiple Reports of Long-Term Outcomes in the Multimodal Treatment Study of Children with ADHD (MTA): Part I: Executive Summary,"

Journal of Attention Disorders 12, no. 1 (July 2008): 4-14, https://doi.org/10.1177/1087054708319345

237 Lisa Cosgrove and Sheldon Krimsky, "A Comparison of DSM-IV and DSM-5 Panel Members' Financial Associations with Industry: A Pernicious Problem Exists," *PLoS Medicine* 9, no. 3 (March 2012): 1-4, https://doi.org/10.1371//journal/pmed.1001190

238 See Chapter Twelve of this volume.

239 Michael W. Corrigan, *Debunking ADHD: 10 Reasons to Stop Drugging Kids for Acting Like Kids* (Lanham: Rowman and Littlefield, 2015), 31.

240 Ibid., 33.

241 Jack Parker et al., "The Long-Term Outcomes of Interventions for the Management of Attention-Deficit Hyperactivity Disorder in Children and Adolescents: A Systematic Review of Randomized Controlled Trials," *Psychology Research and Behavior Management* 6, (2013): 87-99, https://doi.org/10.2147/PRBM.S49114

242 Stephen P. Hinshaw and Richard M. Scheffler, *The ADHD Explosion: Myths, Medication, Money, and Today's Push for Performance* (Oxford: Oxford University Press, March 3, 2014), 10.

243 Richard Saul, "ADHD Does Not Exist," *Time*, March 14, 2014, https://time.com/25370/doctor-adhd-does-not-exist/

244 James M. Swanson et al., "Young Adult Outcomes in the Follow-Up of the Multimodal Treatment Study of Attention-Deficit/Hyperactivity Disorder: Symptom Persistence, Source Discrepancy, and Height Suppression," *Journal of Child Psychology and Psychiatry* 58, no. 6 (June 2017): 663-678, https://doi.org/10.1111/jcpp.12684

245 Samuele Cortese et al., "Comparative Efficacy and Tolerability of Medications for Attention-Deficit Hyperactivity Disorder in Children, Adolescents, and Adults: A Systematic Review and Network Analysis," *Lancet Psychiatry* 5, no. 9 (September 2018): 727-737, https://doi.org/10.1016/S2215-0366(18)30269-4

246 Ibid., 735.

247 John B. Warren, "Unbalanced Risk-Benefit Analysis of ADHD Drugs,"
Lancet Psychiatry 5, no. 11 (November 2018): 871, https://doi.
org/10.1016/S2215-0366(18)30349-3

248 Ibid., 871.

249 Josephine Holland and Kapil Sayal, "Relative Age and ADHD Symptoms,
Diagnosis, and Medication—A Systematic Review," *European Child
and Adolescent Psychology* 28, (November 2019): 1417-1429, https://doi.
org/10.1007/s00787-1229-6

250 Todd E. Elder, "The Importance of Relative Standards in ADHD
Diagnosis: Evidence Based on Exact Birth Dates," *Journal of
Health Economics* 29, (2010): 641-656, https://doi.org/10.1016/j.
jhealeco.2010.06.003; William N. Evans, Melinda S. Morrill, and Stephen
T. Parente, "Measuring Inappropriate Medical Diagnosis and Treatment
in Survey Data: The Case of ADHD among School-Age Children,"
Journal of Health Economics 29, (2010): 657-673, https://doi.org/10.1016/j.
jhealeco.2010.07.005; E.E. Krabbe et al., "Birth Month Indicator as a
Predictor of ADHD Medication Use in Dutch School Classes," *European
Journal of Special Needs Education* 29, no. 4 (2014): 571-578, https://doi.
org/10.1080/08856257.2014.943564; Martin Whitely et al., "Attention
Deficit Hyperactivity Disorder Late Birthdate Effect Common in Both
High and Low Prescribing International Jurisdictions: A Systematic
Review," *Journal of Child Psychology and Psychiatry* 60, no. 4 (April 2019):
380-391, https://doi.org/10.1111/jcp12991p

251 David Healy, *Shipwreck of the Singular: Healthcare's Castaways* (Toronto:
Samizdat Health Writer's Co-operative, 2021), 254.

252 Ibid., 274.

253 David Healy, *The Decapitation of Care* (Toronto: Samizdat Health Writer's
Co-operative, 2021), 34.

254 Healy, *Shipwreck*, 292.

255 Ibid., 241.

256 Ibid., 302.

257 William E. Schmidt, "Sales of Drug Are Soaring for Treatment of Hyperactivity," *New York Times*, May 5, 1987.

258 Ibid.

259 Connie Lenz, "Prescribing a Legislative Response: Educators, Physicians, and Psychotropic Medication for Children," *Journal of Contemporary Health Law and Policy* 22, no. 1 (2006): 77-78.

260 Andrew Blum, "Legal Attack on Ritalin Expands," *National Law Journal*, November 23, 1987.

261 David Treadwell, "Ritalin Controversy: A 'Miracle Drug' Gets Closer Look," *Los Angeles Times*, December 28, 1987, https://www.latimes.com/archives/la-xpm-1987-12-28-mn-21365-story.html

262 Ibid.

263 Virginia S. Cowart, "The Ritalin Controversy: What's Made This Drug's Opponents Hyperactive?" *JAMA* 259, no. 17 (May 6, 1988): 2521-2523.

264 Deborah Cassens Moss, "Ritalin under Fire," *ABA Journal*, November 1, 1988, 19.

265 Eileen M. Ouellette, "Legal Issues in the Treatment of Children with Attention-Deficit Hyperactivity Disorder," *Journal of Child Neurology* 6, (Supplement 1991): S68-S75.

266 Ibid., S68.

267 Cowart, "Controversy," 2523.

268 Moss, "Fire," 19.

269 Thomas H. Maugh, "Use of Drug to Calm Children Rises Sharply, Study Reports," *Los Angeles Times*, October 21, 1988, https://www.latimes.com/archives/la-xpm-1988-10-21-mn-4509-story.html

270 Diane Divoky, "Ritalin: Education's Fix-It Drug?" *Phi Delta Kappan* 70, no. 8 (April 1989): 599-605.

271 Ibid., 600.

272 Ibid., 600.

273 Ibid., 600.

274 Lenz, "Response," 79.

275 Daniel J. Safer, "The Impact of Recent Lawsuits on Methylphenidate Sales," *Clinical Pediatrics* 33, no. 3 (March 1994): 166-168, https://doi.org/1177/000992289403300309

276 Daniel J. Safer, Julie M. Zito, and Eric M. Fine, "Increased Methylphenidate Usage for Attention-Deficit Disorder in the 1990s," *Pediatrics* 98, no. 6 (December 1996): 1084-1088.

277 Vinod S. Bhatara et al., "Trends in Combined Pharmacotherapy with Stimulants for Children," *Psychiatric Services* 53, no. 3 (March 2002): 244, https://doi.org/10.1176/appi.ps.53.3.244

278 Joe Sexton and Rachel L. Swarns, "A Slide into Peril, with No One to Catch Her," *New York Times*, November 15, 1997, A1.

279 Ibid.

280 Ibid.

281 Ibid.

282 Ibid.

283 Ibid.

284 Ibid.

285 Ibid.

286 Carey Goldberg, "For the School Nurses, More Than Tending the Sick," *New York Times*, January 28, 1999.

287 Mark Long and Paul Barrett, "Lawsuit Is Filed Against Novartis over Children's Use of Ritalin in Texas," *Wall Street Journal*, May 15, 2000, B19.

288 Barry Meier, "Suits Charge Conspiracy by Maker and Doctors' Group to Expand Ritalin Use," *New York Times*, September 14, 2000, A16; Toni Locy, "Fight over Ritalin is Heading to Court," *USA Today*, September 15, 2000, A3; *Frontline*, "ADHD Lawsuits," 2001, pbs.org/wgbh/pages/frontline/shows/medicating/backlash/lawsuits.html

289 *Frontline*, "Lawsuits."

290 Ibid.

291 EXPERT REPORTS, "Family Mental Health: Unlocking the Brain's Secrets," *Family Circle*, November 20, 2001.

292 Ibid.

293 Ibid.

294 Ibid.

295 Novartis, "Plaintiffs Withdrawal in New Jersey Marks Fifth and Final Dismissal of All Class Actions Filed against Maker of Ritalin in 2000," March 7, 2002, webarchive.org/web/20030628102148/http://pharma. us.novartis.com/newsroom/pressReleases/releeaseDetail/jsp?PRID=187

296 Douglas Montero, "I Was Told to Dope," *New York Post*, August 7, 2002.

297 Ibid.

298 Ibid.

299 Lenz, "Response," 83.

300 Montero, "Dope."

301 Douglas Montero, "School Pill-oried: Parents Forced to Drug Kids," *New York Post*, August 9, 2002.

302 Gretchen LeFever Watson et al., "Shooting the Messenger: The Case of ADHD," *Journal of Contemporary Psychotherapy* 44, no. 1 (March 2014): 43-52, https://doi.org/10.1007/s10879-013-9244-x

303 Ibid., 44.

304 Ibid., 44-45.

305 Gretchen B. LeFever, Keila V. Dawson, and Ardythe L. Morrow, "The Extent of Drug Therapy for Attention Deficit-Hyperactivity Disorder among Children in Public Schools," *American Journal of Public Health* 89, no. 9 (September 1999): 1359-1364, https://doi.org/10.2105/ ajph.89.9.1359

306 Gretchen B. LeFever, Margaret S. Villers, and Ardythe L. Morrow, "Parental Perceptions of Adverse Educational Outcomes among Children Diagnosed and Treated for ADHD: A Call for Improved School/ Provider Collaboration," *Psychology in the Schools* 39, no. 1 (January 2002): 63-69, https://doi.org/10.1002/pits.10000

307 Russell A. Barkley et al., "International Consensus Statement on ADHD," *Clinical Child and Family Psychology Review* 5, no. 2 (June 2002): 89-111, https://doi.org/10.1023/a:1017494719205

308 Ibid., 90.

309 Sammi Timimi et al., "A Critique of the International Consensus Statement on ADHD," *Clinical Child and Family Psychology Review* 7, no. 1 (March 2004): 59-63, https://doi.org/10.1023/b:ccfp.0000020192.49298.7a

310 Ibid., 59.

311 Ibid., 60.

312 Russel A. Barkley et al., "Critique or Misrepresentation? A Reply to Timimi et al.," *Clinical Child and Family Psychology Review* 7, no. 1 (March 2004): 64-69, https://doi.org/10.1023/b:ccfp.0000020193.48817.30

313 Ibid., 68.

314 Watson et al., "Shooting," 47.

315 Ibid., 45.

316 Ibid., 45.

317 Ibid., 47.

318 Jeanne Lenzer, "Researcher to be Sacked After Reporting High Rates of ADHD," *BMJ* 330, no. 7943 (March 26, 2005): 691, https://doi.org/10.1136/bmj.330.7493.691

319 Jeanne Lenzer, "Researcher Cleared of Misconduct Charges," *BMJ* 331, no. 7521 (October 15, 2005): 865.

320 *Psychology in the Schools*, "Erratum," 42, no. 2 (February 2005): 227.

321 Gretchen LeFever Watson, interview December 3, 2021.

322 Ibid.

323 Ibid.

324 Watson et al., "Shooting," 48.

325 Susanna N. Visser et al., "Trends in the Parent-Report of Health Care Providers Diagnosed and Medicated ADHD: United States, 2003-2011,"

Journal of the American Academy of Child and Adolescent Psychiatry 53, no. 1 (January 2014): 34-46, https://doi.org/10.1016/j.jaac.2013.09.001

326 L. Alan Sroufe, "Ritalin Gone Wrong," *New York Times,* January 28, 2012.

327 Megan Brooks, "FDA Clears Chewable Methylphenidate (QuilliChew) for ADHD," MedScape, December 7, 2015, https://www.medscape.com/viewarticle/855572

328 Meghana Keshavan, "Tasty and Easy to Take, a New ADHD Drug Alarms Some Psychiatrists," *STAT*, May 23, 2016, https://www.statnews.com/2016/05/23/adhd-drug-concerns/

329 Piper et al., "Trends," 6.

330 P. Pichot, "Circular Insanity, 150 Years on," *Bulletin of the National Academy of Medicine* 188, no. 2 (2004): 275-284.

331 Jacob Kasanin, "The Affective Psychoses in Children," *American Journal of Psychiatry* 10, no. 6 (May 1931): 897-926.

332 Whitaker, *Epidemic*, 232-246.

333 Warren A. Weinberg and Roger A. Brumback, "Mania in Childhood," *American Journal of Diseases of Childhood* 130, no. 4 (April 1976): 380-385.

334 Ibid., 383.

335 Ibid., 383.

336 Ibid., 384.

337 Joseph Biederman et al., "Attention-Deficit Hyperactivity Disorder and Juvenile Mania: An Overlooked Comorbidity?" *Journal of the American Academy of Child and Adolescent Psychiatry* 35, no. 8 (August 1996): 997-1008, https://doi.org/10.1097/00004583-199608000-00010

338 Martha E. Hellander, "Children with Bipolar Disorder," *Journal of the American Academy of Child and Adolescent Psychiatry* 38, no. 5 (May 1999): 495.

339 Demitri Papolos and Janice Papolos, *The Bipolar Child* (New York: Broadway Books, 1999), xvi.

340 Ibid., xvi.

341 Ibid., xvii.

342 Carmen Moreno et al., "National Trends in the Outpatient Diagnosis and Treatment of Bipolar Disorder in Youth," *Archives of General Psychiatry* 64, no. 9 (September 2007): 1032-1039, https://doi.org/10.1001/archpsyc.64.9.1032

343 Jeffrey Kluger et al., "Young and Bipolar," *Newsweek*, August 19, 2002.

344 Jennifer Lish et al., "The National Depressive and Manic-Depressive Association (DMDA) Survey of Bipolar Members," *Journal of Affective Disorders* 31, no. 4 (August 1994): 281-294, https://doi.org/10.1016/0165-0327(94)90104-x; Giovanni L. Faedda et al., "Pediatric-Onset Bipolar Disorder: A Neglected Clinical and Public Health Problem," *Harvard Review of Psychiatry* 3, no. 4 (November-December 1995): 171-195, https://doi.org/10.3109/10673229509017185; Franck Schürhoff et al., "Early and Late-Onset Bipolar Disorders: Two Different Forms of Manic-Depressive Illness?" *Journal of Affective Disorders* 58, no. 3 (2000): 215-221, https://doi.org/10.1016/s0165-0327(99)00111-1; Roy H. Perliss et al., "Long-Term Implications of Early Onset in Bipolar Disorder: Data from the First 1000 Participants in the Systematic Treatment Enhancement Program for Bipolar Disorder (STEP-BD)," *Biological Psychiatry* 55, no. 9 (May 1, 2004): 875-881, https://doi.org/10.1016/j.biopsych.2004.01.022; Boris Birmaher, "Longitudinal Course of Pediatric Bipolar Disorder," *American Journal of Psychiatry* 164, no. 4 (April 2007): 537-539, https://doi.org/10.1176/ajp.2007.164.4.537; Eric A. Youngstrom, Boris Birmaher, and Robert L. Findling, "Pediatric Bipolar Disorder: Validity, Phenomenology, and Recommendations for Diagnosis," *Bipolar Disorders* 10, no. 1 pt 2 (February 2008): 194-214, https://doi.org/10.1111/j.1399-5618.2007.00563.x

345 Eliot Valenstein, *Blaming the Brain: The Truth About Drugs and Mental Health* (New York: Free Press, October 5, 1998), 43-47.

346 Faedda et al., "Pediatric-Onset Bipolar Disorder," 184-185.

347 David Healy, *Mania: A Short History of Bipolar Disorder* (Baltimore: Johns Hopkins University Press, 2008).

348 David Healy, "Shaping the Intimate: Influences on the Experience of Everyday Nerves," *Social Studies of Science* 34, no. 2 (April 2004): 219-245, https://doi.org/10.1177/0306312704042620

349 Healy, *Mania*, 132.

350 Youngstrom et al., "Pediatric Bipolar Disorder," 11.

351 Janet Wozniak et al., "A Pilot Study of Childhood-Onset Mania," *Journal of the American Academy of Child and Adolescent Psychiatry* 34, no. 12 (December 1995): 1577-1583, 10.1097/00004583-199512000-00007

352 Stephen V. Faraone et al., "Is Comorbidity with ADHD a Marker for Juvenile-Onset Mania?" *Journal of the American Academy of Child and Adolescent Psychiatry* 36, no. 8 (August 1997): 1046-1055, https://doi.org/10.1097/00004583-199708000-00012; Youngstrom et al., "Pediatric Bipolar Disorder," 11; Christine Demeter et al., "Current Research in Child and Adolescent Bipolar Disorder," *Dialogues in Clinical Neuroscience* 10, no. 2 (June 2008): 215-228; Florian D. Zepf, "Attention-Deficit-Hyperactivity Disorder and Early-Onset Bipolar Disorder: Two Facets of One Entity?" *Dialogues in Clinical Neuroscience* 11, no. 1 (March 2009): 63-72.

353 Mark Olfson et al., "National Trends in the Outpatient Treatment of Children and Adolescents with Antipsychotic Drugs," *Archives of General Psychiatry* 63, (June 2006): 679-685, https://doi.org/10.1001/archpsyc.63.6.679

354 Margaret Harris et al., "The Impact of Mood Stabilizers on Bipolar Disorder: The 1890's and 1990's Compared," *History of Psychiatry* 16, no. 4 (2005): 423-434, https://doi.org/10.1177/0957154X05052088

355 Ibid., 427-430.

356 Nancy J. Huxley and Ross J. Baldessarini, "Disability and Its Treatment in Bipolar Disorder Patients," *Bipolar Disorders* 9, no. 1-2 (2007): 183-196, https://doi.org/10.1111/j.1399-5618.2007.00430.x

357 Ibid., 183.

358 Ibid., 184.

359 Ibid., 183.

360 Karen Brooks, "No Small Burden," *Fort Worth Star-Telegram*, July 17, 2000.

361 Ibid.

362 Ibid.

363 Ibid.

364 Ibid.

365 Mary Ann McDonnell and Janet Wozniak, *Is Your Child Bipolar?* (New York: Bantam Books, 2008).

366 Ibid., xiii.

367 Ibid., 1, 212.

368 Ibid., 17.

369 Ibid., 159.

370 Ibid., 142.

371 Ibid., 143.

372 Ibid., 188-189.

373 Ibid., 188-189.

374 Ibid., 180.

375 Ibid., 180-183.

376 Ibid., 182-183.

377 Ibid., 184.

378 Ibid., 184.

379 Ibid., 184-185.

380 Ibid., 185.

381 Ibid., 185-186.

382 Ibid., 186.

383 Judith Warner, *We've Got Issues: Children and Parents in the Age of Medication* (New York: Riverhead Books, 2010).

384 Ibid., 93.

385 Ibid., 45.

386 Ibid., 45.

387 Ibid., 52.

388 Ibid., 52.

389 *Fifth Estate*, "Chazz Petrella: The Boy Who Should Have Lived," Narr. Gillian Findlay, CBC, March 27, 2015.

390 Alex M. Cressman et al., "Prescription Stimulant Use and Hospitalization for Psychosis and Mania," *Journal of Clinical Psychopharmacology* 35, no. 6 (December 2015): 667-671, https://doi.org/10.1097/JCP.0000000000000406

391 Ibid., 668.

392 Austin Bradford Hill, "The Environment and Disease: Association or Causation?" *Proceedings of the Royal Society of Medicine* 58, no. 5 (May 1965): 295-300.

393 Cressman et al., "Mania," 667-668.

394 Juvenile Bipolar Research Foundation, https://www.jbrf.org/, 2015.

395 Scott Allen, "Backlash on Bipolar Diagnosis in Children," *Boston Globe*, June 17, 2007, A1, A8.

396 Lambert, "Defense."

397 Maria Cramer, "DSS Dropped Inquiry Before Girl, 4, Was Found Dead," *Boston Globe*, February 8, 2007, A1, B4.

398 Lane Lambert, "Case Closed: Carolyn Riley's Murder Conviction Also Upheld in Rebecca Riley's Death," *Patriot-Ledger*, May 2, 2014, https://www.patriotledger.com/article/20140502/NEWS/140508819

399 Patricia Wen, "Tufts Settles Suit Against Doctor in Girl's Death for $2.5m," *Boston Globe*, January 25, 2011, http://archive.boston.com/lifestyle/health/articles/2011/01/25/tufts_settles_suit_against_doctor_in_girls_death_for_25m/

400 Lester Grinspoon and Peter Hedblom, *The Speed Culture: Amphetamine Use and Abuse in America* (Cambridge: Harvard University Press, 1974).

401 Dominic Streatfield, *Cocaine: An Unauthorized Biography* (London: Virgin, 2003).

402 Nora D. Volkow et al., "Is Methylphenidate Like Cocaine?" *Archives of General Psychiatry* 52, (June 1995): 456-463, https://doi.org/10.1001/archpsych.1995.03950180042006; Brian Vastag, "Pay Attention: Ritalin

Acts Much Like Cocaine," *JAMA* 286, no. 8 (August 22/29, 2001): 905-906, https://doi.org/10.1001/jama.286.8.905

403 Francis C. Colpaert et al., "Discriminative Properties of Cocaine: Neuro-pharmacological Characteristics as Derived from Stimulus Generalization Experiments," *Pharmacology, Biochemistry, and Behavior* 10, no. 4 (April 1979): 535-546, https://doi.org/10.1016/0091-3057(79)90229-6

404 Shannon M. Smith et al., "Classification and Definition of Misuse, Abuse, and Related Events in Clinical Trials: ACTTION Systematic Review and Recommendations," *Pain* 154, no. 11 (November 2013): 2287-2296, https://doi.org/10.1016//j.pain.2013.05.053

405 Einar S. Perman, "Speed in Sweden," *NEJM* 283, (October 1, 1970): 760-761, https://doi.org/10.1056/NEJM197010012831410

406 Gene R. Haslip, "ADD/ADHD Statement of Drug Enforcement Admin-istration at the Conclusion of the Conference on Stimulant Use in the Treatment of ADHD," Drug Enforcement Administration, December 10-12, 1996.

407 United Nations Information Service, "INCB Sees Continuing Risk in Stimulant Prescribed for Children," March 4, 1997, incb.prg/incb/en/news/press-releases-1996.html

408 John Bacon, "Ritalin Drug Abuse on the Rise," *USA Today*, August 3, 1988, D1.

409 K. Graff Low and A.E. Gendaszek, "Illicit Use of Psychostimulants among College Students: A Preliminary Study," *Psychology, Health, and Medicine* 7, no. 3 (2002): 283-287, https://doi.org/10.1080/13548500220139386

410 Alan D. DeSantis, Elizabeth M. Webb, and Seth M. Noar, "Illicit Use of Prescription ADHD Medications on a College Campus: A Multi-methodological Approach," *Journal of American College Health* 57, no. 3 (November-December 2008): 315-324, https://doi.org/10.3200/JACH.57.3.315-324; Alan D. DeSantis and Audrey Curtis Hane, "'Adderall is Definitely Not a Drug': Justifications for the Illegal Use of ADHD Stimulants," *Substance Use and Misuse* 45, (2010): 31-46, 10.3109/10826080902858334; Alan D. DeSantis, Seth M. Noar, and Elizabeth M. Webb, "Speeding Through the Frat House: A Qualita-

tive Exploration of Nonmedical ADHD Stimulant Use in Fraternities," *Journal of Drug Education* 40, no. 2 (2010): 157-170, https://doi.org/10.2190/DE.40.2.d

411 DeSantis et al., "Illicit Use," 321.

412 DeSantis et al., "Speeding," 160-161.

413 DeSantis et al., "Illicit Use," 317-320.

414 DeSantis et al., "Illicit Use," 320; DeSantis et al., "Speeding," 164.

415 DeSantis et al., "Speeding," 164.

416 DeSantis et al., "Illicit Use," 320.

417 Jennifer Setnik, G. Randall Bond, and Mona Ho, "Adolescent Prescription ADHD Medication Abuse is Rising Along with Prescriptions for These Medications," *Pediatrics* 124, no. 3 (September 2009): 875-880, https://doi.org/10.1542/peds.2008-0931

418 Substance Abuse and Mental Health Services Administration, "Emergency Department Visits Involving Nonmedical Use of Stimulants among Adults Aged 18 to 34 Increased between 2005 and 2011," *DAWN Report*, August 8, 2013, samhsa.gov/data/sites/default/files/spot103-cns-stimulants-adults/spot103-cns-stimulants-adults.pdf

419 Susan Donaldson James, "Adderall Abuse Alters Brain, Claims a Young Life," ABC News, November 5, 2010, abcnews.go.com/Health/MindMoodNews/Adderall-psychosis-suicide-college-students-abuse-study-drugs/story?id=12066619

420 Brianna Gurciullo, "Law Student Died from Lethal Mix of Heroin and Adderall," *GW Hatchet*, March 7, 2013, gwhatchet.com/2013/03/07/law-student-died-from-lethal-mix-of-heroin-adderall

421 Lev Facher, "One Night, One Pill, One Tragedy—and a Mother's Mission," *Michigan Daily*, September 8, 2015, michigandaily.com/section/statement/one-night-one-pill-one-tragedy---and-mother's-mission

422 Luke Henkhaus, "Autopsy Reveals Details in Phi Gamma Delta Student's Death," *Battalion*, December 13, 2018, thebatt.com/news/autopy-reveals-details-in-phi-gamma-delta-student-death/article_0b91df28-ff0d-11e8-bf03-0bddd1d01ea3.html

423 Sean Esteban McCabe et al., "Non-Medical Use of Prescription Stimulants among US College Students: Prevalence and Correlates from
a National Survey," *Addiction* 99, (2005): 96-106, 10.1111/j.1360-
0443.2005.00944.x; Audrey M. Shillington et al., "College Undergraduate
Ritalin Abusers in Southwestern California: Protective and Risk Factors,"
Journal of Drug Issues 36, no. 4 (October 1, 2006): 999-1014, https://doi.
org/10.1177/002204260603600411; Amelia M. Arria et al., "Nonmedical
Use of Prescription Stimulants and Analgesics: Associations with Social
and Academic Behaviors among College Students," *Journal of Drug Issues*
38, no. 4 (Fall 2008): 1045-1060.

424 Gretchen LeFever Watson, Andrea Powell Arcona, and David O.
Antonuccio, "The ADHD Drug Abuse Crisis on American College
Campuses," *Ethical and Human Psychology and Psychiatry* 17, no. 1
(October 2015): 1-16, https://doi.org/10.1891/1559-4343.17.1.5

425 James Butcher, "Cognitive Enhancement Raises Ethical Concerns,"
Lancet 362, no. 9378 (July 12, 2003): 132-133, https://doi.org/10.1016/
s0140-6736(03)13897-4; Gina Jachimowicz and R. Edward Geiselman,
"Comparison of Ease of Falsification of Attention Deficit Hyperac-
tivity Disorder Diagnosis Using Standard Behavioral Scales," *Cognitive
Sciences Online* 2, (2004): 6-20; Jessica Feinstein, "Adderall: The Academic
Steroid," *Yale Daily News*, January 24, 2005, https://yaledailynews.com/
blog/2005/01/24/adderall-the-academic-steroid;. Alysson Granger
Harrison, "Adults Faking ADHD? You Must Be Kidding!" *ADHD Report*
14, no. 4 (August 2006): 1-7, https://doi.org/10.1521/adhd.2006.14.4.1;
Allyson G. Harrison, Melanie J. Edwards, and Kevin C.H. Parker,
"Identifying Students Faking ADHD: Preliminary Findings and Strat-
egies for Detection," *Archives of Clinical Neuropsychology* 22, (2007):
577-588, https://doi.org/10.1016/j.acn.2007.03.008

426 Nadine M. Lambert and Carolyn S. Hartsough, "Prospective Study of
Tobacco Smoking and Substance Dependencies among Samples of
ADHD and Non-ADHD Participants," *Journal of Learning Disabilities* 31, no 6 (November/December 1998): 533-544, https://doi.
org/10.1177.00222194980310060 3

427 Ibid., 540.

428 Ibid., 540.

429 Peter R. Breggin, *Talking Back to Ritalin* (Cambridge, MA: Perseus Publishing, 2001).

430 Joseph Biederman et al., "Pharmacotherapy of Attention-Deficit/Hyperactivity Disorder Reduces Risk for Substance Use Disorder," *Pediatrics* 104, no. 2 (August 1999): 1-5, https://doi.org/10.1542/peds.104.2.e20

431 Ibid., 1.

432 Ibid., 3.

433 Ibid., 2.

434 James A. Halikas et al., "Predicting Substance Abuse in Juvenile Offenders: Attention Deficit Disorder versus Aggressivity," *Child Psychiatry and Human Development* 21, no. 1 (Fall 1990): 49-55, https://doi.org/10.1007/bf00709927

435 Lydia Furman, "What is Attention-Deficit Hyperactivity Disorder?" *Journal of Child Neurology* 20, no. 12 (December 2005): 994-1002, https://doi.org/10.10.1177/088307380502001301

436 Timothy E. Wilens et al., "Does Stimulant Therapy of Attention-Deficit/Hyperactivity Disorder Beget Later Substance Abuse? A Meta-Analytic Review of the Literature," *Pediatrics* 111, no. 1 (January 2003): 179-185, https://doi.org/10.1542.peds.111.1.179

437 Ibid., 182.

438 Lawrence H. Diller, "Bitter Pill," *Psychotherapy Networker*, January/February 2005, 55-61.

439 Kathleen Maclay, "Educator Nadine Lambert Dies in Accident," UC Berkeley, May 4, 2006, Berkeley.edu/news/media/releases/2006/05/04_Lambertobit.shtml

440 Brooke S.G. Molina et al., "Delinquent Behavior and Emerging Substance Use in the MTA at 36 Months: Prevalence, Course, and Treatment Effects," *Journal of the American Academy of Child and Adolescent Psychiatry* 46, no. 8 (August 2007): 1028-1040, https://doi.org/10.1097/chi.0b013e318068d96; these findings were confirmed at the eight-year follow up: Brooke S.G. Molina et al., "Adolescent Substance Use in

the Multimodal Treatment Study of Attention-Deficit/Hyperactivity Disorder (ADHD) (MTA) as a Function of Childhood ADHD, Random Assignment to Childhood Treatments, and Subsequent Medication," *Journal of the American Academy of Child and Adolescent Psychiatry* 52, no. 3 (March 2013): 250-263, https://doi.org/10.1016/jaac.2012.12.014

441 Joseph Biederman et al., "Stimulant Therapy and Risk for Subsequent Substance Use Disorders in Male Adults with ADHD: A Naturalistic Controlled 10-Year Follow-Up Study," *American Journal of Psychiatry* 165, no. 5 (May 2008): 597-603, https://doi.org/10.1176/appi.ajp.2007.07091486

442 Ibid., 602.

443 See Chapter Twelve for a discussion of the financial relationship between the drugmakers and Joseph Biederman and his associates.

444 K. Bergstrom and B. Bille, "Computed Tomography of the Brain in Children with Minimal Brain Damage: A Preliminary Study of 46 Children," *Neuropädiatrie* 9, no. 4 (November 1978): 378-384, https://doi.org/10.1055/s-0028-1091497

445 Ibid., 382.

446 J.S. Thompson, Ronald J. Ross, and Samuel J. Horowitz, "The Role of Computed Axial Tomography in the Study of the Child with Minimal Brain Dysfunction," *Journal of Learning Disabilities* 13, no. 6 (June/July 1980): 334-337, https://doi.org/10.1177/00222/1948001300608

447 Bennet A. Shaywitz et al., "Attention-Deficit Disorder: Quantitative Analysis of CT," *Neurology* 33, (November 1983): 1500-1503, https://doi.org/10.1212/wnl.33.11.1500

448 Eric Taylor, "Syndromes of Attention Deficit and Hyperactivity," in *Child and Adolescent Psychiatry: Modern Approaches*, ed. Michael Rutter, Eric Taylor, and Lionel Hersov (Oxford: Blackwell Science, 1994), 285-307.

449 James J. McGough and James T. McCracken, "Assessment of Attention Deficit Hyperactivity Disorder: A Review of Recent Literature," *Current Opinion in Pediatrics* 12, no. 4 (August 2000): 319-324, https://doi.org/10.1097/00008480-200008000-00006

450 Alan Baumeister and Mike F. Hawkins, "Incoherence of Neuroimaging Studies of Attention Deficit/Hyperactivity Disorder," *Clinical Neuropharmacology* 24, no. 1 (2001): 2-10, https://doi.org/10.1097/00002826-200101000-00002

451 Jay N. Giedd et al., "Brain Imaging of Attention Deficit/Hyperactivity Disorder," *Annals of the New York Academy of Sciences* 931, (June 2001): 33-49, https://doi.org/10.1111/j.1749-6632.2001.tb05772.x

452 Ibid., 45.

453 Francis Xavier Castellanos et al., "Developmental Trajectories of Brain Volume Abnormalities in Children and Adolescents with Attention-Deficit/Hyperactivity Disorder," *JAMA* 288, no. 14 (October 9, 2002): 1740-1748, https://doi.org/10.1001/jama.288.14.1740

454 Erica Goode, "Brain Size Tied to Attention Deficit Hyperactivity Disorder," *New York Times*, October 9, 2002.

455 Lisa Fine Goldstein, "Study: ADHD Drugs Unrelated to Smaller Brain Sizes," *Education Week* 22, no. 7 (October 16, 2002).

456 *Detroit News*, "Ritalin Is Safe—and It Works," December 12, 2002.

457 Castellanos et al., "Trajectories," 1743.

458 Ibid., 1745.

459 Jonathan Leo and David Cohen, "Broken Brains or Flawed Studies? A Critical Review of ADHD Neuroimaging Research," *Journal of Mind and Behavior* 24, no. 1 (Winter 2003): 29-55.

460 Ibid., 47.

461 Ibid., 34-41.

462 Francis Xavier Castellanos and Erica Proal, "Large-Scale Brain Systems in ADHD: Beyond the Prefrontal-Striatal Model," *Trends in Cognitive Science* 16, no. 1 (January 2012): 17-26, https://doi.org/10.1016/j.tics.2011.11.007

463 Ibid., 17.

464 ADHD-200 Consortium, "The ADHD-200 Consortium: A Model to Advance the Translational Potential of Neuroimaging in Clinical Neuro-

science," *Frontiers in Systems Neuroscience* 6, Article 62 (September 2012): 1-5, https://doi.org/10.3389/fnsys/2002.00062

465 Ibid., 2.

466 Matthew R.G. Brown et al., "ADHD-200 Global Competition: Diagnosing ADHD Using Personal Characteristic Data Can Outperform Resting State fMRI Measurements," *Frontiers in Systems Neuroscience* 6, (September 28, 2012): 1-22, https://doi.org/10.3389/fnsys.2012.00069

467 ADHD-200 Consortium, "Neuroimaging," 3.

468 Brown et al., "Diagnosing," 13.

469 ADHD-200 Consortium, "Neuroimaging," 4.

470 Martine Hoogman et al., "Subcortical Brain Volume Differences in Participants with Attention Deficit Hyperactivity Disorder in Children and Adults: A Cross-Sectional Mega-Analysis," *Lancet Psychiatry*, published online February 15, 2017, https://doi.org/10.1016/S2215-0366(17)30049-4

471 Hoogman et al., "Brain Volumes," 316.

472 Conor Gaffey, "Study Finds Brains of ADHD Sufferers Are Smaller," *Newsweek*, February 16, 2017, https://www.newsweek.com/brains-adhd-sufferers-are-smaller-suggesting-it-physical-disorder-study-557372

473 Susan Scutti, "Brains of Those with ADHD Show Smaller Structures Related to Emotion," CNN, February 16, 2017, https://www.cnn.com/2017/02/15/health/adhd-brain-scans-study/index.html

474 Henry Bodkin, "ADHD is a Brain Disorder, not a Label for Poor Parenting," *Daily Telegraph*, February 16, 2017, https://www.telegraph.co.uk/science/2017/02/15/adhd-brain-disorder-not-label-poor-parenting-say-scientists/

475 Vic Adhopia, "Children with ADHD Have Some Smaller Brain Regions, Study Shows," Canadian Broadcasting Corporation, February 16, 2017, cbc.ca/news/health/adhd-brain-structures-1.3983919

476 Jennifer Lea Reynolds, "Are Brains Different for Kids Who Have ADHD?" *US News and World Report*, June 16, 2017, https://usnews677-ya-

hoopartner.tumblr.com/post/161890476983/are-brains-different-for-kids-who-have-adhd

477 Robert Whitaker and Michael W. Corrigan, "*Lancet Psychiatry* Needs to Retract ADHD Brain Scan Study," Mad in America, April 15, 2017, https://www.madinamerica.com/2017/04/lancet-psychiatry-needs-to-retract-the-adhd-enigma-study/

478 Hoogman et al., "Brain Volumes," 316.

479 Fateme Samea et al., "Brain Alterations in Children/Adolescents with ADHD Revisited: A Neuroimaging Meta-Analysis of 96 Structural and Functional Studies," *Neuroscience and Biobehavioral Reviews* 100, (May 2019): 1-8, https://doi.prg/10.1016/j.neubiorev.2019.02.011

480 Russell Barkley, "This is How You Treat ADHD Based off Science," September 23, 2014, https://www.youtube.com/watch?v=_tpB-B8BX-k0&t=189s

481 Steven V. Faraone, "Discussion of 'Genetic Influence on Parent-Reported Attention-Related Problems in a Norwegian General Population Twin Sample,'" *Journal of the American Academy of Child and Adolescent Psychiatry* 35, no. 5 (May 1996): 596-598.

482 Harold S. Koplewicz, *It's Nobody's Fault: New Hope and Help for Difficult Children* (New York: Times Books, 1996).

483 Ibid., 5-6.

484 Ibid., 14.

485 Ibid., 79.

486 Ibid., 79.

487 Ibid., 79.

488 Ibid., 80.

489 Ibid., xv.

490 Ibid., xvi.

491 Ibid., 84.

492 David Healy, Joann LeNoury, and Julie Wood, *Children of the Cure: Missing Data, Lost Lives, and Antidepressants* (Toronto: Samizdat Health Writer's Co-operative, 2020).

493 Stephen V. Faraone et al., "Segregation Analysis of Attention Deficit Hyperactivity Disorder," *Psychiatric Genetics* 2, no. 4 (1992): 257-275, https://doi.org/10.1097/00041444-199210000-00004

494 Stephen V. Faraone and Henrik Larsson, "Genetics of Attention Deficit Hyperactivity Disorder," *Molecular Psychiatry* 24, (2019): 562-575, https://doi.org/10.1038/s41380-018-0070-0

495 E.g., Dawei Li et al., "Meta-Analysis Shows Significant Association between Dopamine System Genes and Attention Deficit Hyperactivity Disorder (ADHD)," *Human Molecular Genetics* 15, no. 14 (2006): 2276-2284, https://doi.org/10.1093/hmg/ddl152; J. Gordon Millchap, "Etiologic Classification of Attention-Deficit Hyperactivity Disorder," *Pediatrics* 121, no. 2 (February 2008): 358-365, https://doi.org/10.1542/peds/2007-1332; Ian R. Gizer, Courtney Ficks, and Irwin D. Waldman, "Candidate Gene Studies of ADHD: A Meta-Analytic Review," *Human Genetics* 126, (2009): 51-90, https://doi.org/10.1007/s00439-009-0694-x; Oussama Kebir et al., "Candidate Genes and Neuropsychological Phenotypes in Children with ADHD: Review of Association Studies," *Journal of Psychiatry and Neuroscience* 34, no. 2 (2009): 88-101; Benjamin M. Neale, "Meta-Analysis of Genome-Wide Association Studies of Attention-Deficit/Hyperactivity Disorder," *Journal of the American Academy of Child and Adolescent Psychiatry* 49, no. 9 (September 2010): 884-897, https://doi.org/10.1016/j.jaacp.2010.06/008; Mauricio Arcos-Burgos and Maximillian Muenke, "Toward a Better Understanding of ADHD: *LPHN3* Gene Variants and the Susceptibility to Develop ADHD," *ADHD Attention Deficit Hyperactivity Disorder* 2, no. 3 (November 2010): 139-147, https://doi.org/10.1007/s12402-0030-2; Stephen V. Faraone, "Epidemiology of Attention Deficit Hyperactivity Disorder," in *Textbook in Psychiatric Epidemiology 3rd Edition* ed. Ming T. Tsuang, Mauricio Tohen, and Peter Jones (New York: John Wiley and Sons, 2011), 449-467; B. Franke et al., "The Genetics of Attention-Deficit/Hyperactivity Disorder in Adults, a Review," *Molecular Psychiatry* 17, no. 10 (October 2012): 960-987, https://doi.org.10.1038//mp/2011/138

496 The fundamental assumption of family studies—that familial equals genetic—is false. The fundamental assumption of twin studies—the Equal Environment Assumption—is false. The fundamental assumption of adoption studies—that adoption randomizes environmental variation—is false. See chapters 2-5 of my book, *Madness and Genetic Determinism*. On these matters I am deeply indebted to Jay Joseph, a clinical psychologist who has been writing and publishing critiques of psychiatric genetics for the past more than twenty years. For Dr. Joseph's devastating review of family, twin, and adoption studies of ADHD, see "Not in Their Genes: A Critical View of the Genetics of Attention-Deficit Hyperactivity Disorder," *Developmental Review* 20, (2000): 539-567, https://doi.org.10.1006/drev/2000/0511; see also his follow-up paper, "ADHD and Genetics: A Consensus Reconsidered," in *Rethinking ADHD: From Brain to Culture*, ed. Sami Timimi and Jonathan Leo (New York: Palgrave MacMillan, 2009), 58-91; for a discussion of the inherent problems of psychiatric genetics studies in general, see his other voluminous writings on the subject.

497 Barkley, Russell A., "Attention-Deficit Hyperactivity Disorder," *Scientific American* 279, no. 3 (September 1998): 66-71.

498 I have elected to omit linkage studies and candidate-gene studies, which have failed to produce any clinically significant findings and which now are considered obsolescent modes of inquiry anyway. For a review of these studies, see Faraone and Larsson, "Genetics of Attention Deficit Hyperactivity Disorder."

499 Nigel M. Williams et al., "Rare Chromosomal Deletions and Duplications in Attention-Deficit Hyperactivity Disorder: A Genome-Wide Study," *Lancet* 376, no. 9750 (October 23, 2010): 1401-1408, https://doi.org/10.1016/S0140-6736(10)61109-9

500 CNN, "ADHD is a Genetic Condition, Study Says," September 29, 2010, thechart.blogs.cnn.com/2010/09/29/adhd-is-a-genetic-condition-study-says/

501 Sarah Boseley, "Hyperactive Children May Suffer from Genetic Disorder, Says Study," *Guardian*, September 29, 2010, https://www.theguardian.com/society/2010/sep/30/hyperactive-children-genetic-disorder-studya

502 Kate Kelland, "Study Finds Genetic Link to ADHD," Australian Broad-
      casting Company, September 30, 2010, abc.net.au/news/2010-09-30/
      study-finds-genetic-link-to-adhd/228092

503 Boseley, "Hyperactive Children."

504 Kelland, "Study."

505 Williams et al., "Chromosomal Deletions," 1404.

506 Ibid., 1404.

507 Julia J. Rucklidge and Rosemary Tannock, "Psychiatric, Psychosocial, and
      Cognitive Functioning of Female Adolescents with ADHD," *Journal of
      the American Academy of Child and Adolescent Psychiatry* 40, no. 5 (May
      2001): 530-540, https://doi.org/10.1097/00004583-200105000-00012

508 Klaus-Peter Lesch et al., "Genome-Wide Copy Number Variation Analysis
      in Attention Deficit/Hyperactivity Disorder: Association with Neuro-
      peptide Y Gene Dosage in an Extended Pedigree," *Molecular Psychiatry*
      16, no. 5 (May 2011): 491-503, https://doi.org/10.1038/mp.2010.29; J.
      Elia et al., "Genome-Wide Copy Number Variation Study Associates
      Metabotropic Glutamate Receptor Gene Networks with Attention
      Deficit Hyperactivity Disorder," *Nature Genetics* 44, no. 1 (December
      4, 2011): 78-84, http://doi.org/10.1038/ng.1013; Nigel M. Williams et
      al., "Genome-Wide Analysis of Copy Number Variants in Attention
      Deficit Hyperactivity Disorder: The Role of Rare Variants and Dupli-
      cations at 15q13.3," *American Journal of Psychiatry* 169, no. 2 (February
      2012): 195-204, https://doi.org/10.I1176/appi.ajp.2011.11060822; I.
      Jarick et al., "Genome-Wide Analysis of Rare Copy Number Variations
      Reveals *PARK2* as a Candidate Gene for Attention-Deficit/Hyperactivity
      Disorder," *Molecular Psychiatry* 19, no. 1 (January 2014): 115-121, https://
      doi.org/10.1038/mp/2010.29; Joseph T. Glessner et al., "Copy Number
      Variation Meta-Analysis as Novel Duplication at 9p24 Associated with
      Multiple Neurodevelopmental Disorders," *Genome Medicine* 9, no. 1
      (September 2017) 1-11, https://doi.org/10.1186/s13073-017-0494-1.

509 Glessner et al., "Meta-Analysis," 6.

510 Benjamin M. Neale et al., "Meta-Analysis."

511 Ditte Demontis et al., "Discovery of the First Genome-Wide Significant Risk Loci for ADHD," *Nature Genetics* 51, no. 1 (January 2019): 63-75, https://doi.org.10/1038/s41588-018-0269-7

512 *Daily Mail*, "Don't Blame the Parents. ADHD is in Our Genes," November 27, 2018, 5.

513 Nicola Davis, "Scientists Find Genetic Variants That Increase the Risk of ADHD," *Guardian*, November 26, 2018, https://amp.theguardian.com/society/2018/nov/26/scientists-find-genetic-variants-that-increase-risk-of-adhd

514 *Economist*, "Attention Please: Psychiatric Genetics," 429, no. 9120 (December 1, 2018).

515 Guilherme Polanczyk et al., "The Worldwide Prevalence of ADHD: A Systematic Review and Metaregression Analysis," *American Journal of Psychiatry* 164, no. 6 (June 2007): 942-948, https://doi.org/10.1176/ajp.2007.164.6.942

516 Davis, "Genetic Variants."

517 Ibid.

518 Kenneth S. Kendler, "'A Gene For…': The Nature of Gene Action in Psychiatric Disorders," *American Journal of Psychiatry* 162, no. 7 (July 2005): 1243-1252, https://doi.org/10.1176/appi.ajp.162.7.1243

519 Jay Joseph, "Problems in Psychiatric Genetic Research: A Reply to Faraone and Biederman," *Developmental Review* 20, (2000): 582-593, https://doi.org/10.1006/drev.2000.0518

520 Joseph, "Consensus," 75.

521 Joseph Biederman and Steven V. Faraone, "The Johnson and Johnson Center for Pediatric Psychopathology at the Massachusetts General Hospital," 2002.

522 Allen, "Backlash," A8.

523 Ibid.

524 Gardiner Harris and Benedict Carey, "Researchers Fail to Reveal Full Drug Pay," *New York Times*, June 8, 2008, A1.

525 Ibid.

526 Ibid.

527 Ibid.

528 Marcia Angell, "Drug Companies and Doctors: A Story of Corruption," *New York Review of Books*, January 15, 2009, nybooks.com/articles/2009/01/15/drug-companies-doctorsa-story-of-corruption

529 Marcia Angell, *The Truth About the Drug Companies* (New York: Random House, August 24, 2004).

530 Angell, "Corruption."

531 Ibid.

532 Eric Convey, "Mass. General Disciplines Three Psychiatrists," *Boston Business Journal*, July 1, 2011, bizjournals.com//boston/news/2011/07/01/mass-general-punishes-three-html

533 Ibid.

534 United States Department of Justice, "Johnson and Johnson to Pay More Than \$2.2 Billion to Resolve Criminal and Civil Investigations," November 4, 2013, justice.gov/opa/pr/johns-johns-pay-more—22-billion-resolve-criminal-and-civil-investigations

535 Brendan Pierson and Nate Redmond, "Jury Says J&J Must Pay \$8 Billion in Case over Male Breast Growth Linked to Risperdal," Reuters, January 17, 2018, reuters.com/article/us-johnson-johnson-risperdal-verdict/jury-says-jj-must-pay-8-billion-in-case-over-male-breast-growth-linked-to-risperdal-idUSKBN1WN2HK

536 Massachusetts General Hospital, "About Joseph Biederman, MD," massgeneral.org/psychiatry/doctors/17789/Joseph-Biederman

537 Ibid.

538 David Healy, *Pharmageddon* (Berkeley and Los Angeles: University of California Press, 2012).

539 David Cohen, Shannon Hughes, and David J. Jacobs, "The Deficiencies of Drug Treatment Research: The Case of Strattera™," in *Rethinking*

ADHD: From Brain to Culture, ed. Sami Timimi and Jonathan Leo (New York: Palgrave MacMillan, 2009), 313-333.

540 G. Chouinard et al., "An Early Phase II Clinical Trial with Followup of Tomoxetine (LY139603) in the Treatment of Newly Admitted Depressed Patients," *Psychopharmacology Bulletin* 21, no. 1 (1985): 73-76, https://doi.org/10.1007/BF00427436

541 Cohen et al., 315.

542 Ibid., 316.

543 Martin T. Stein, "FDA Alert: Pemoline Market Withdrawal," NEJM Journal Watch, December 9, 2005, jwatch.org/pa200512090000003/2005/12/09/fda-alert-pemoline-market-withdrawal

544 Joseph Biederman et al., "Efficacy of Atomoxetine versus Placebo in School-Age Girls with Attention-Deficit/Hyperactivity Disorder," *Pediatrics* 110, no. 6 (December 2002): 1-7, https://doi.org/10.1542/peds.110.6.e75

545 Cohen et al., "Deficiencies."

546 Ibid., 326.

547 Theodore Henderson and Keith Hartman, "Aggression, Mania, and Hypomania Induction Associated with Atomoxetine," *Pediatrics* 114, no. 3 (September 2004): 895, https://doi.org/10.1542/peds.2004-1140

548 Miranda Hitti, "FDA Issues Advisory on ADHD Drug Strattera," WebMD, September 29, 2005, webmd.com/add-adhd/childhood-adhd/news/20050929/fda-issues-advisory-on-adhd-drug-strattera#1

549 Martin Whitely, *Overprescribing Madness*, Chapter Nine, Kindle.

550 Ibid.

551 Eli Lilly and Company, "Strattera Posts Fastest Launch Ever for a New ADHD Medicine with 1 Million Prescriptions in First Six Months," July 22, 2003, businesswire.com/news/home/20030722005458/Eli-Lilly-Company-Strattera-Posts-Fastest-Launch

552 Eric Sagonosky, "Stampeding Generics Expected to Trample Lilly's Now-Off-Patent ADHD Med Strattera," May 31, 2017, fiercepharma.

com/lilly-s-adhd-med-strattera-faces-new-generic-competition-from-te-va-and-others

553 Linda Logdberg, "Being a Ghost in the Machine: A Medical Ghostwriter's Point of View," *PLoS Medicine* 8, no. 8 (August 2011): 1-2, https://doi.org/10.1371/journal.pmed.1001071

554 C. Lee Ventola, "Direct-to-Consumer Pharmaceutical Advertising: Therapeutic or Toxic?" *Pharmacy and Therapeutics* 36, no. 10 (October 2011): 669-684.

555 Amanda L. Connors, "Big Bad Pharma: An Ethical Analysis of Physician-Directed and Consumer-Directed Marketing Tactics," *Albany Law Review* 73, no. 1 (September 2009): 243-282, https://doi.org/10.1162/156265160360706615

556 Alan Schwarz, "The Selling of Attention Deficit Disorder," *New York Times*, December 15, 2013.

557 Ibid.

558 Meredith Waldman, "Drug Ads Move Online, Creating a Web of Regulatory Challenges," *Nature Medicine* 16, no. 1 (January 2010): 22, https://doi.org/10.1038/nm0110-22

559 Shire plc, "Full Year and Fourth Quarter Results Ended 31 December 2002," accessed May 23, 2020, investors.shire.com/~/media/Files/S/Shire-IR/presentations-webcast/year-2003/q4-presentation-27-02-03.pdf; Shire plc, "Annual Review 2008," accessed May 23, 2020, investors.shire.com/~/media/Files/S/Shire-IR/annual-interim-reports/archive/shireannualreviewandsummary2008.pdf

560 Pew Research Center, "Despite Subscription Surges for Largest U.S. Newspapers, Circulation and Revenue Fall for Industry Overall," June 1, 2017, pewresearch.org/fact-tank/2017/06/01/circulation-and-revenue-fall-for-newspaper-industry/

561 *Frontline*, "Federal Laws Pertaining to ADHD Diagnosed Children," accessed April 28, 2020, pbs.org/wgbh/pages/frontline/shows/medicating/schools/feds.html

562 Ibid.

563 Robert Reid and Antonis Katsiyannis, "Attention-Deficit/Hyperactivity Disorder and Section 504," *Remedial and Special Education* 16, no. 1 (January 1995): 44-5, https://doi.org/10.1177/074193259501600106

564 Sam Dillon, "Special Education Absorbs Resources," *New York Times*, April 7, 1994, A1; Sam Dillon, "Comptroller Report Faults Special Education Policy," *New York Times*, June 27, 1994, B3.

565 House of Commons, "Education and Skills: Third Report," July 6, 2006, https://publications.parliament.uk/pa/cm200506/cmselect/cmeduski/478/47802.htm; Department for Education, "Statistical First Release: Special Educational Needs in England, January 2010," June 23, 2010, https://www.gov.uk/government/statistics/special-education-al-needs-in-england-january-2010; Department for Education, "Support and Aspiration: A New Approach to Special Educational Needs and Disability," March 9, 2011, https://www.gov.uk/government/publica-tions/support-and-aspiration-a-new-approach-to-special-education-al-needs-and-disability-consultation

566 Raphaelle Beau-Lejdstrom, Ian Douglas, Stephen J.W. Evans, and Liam Smeeth, "Latest Trends in ADHD Drug Prescribing Patterns in Children in the UK: Prevalence, Incidence, and Persistence," *BMJ Open* 6, June 13, 2016, https://doi.org/10.1136/bmjopen-2015-010508

567 Lawrence H. Diller, *Running on Ritalin: A Physician Reflects on Children, Society, and Performance in a Pill* (New York: Bantam Books, 1998).

568 Michael Griffith, "A Look at Funding for Students with Disabilities," *The Progress of Education Reform* 16, no. 1 (March 2015): 1-6.

569 Ibid., 3.

570 Jess Staufenberg, "Private Special School Places Cost £480 Million Per Year," *Schools Week*, March 4, 2017, https://schoolsweek.co.uk/private-spe-cial-school-places-cost-480-million-per-year/

571 James M. Perrin et al., "Changing Patterns of Conditions among Children Receiving Supplemental Security Income Disability Benefits," *Archives of Pediatrics and Adolescent Medicine* 153, no. 1 (January 1999): 80-84, https://doi.org/10.1001/archpedi.153.1.80

572 Reid and Katsiyannis, "Section 504," 48-49.

573 Adam Clymer, "Senate Passes Bill on Teaching the Disabled," *New York Times*, May 15, 1997, B14.

574 Ruth Shalit, "Defining Disability Down," *New Republic*, August 25, 1997, 16-22.

575 Ibid.

576 See Chapter Three of this volume for the story of Sabrina Green.

577 Mitchell Kline, "ADHD Case Grabs Attention," *Tennessean*, September 25, 2009.

578 Darios Getahun and Stephen J. Jacobsen, "Recent Trends in Childhood Attention Deficit-Hyperactivity Disorder," *JAMA Pediatrics* 167, no. 3 (March 2013): 282-288, https://doi.org/10.1001/2013.jamapediatrics.401; CDC, "Mental Health Surveillance Among Children—United States, 2005-2011," May 17, 2013, https://www.cdc.gov/mmwrhtml/su6202a1.htm

579 Alison Leigh Cowan, "Amid Affluence, a Struggle over Special Education," *New York Times*, April 24, 2005.

580 Elissa Gootman, "In Special Education Cases, City is Fighting Harder Before Paying for Private School," *New York Times*, December 12, 2007, B3.

581 Jeff Bercovici, "Fired Yahoo Exec's $109M Golden Parachute Was One of the Biggest Ever," *Forbes*, January 16, 2014, https://www.forbes.com/sites/jeffbercovici/2014/01/16/fired-yahoo-execs-109m-golden-parachute-was-one-of-the-biggest-ever/#73e36b094a4f

582 Warner, *Issues*, 104.

583 Craig S. Lerner, "Accommodations for the Learning Disabled: A Level Playing Field or Affirmative Action for Elites?" *Vanderbilt Law Review* 57, no. 3 (2019): 1108-1109.

584 Shalit, "Disability."

585 CHADD, "Annual Report FY18," accessed April 27, 2020, chadd.org/wp-content/uploads/2019/01/AnnReport-FY18.pdf

586 John Merrow, "Reading, Writing, and Ritalin," *New York Times*, October 21, 1995, A21.

587 CHADD, "About ADHD," accessed April 27, 2020, chadd.org/about-adhd/overview

588 CHADD, "Position Paper on Controlled Substance Measures," accessed April 27, 2020, chadd.org/about-adhd/overview/

589 CHADD, "Public Policy Agenda for Children and Adolescents," accessed April 27, 2020, chadd.org/wp-content/uploads2018/06/Public-Policy-Agenda-for-Children-Adolescents.pdf

590 Maurice W. Laufer and Eric Denhoff, "Hyperkinetic Behavior Syndrome in Children," *Journal of Pediatrics* 50, no. 4 (April 1957): 463-474, https://doi.org/10.1016/S0022-3476(57)80257-1

591 Stella Chess, "Diagnosis and Treatment of the Hyperactive Child," *New York State Journal of Medicine* 60, (1960): 2382.

592 Pincus and Glaser, "Minimal Brain Damage," 32.

593 Daniel J. Safer and Mark A. Stewart, "Hyperactivity in Children," in *Hyperactive Children: Diagnosis and Management*, ed. Daniel J. Safer and Richard P. Allen (Baltimore: University Park Press, 1970), 21.

594 Wender, *Hyperactive Child*, 28.

595 Paul H. Wender, "The Concept of Adult Minimal Brain Dysfunction," in *Psychiatric Aspects of Minimal Brain Dysfunction*, ed. Leopold Bellak (New York: Grune and Stratton, 1979), 1-15.

596 Ibid., 2.

597 Ibid., 2.

598 Ibid., 2-3.

599 Ibid., 3.

600 Ibid., 3.

601 Paul H. Wender, David R. Wood, and Fred W. Reimherr, "Pharmacolgical Treatment of Attention Deficit Disorder, Residual Type (ADD-RT) in Adults," *Psychopharmacology Bulletin* 21, no. 2 (1985): 222-231.

602 Ibid., 229.

603 Frank Wolkenberg, "Out of a Darkness," *New York Times*, October 11, 1987.

604 Ibid.

605 Ibid.

606 Ibid.

607 Geoffrey Cowley, "The Not-Young and the Restless," *Newsweek*, July 26, 1993, 48.

608 Geoffrey Cowley, "The Promise of Prozac," *Newsweek*, March 26, 1990, 38-41.

609 D. Hales and R. Hales, "Pay Attention," *American Health*, September 1993, 62-65.

610 Ibid., 64.

611 Ibid., 65.

612 Ibid., 65.

613 Joseph Biederman et al., "Patterns of Psychiatric Comorbidity, Cognition, and Psychosocial Functioning in Adults with Attention Deficit Hyperactivity Disorder," *American Journal of Psychiatry* 150, no. 12 (December 1993): 1792-1798, https://doi.org/10.1176/ajp.150.12.1792; Joseph Biederman et al., "Young Adult Outcome of Attention Deficit Hyperactivity Disorder: A Controlled 10-Year Follow-Up Study," *Psychological Medicine* 36, no. 2 (February 2006): 167-179, http://doi.org/10.1017/S0033291705006410; Joseph Biederman et al., "Functional Impairments in Adults with Self-Reports of Undiagnosed ADHD: A Controlled Study of 1001 Adults in the Community," *Journal of Clinical Psychiatry* 67, no. 4 (April 2006): 524-540, https://doi.org/10.4088/jcp.v67n0403; Thomas J. Spencer, Joseph Biederman and Eric Mick, "Attention-Deficit/Hyperactivity Disorder: Diagnosis, Lifespan, Comorbidities, and Neurobiology," *Ambulatory Pediatrics* 7, no. 1S (January-February 2007): 73-81, https://doi.org/10.1016/j.ambp.2006.07.006; Joseph Biederman et al., "Educational and Occupational Underattainment in Adults with Attention-Deficit/Hyperactivity Disorder: A Controlled Study," *Journal of Clinical Psychiatry* 69, no. 8 (August 2008): 1217-1222, https://doi.org/10.4088/jcp.v69n0803

614 Spencer et al., "Life Cycle," 410.

615 Leonard A. A. Adler et al., "Functional Outcomes in the Treatment of Adults with ADHD," *Journal of Affective Disorders* 11, no. 6 (May 2008): 720-727, https://doi.org/10.1177/1087054707308490

616 Ibid., 725.

617 Edward M. Hallowell and John J. Ratey, *Driven to Distraction* (New York: Pantheon Books, 1994).

618 Ibid., 151, 197, 212.

619 Ibid., 1.

620 Ibid., 42.

621 Ibid., 20.

622 Ibid., 274.

623 Ibid., 192, 218.

624 Ibid., 100.

625 Ibid., 102.

626 Ibid., 108.

627 Ibid., 91.

628 Ibid., 99.

629 See for example Claudia Wallis, "Life in Overdrive," *Time*, Monday, July 18, 1994; Marianne Szegedy-Maszak, "Driven to Distraction," *US News and World Report*, April 26, 2004; Daniel Lavelle, "'I Assumed It Was All My Fault': The Adults Dealing with Undiagnosed ADHD," *Guardian*, Tuesday September 5, 2017, https://www.theguardian.com/society/2017/sep/05/i-assumed-it-was-all-my-fault-the-adults-dealing-with-undiag-nosed-adhd; Daniel Lavelle, "'People with ADHD Can Be Incredibly Valuable at Work,'" *Guardian*, Sunday March 18, 2018, https://www.theguardian.com/society/2018/mar/18/people-with-adhd-incredi-bly-valuable-at-work-diagnosis-support; Tom Hawking, "Tuning Out the Static: It Took 40 Years before I Found Out That I Have ADHD," *Guardian*, July 9, 2019, https://www.theguardian.com/commentis-free/2019/jul/10/tuning-out-the-static-it-took-40-years-before-I-found-out-that-i-have-adhd; Kate Aubusson, "'I Thought I Was a Loser, Now

I Have the Answer': Rise in Adult ADHD," *Sydney Morning Herald*, November 3, 2019, https://www.smh.com.au/national/i-thought-i-was-a-loser-now-i-have-the-answer-rise-in-adult-adhd-20191101-p536kn.html; Jason Wilson, "A New Life: Being Diagnosed with ADHD in My 40s Has Given Me Something Quite Magical," *Guardian*, January 14, 2020, https://www.theguardian.com/society/commentisfree/2020/jan/15/a-new-life-being-diagnosed-wth-adhd-in-my-40s-has-given-me-something-quite-magical; Adrian Chiles, "My Treatment for ADD Changed My Life, so Why Can't I Stop Worrying About It?" *Guardian*, September 30, 2020, https://www.theguardian.com/society/2020/sep/30/my-treatment-for-add-changed-my-life-so-why-cant-i-stop-worrying-about-it; Jill Foster, "Woman Diagnosed with ADHD at 44: 'I Thought It Only Affected Young Boys,'" *Yahoo! Life*, March 15, 2021, https://www.yahoo.com/lifestyle/wioman-diagnosed-adhd-at-44-100037439.html; Matilda Bosely, "Tik Tok Accidently Detected My ADHD. For 25 Years Everyone Missed the Warning Signs," *Guardian*, June 3, 2021, https://www.theguardian.com/commentisfree/2021/jun/04/tiktok-accidently-detected-my-adhd-for-23-years-everyone-missed-the-warning-signs

630 In fact there is no neurological or genetic test that can be used to distinguish ADHD kids or adults from their "normal" age-mates. See Chapter Eleven of this volume.

631 Reddy Sumathi, "An Unexpected Diagnosis in Seniors—Doctors Are Identifying ADHD in Older Adults More Often," *Wall Street Journal*, February 25, 2020.

632 J.J.S. Kooij et al., "Updated European Consensus Statement on Diagnosis and Treatment of Adult ADHD," *European Psychiatry* 56, (2019): 14-34, https://doi.org/10.1016.j.europsy.2018.11.001

633 "FDA Permits Marketing of First Medical Device for Treatment of ADHD," FDA, April 19, 2019, https://www.fda.gov/news-events/press-announcements/fda-permits-marketing-first-medical-device-treatment-adhd

634 James J. McGough et al., "Double-Blind, Sham-Controlled, Pilot Study of Trigeminal Nerve Stimulation for Attention-Deficit/Hyperactivity Disorder," *Journal of the American Academy of Child and Adolescent*

Psychiatry 58, no. 4 (April 2019): 403-411, https://doi.org/10.1016/j.jaac.2018.11.013

635 FDA, "Marketing."

636 McGough et al., "Pilot Study," 408.

637 Ibid., 408-409.

638 NeuroSigma, "Monarch External Trigeminal Nerve Stimulation System (eTNS) for ADHD," November 26, 2019, https://www.youtube.com/watch?v=qP2l5wU0Zb8

639 Ibid.

640 Deborah J. Rhea, "Recess: The Forgotten Classroom," *Instructional Leader* 29, no. 1 (January 2016): 1-4, http://liinkproject.tcu.edu/wp-content/uploads/2014/11/Rhea-Instructional-Leader-Journal-2016-pub-Recess-LiiNK.pdf; Deborah J. Rhea, Alexander P. Rivchun, and Jacqueline Pennings, "The LiiNK Project: Implementation of a Recess and Character Development Pilot Study with Grades K & 1 Children," *TAHPERD Journal*, Summer 2016, 14-17, 35, http://liinkproject.tcu.edu/wp-content/uploads/2016/11/TAHPERD-Journal-LiiNK-article-2016.pdf; Valerie Strauss, "Why Some Schools Are Sending Kids Out to Recess Four Times a Day," *Washington Post*, September 13, 2016, https://www.washingtonpost.com/news/answer-sheet/wp/2016/09/13/recess-four-times-a-day-why-some-schools-are-now-letting-kids-play-an-hour-a-day/; Laura E. Clark and Deborah J. Rhea, "The LiinNK Project: Comparisons of Recess, Physical Activity, and Positive Emotional States in Grades K-2 Children," *International Journal of Child Health and Nutrition* 6, no. 6 (2017): 54-61, https://www.frontiersin.org/articles/10.3389/feduc.2018.00009/full; Deborah J. Rhea and Alexander P. Rivchun, "The LiiNK Project: Effects of Multiple Recesses and Character Curriculum on Classroom Behaviors and Listening Skills in Grades K-2 Children," *Frontiers in Education* 3, (February 15, 2018): 1-10, https://doi.org/10.3389/feduc.2018.00009; Deborah J. Rhea and Michelle Baumi, "An Innovative Whole Child Approach to Learning: The LiiNK Project," *Childhood Education* 94, no. 2 (March/April 2018): 56-63, https://doi.org/10.1080/00094056.2018.1451691; Jake Whitney, "This Researcher Thinks Recess is the Key to Better Test Scores," *D Magazine*, July 10,

2019, https://www.dmagazine.com/frontburner/2019/07/more-recess-better-test-scores-liink-tcu/; LiiNK Project, "What Is Link Project?" 2020, https://liinkproject.tcu/about-us/what-is-liink-project/; LiiNK Project, "Logic Behind LiiNK," 2020, https://liinkproject.tcu.edu/about-us/logic-behind-liink

641 Strauss, "Four Times a Day."

642 Rhea, "Recess," 1.

643 LiiNK Project, "What is LiiNK Project?"

644 Rhea et al., "Implementation," 14.

645 Clark and Rhea, "Comparisons," 55.

646 LiiNk Project, "Logic Behind LiiNK."

647 Clark and Rhea, "Comparisons," 56-58; Rhea and Rivchun, "Effects," 5-8.

648 Rhea and Baumi, "Whole-Child," 62.

649 Heidi Boland et al., "A Literature Review and Meta-Analysis on the Effects of ADHD Medications on Functional Outcomes," *Journal of Psychiatric Research* 123, (April 2020): 21-30, https://doi.org/10.1016/j.jpsychires.2020.01.006

650 Ibid., 30.

651 Ibid., 22-23.

652 William Shrank et al., "Healthy User and Related Biases in Observational Studies of Preventive Interventions: A Primer for Physicians," *Journal of General Internal Medicine* 26, no. 5 (May 2011): 546-550, https://doi.org/10.1007/s11606-010-1609-1

653 Ibid., 547.

654 Ibid., 547.

655 Colin R. Dormuth et al., "Statin Adherence and Risk of Accidents: A Cautionary Tale," *Circulation* 119, no. 15 (April 21, 2009): 2051-2057, https://doi.org/10.1161.CIRCULATIONAHA.108.824151

656 Jeffrey Curtis et al., "Placebo Adherence, Clinical Outcomes and Mortality in the Women's Health Initiative Randomized Hormone Therapy Trials,"

Medical Care 49, no. 5 (May 2011): 427-435, https://doi.org/10.1097/
MLR.0b013e18207ed9c

657 Shrank et al., "Biases," 546.

658 Boland et al., "Outcomes," 21.

659 Ibid., 23-26.

660 Ibid., 26.

661 Ibid., 23.

662 Ibid., 23.

663 See Chapter Three of this volume.

664 Lauren Hodges, "A Quiet and 'Unsettling' Pandemic Toll: Students Who've
Fallen Off the Grid," National Public Radio, December 29, 2020, https://
www.npr.org/2020/12/29/948866982/1-quiet-and-unsettling-panedmic-
toll-students-whove-fallen-off-thegrid

665 Farida B. Amhad and Robert N. Anderson, "The Leading Causes of Death
in the US for 2020," *JAMA,* published online March 31, 2021, https://doi.
org/10.1001.jama.2021.5649

666 Lia Novotny, "More Pediatricians Talking About ADHD During COVID-
19," athenahealth, May 29, 2020, https://athenahealth.com/knowl-
edge-hub/clinical-trends/more-pediatricians-talking-about-ADHD-
during-COVID-19

667 See Chapter Eleven of this volume for a discussion of Dr. Koplewicz's work.

668 Olivia Solon, "The Great Attention Deficit: More Parents Seek ADHD
Diagnosis and Drugs for Kids to Manage Learning," *NBC News,*
February 16, 2021, https://nbcnews.com/tech/tech-news/great-attention-
deficit-more-parents-seek-adhd-diagnosis-drugs-kids-n1257660

669 Ibid.

670 Ibid.

671 Ibid.

672 Solon, "Attention Deficit."

673 Novotny, "Pediatricians."

674 Ibid.

675 Libby Baney et al., "The Future of Telehealth and the Ryan Haight Act Post-Pandemic," National Association of Boards of Pharmacy, April 22, 2021, https://nabp.pharmacy/news/blog/the-future-of-telehealth-and-the-ryan-haight-act-postppandemic/

676 Crunchbase, "Cerebral," accessed March 14, 2022, https://www.crunchbase.com/organization/cerebral

677 Cerebral: Expert Help for Your Emotional Health, 2022, https://cerebral.com

678 Ibid.

679 Polly Mosendz and Caleb Melby, "ADHD Drugs are Convenient to Get Online. Maybe Too Convenient," *Bloomberg Businessweek*, March 11, 2022, https://apple.news/AOO9s4XqrSb6GSEbpcvALJg

680 Ibid.

681 Ibid.

682 Ibid.

683 Nisha Basu and Jonathan Bush, "Archaic In-Person Exam for Digital Prescribing is Holding Back Health Care Innovation," *STAT*, December 8, 2021, https://www.statnews.com/2021/12/08/archaic-in-person-exam-law-barrier-digital-prescribing-health-care-innovation/

684 Richard M. Scheffler et al., "The Global Market for ADHD Medications," *Health Affairs* 26, no. 2 (March/April 2007): 450-457, https://doi.org/10.1377/hltaff.26.2.450

685 Ibid., 451.

686 Ibid., 453.

687 International Narcotics Control Board, "Report 2014," Tuesday, March 3, 2015, https://www.incb.org/incb/en/publications/annual-reports/annual-report-2014.html. Actually, the United States no longer is the world leader in terms of per capita consumption of methylphenidate. That honor belongs to Iceland. However, the majority of prescriptions in that country are written for patients over twenty years of age, and the desire of

the inhabitants of that cold dark gloomy isle for a pick-me-up is perhaps understandable.

688 Sami Timimi, "ADHD is Best Understood as a Cultural Construct," *British Journal of Psychiatry* 184, no. 1 (January 2004): 8, https://doi.org/10.1192/bjp.184.1.8

689 E.M. Mann et al., "Cross-Cultural Differences in Rating Hyperactive-Disruptive Behaviors in Children," *American Journal of Psychiatry* 149, no. 11 (November 1992): 1539-1542, https://doi.org/10.1176/ajp.149.11.1539

690 Polanczyk et al., "Prevalence."

691 Benjamin B. Lahey et al., "Predictive Validity of ICD-10 Hyperkinetic Disorder Relative to DSM-IV Attention Deficit Hyperactivity Disorder Among Younger Children," *Journal of Child Psychology and Psychiatry* 47, no. 5 (2006): 472-479, https://doi.org/10.1111/j.1469-7610.2005.015900.x

692 Polanczyk et al., "Prevalence," 945.

693 Ibid., 945-946.

694 Erik G. Wilcutt, "The Prevalence of *DSM-IV* Attention-Deficit Hyperactivity Disorder: A Meta-Analytic Review," *Neurotherapeutics* 9, no. 3 (July 2012): 490-499, https://doi.org/10.1007/s13311-012-0135-8; Guilherme V. Polanczyk, Erik G. Wilcutt, Giovanni A. Salum, Christian Kieling, and Luis A. Rohde, "ADHD Prevalence Estimates Across Three Decades: An Updated Systematic Review and Meta-Regression Analysis," *International Journal of Epidemiology* 43, no. 2 (April 2014): 434-442, https://doi.org/10.1093/ije/dyt262

695 Scheffler et al., "Global Market," 451.

696 Peter Conrad and Meredith R. Bergey, "The Impending Globalization of ADHD: Notes on the Expansion and Growth of a Medicalized Disorder," *Social Science and Medicine* 122, (December 2014): 31-43, https://doi.org/10.1016/j.socscimed.2014.10.019

697 Ibid., 36.

698 Ibid., 36.

699 ADHD Institute, accessed September 10, 2021, https://adhd-institute.com

700 Xian Janssen, "Attention Deficit Hyperactivity Disorder," accessed
September 10, 2021, https://www.xian-janssen.com.cn/en/therapy/adhd

701 Christine B. Phillips, "Medicine Goes to School: Teachers as Sickness
Brokers for ADHD," *PLoS Medicine* 3, no. 4 (April 2006): 433-435,
https://doi.org/10.1371/journal.pmed.0030182

702 ADHD Europe, "ADHD Myths and Facts," accessed September 10, 2021,
https://adhdeurope.eu/awareness/myths-and-facts

703 ADHD Australia, "What is ADHD," accessed September 10, 2021, https://
www.adhdaustralis.org/about-adhd/what-is-attention-deficit-hyperactivi-
ty-disorder-adhd/

704 Center for ADHD Awareness Canada, "ADHD Facts—Dispelling the
Myths," accessed September 10, 2021, https://caddac.ca/understand-
ing-adhd/in-general/facts-stats-myths/

705 ADHD New Zealand, "Managing ADHD in Schools," accessed September
10, 2021, https://www.adhd.org/nz/adhd-in-schools.html

706 ADHD UK, "Adult ADHD Self-Screening Tool," accessed September 10,
2021, https://adhduk.co.uk/adult-adhd-screening-survey/

707 R. Rao Gogineni, April E. Fallon, and Nyapati R. Rao, "International
Medical Graduates in Child and Adolescent Psychiatry: Adaptation,
Training, and Contributions," *Child and Adolescent Psychiatric Clinics
of North America* 19, no. 4 (October 2010): 833-853, https://doi.
org/10.1016/j.chc.2010.07.009

708 Persistence Market Research, "ADHD Therapeutics Market to Expand
Twofold by 2030, Deprioritized Status of ADHD in Hospitals Due to
Covid-19 Pandemic Surging Market Growth," April 2020, https://www.
persistencemarketresearch.com/market-research/attention-deficit-hyper-
activity-disorder-therapeutics-market.asp

709 Virginia I. Douglas, "Stop, Look, and Listen: The Problem of Sustained
Attention and Impulse Control in Hyperactive and Normal Children,"
Canadian Journal of Behavioural Science 4, no. 4 (1972): 259-282.

710 Ibid., 263-264.

711 Ibid., 262.

712 Claudia Malacrida and Tiffani Semach, "In the Elephant's Shadow: The Canadian ADHD Context," in *Global Perspectives on ADHD: Social Dimensions of Diagnosis and Treatment in Sixteen Countries*, ed. Meredith R. Bergey et al., (Baltimore: Johns Hopkins University Press, 2018), 34-53.

713 Ibid., 35.

714 Ibid., 36.

715 Ibid., 46.

716 ADD Vancouver Support Group, accessed September 19, 2021, addvancouversupport.ca

717 CADDAC, accessed September 19, 2021.

718 Jan Hoffmann, "Purdue Pharma is Dissolved and Sacklers Pay $4.5 Billion to Settle Opioid Claims," *New York Times*, September 2, 2021.

719 Malacrida and Semach, "Context," 36.

720 Canadian ADHD Resource Alliance, accessed September 19, 2021, https://www.caddra.ca

721 Malacrida and Semach, "Context," 42.

722 Canadian Press, "Poll: Canadians are Most Proud of Universal Medicare," Sunday, November 25, 2012, https://www.ctvnews.ca/canada/poll-canadians-are-most-proud-of-universal-medicare-1.1052929

723 Stephen P. Hinshaw et al., "International Variation in Treatment Procedures for ADHD: Social Context and Recent Trends," *Psychiatric Services* 62, no. 5 (May 2011): 459-464, https://doi.org/10.1176/ps.62.5.pss6205_0459

724 Malacrida and Semach, "Context," 45.

725 Scheffler et al., "Market."

726 Christian Bröer et al., "Exploring the ADHD Diagnosis in Ghana," in *Global Perspectives on ADHD: Social Dimensions of Diagnosis and Treatment in Sixteen Countries*, ed. Meredith R. Bergey et al., (Baltimore: Johns Hopkins University Press, 2018), 354-375.

727 Ibid., 362-363.

728 Ibid., 363.

729 Ibid., 363.

730 Ibid., 364.

731 Ibid., 369-372; also personal observations.

732 Personal observations.

733 United States Department of Labor, "Child Labor and Forced Labor Reports," 2019, https://dol.gov/agencies/ilab/resources/reports/child-labor/ghana

734 Madeleine Akrich and Vololona Rabeharisoa, "The French ADHD Landscape," in *Global Perspectives on ADHD: Social Dimensions of Diagnosis and Treatment in Sixteen Countries*, ed. Meredith R. Bergey et al., (Baltimore: Johns Hopkins University Press, 2018), 233-260; Manuel Vallée, "The Countervailing Forces Behind France's Low Ritalin Consumption," *Social Sciences and Medicine* 238, (August 15, 2019): 1-8, https://doi.org/10.1016/j.socscimed.2019.112492 [Epub ahead of print]

735 Vallée, "Forces," 3.

736 Ibid., 3.

737 Akrich and Rabeharisoa, "Landscape," 235.

738 Ibid., 235-237.

739 Ibid., 239.

740 Michel Lecendreux, Eric Konofal, and Stephen V. Faraone, "Prevalence of Attention Deficit Hyperactivity Disorder and Associated Features among Children in France," *Journal of Attention Deficit Disorders* 15, no. 6 (August 2011): 516-524, https://doi.org/10.1177/1087054710372491

741 Akrich and Rabeharisoa, "Landscape," 248-249.

742 Ibid., 239.

743 Julien Brygo, "La Pilule de l'Obéissance," *Le Monde Diplomatique*, December 2019, https://www.monde-diplomatique.fr/2019/12/BRYGO/61087

744 Damien Mascret, "Le Ritaline, entre Sous-Prescription et Abus," *Le Figaro*, May 17, 2017, https://sante/lefigaro.fr/article/ritaline-entre-sous-prescription-et-abus

745 Agence Nationale de Sécurité du Médicament et des Produits de Santé, "Méthylphénidate: Données d'Utilisation et de Sécurité d'emploi en France." July 4, 2021, https://ansm.sante.fr/actualities/methylphenidate-donees-dutilisation-et-de-securite-demploi-en-france

746 HyperSupers TDAH France, "Fin de la Prescription Initiale Hospitaliére (PIH) pour le Méthylphenidate," September 13, 2021, https://tdah-france.fr

747 Phillippe Pinel, *A Treatise on Mental Alienation*, trans. Gordon Hickish, David Healy, and Louis C. Charland (Chichester: J. Wiley and Sons, 2008).

748 Ibid., 4.

749 Manuel Vallée, "Resisting American Psychiatry," *Advances in Medical Sociology* 12, (2011): 97-98.

750 Akrich and Rabeharisoa, "Landscape," 238.

751 Claire Edwards et al., "Attention Deficit Hyperactivity Disorder in France and Ireland: Parents' Groups' Scientific and Political Framing of an Unsettled Condition," *Biosocieties* 9, no. 2 (2014): 153-172.

752 Akrich and Rabeharisoa, "Landscape," 253.

753 Ibid., 252-254.

754 Ibid., 254.

755 Ibid., 239.

756 Aude Mazoué, "French Psychiatry Has Gone Downhill in Part Because of American Influence," France24, October 3, 2021, https://www.france24.com/en/france/20211003-french-psychiatry-has-gone-downhill-in-part-because-of-american-influence

757 Carl Jung, *Two Essays on Analytical Psychology*, trans. R.F.C. Hull (Princeton: Princeton University Press), 41-63.

758 Gordon Claridge and David Healy, "The Psychopharmacology of Individual Differences," *Human Psychopharmacology: Clinical and Experimental* 9, no. 4 (July/August 1994): 285-298, https://doi.org/10.1002/hup.470090408

759 Healy, *Shipwreck*, 220.

760 James Davies, *Sedated: How Modern Capitalism Created Our Mental Health Crisis* (London: Atlantic Books, 2021).

761 Antidepressants: see Christian J. Bachmann et al., "Trends and Patterns of Antidepressant Use in Children and Adolescents from Five Western Countries, 2005-2012," *European Neuropsychopharmacology* 26, (2016): 411-419, https://doi.org/10.1016/j.euroneuro.2016.02.001; Laura A. Pratt, Debra J. Brody, and Qiuping Gu, "Antidepressant Use among Persons Aged 12 and over: United States, 2011-2014," NCHS Data Brief, no. 283 (August 2017), cdc.gov/nchs/products/databriefs/db283.htm; antipsychotics: see Olfson et al., "Trends." Between 2006 and 2010, the number of youth prescriptions for antipsychotics dropped somewhat, but it remained far in excess of what it was in 1993; see Mark Olfson, Marissa King, and Michael Schoenbaum, "Treatment of Young People with Antipsychotic Medications in the United States," *JAMA Psychiatry* 72, no. 9 (September 2015): 867-874, https://doi.org/10.1001/jamapsychiatry.2015.0500

762 J.M. Twenge et al., "Increases in Depressive Symptoms, Suicide-Related Outcomes, and Suicide Rates among U.S. Adolescents after 2010 and Links to Increased New Media Screen Time," *Clinical Psychological Science* 6, no. 1 (2017): 3-17, https://doi.org/10.1177.216770026117723376; CDC, "Fatal Injury Reports: National, Regional, and State 1981-2016," page last updated February 19, 2017, https://webappa.cdc.gov/sasweb/ncipc/mortrate.html; Holly Hedegaard, Arialdi M. Miniño, and Margaret Warner, "Drug Overdose Deaths in the United States, 1999-2017," NCHS Data Brief, no. 329 (November 2018), cdc.gov/nchs/data/databriefs/db329-h.pdf

763 Schwarz, "Attention Deficit Disorder."

764 Ibid.

765 Ryan D'Agostino, "The Drugging of the American Boy," *Esquire*, May 27, 2014, https://www.esquire.com/news-politics/a32858/drugging-of-the-american-boy-0414/

766 Stephanie Thompson, "Some Parents Are Turning to Medical Marijuana to Treat ADHD Instead of Adderall," *Business Insider*, January 7, 2020, https://www.businessinsider.com/adhd-marijuana-adderall-alterna-

tive-kids-2020-1?utm_source=feedburner&utm_medium=referral. This alarming news becomes even more alarming in light of mounting evidence that marijuana causes agitation and violence in a small percentage of users. Cf. Alex Berenson, *Tell Your Children: The Truth About Marijuana, Mental Illness, and Violence* (New York: Free Press, 2019).

767 Alan A. Baumeister, "Is Attention Deficit/Hyperactivity Disorder a Risk Syndrome for Parkinson's Disease?" *Harvard Review of Psychiatry* 29, no. 2 (March/April 2021): 142-158, https://doi.org/10.1097. HRP/0000000000000283

768 Supernus, "Supernus Announces FDA Approval of Qelbree," April 2, 2021, https://ir.supernus.com/node/12206/pdf.

769 Supernus, "Highlights of Prescribing Information," April 2, 2021, https://www.supernus.com/sites/default/files/Qelbree-Prescribing-info.pdf.

770 Earl D. Bond and G.E. Partridge, "Post-Encephalitic Behavior Disorders in Boys and Their Management in a Hospital," *American Journal of Psychiatry* 83, no. 1 (July 1926): 25-103, https://doi.org/10.1176/ajp.83.1.25

771 Ibid., 28-30.

772 Earl D. Bond and Lauren H. Smith, "Post-Encephalitic Behavior Disorder: A Ten-Year Review of the Franklin School," *American Journal of Psychiatry* 92. no. 1 (July 1935): 17-33, https://doi.org/10.1176/ajp.92.1.17

773 Ibid., 29-31.

About the Author

Patrick D Hahn is a free-lance writer and independent scholar with a long-standing interest in iatrogenic harm and the medicalization of everyday life.

His first book, *Madness and Genetic Determinism: Is Mental Illness in Our Genes?*, explores how genetic determinist views of so-called "mental illness" have obscured the well-established role of childhood sexual abuse and other adverse childhood experiences in the genesis of those conditions.

His second book, *Prescription for Sorrow: Antidepressants, Suicide, and Violence*, traces the history of how so-called "antidepressants" came on to the market and have stayed on the market, detailing how the drug companies and the mostly compliant mainstream media have exaggerated the benefits and hidden the harms caused these drugs, which include addiction, suicide, and violence.

His writing on mental health and other issues has also appeared in the *Baltimore Sun*, *Mad in America*, the *Canada Free Press*, *Natural News Blogs*, and numerous other venues. Dr. Hahn is an Affiliate Professor of Biology at Loyola University Maryland.

www.ingramcontent.com/pod-product-compliance
Lightning Source LLC
Chambersburg PA
CBHW051455030726
47592CB00006B/1947